ACSM's
Exercise Management for Persons with Chronic Diseases and Disabilities

AMERICAN COLLEGE OF
SPORTS MEDICINE

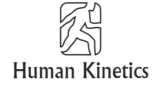

Human Kinetics

Library of Congress Cataloging-in-Publication Data

ACSM's exercise management for persons with chronic diseases and
 disabilities / American College of Sports Medicine.
     p.   cm.
   Includes index.
   ISBN 0-87322-798-0
   1. Exercise therapy. 2. Exercise tests. 3. Chronic diseases-
-Exercise therapy. 4. Handicapped--Rehabilitation. I. American
College of Sports Medicine.
   [DNLM: 1. Exercise Therapy. 2. Exercise Tolerance. 3. Chronic
Disease--therapy. 4. Disabled. WB 541 A187 1997]
RM725.A3 1997
615.8'24--dc21
DNLM/DLC
for Library of Congress   96-48817
                                       CIP

ISBN: 0-87322-798-0

Acquisitions Editor: Scott Wikgren; **Developmental Editor:** Holly Gilly; **Assistant Editors:** Chad Johnson and Coree Schutter; **Editorial Assistant:** Amy Carnes; **Copyeditor:** Joyce Sexton; **Proofreader:** Pam Johnson; **Indexer:** Theresa Schaefer; **Graphic Designer:** Stuart Cartwright; **Graphic Artist:** Denise Lowry; **Photo Editor:** Boyd LaFoon; **Cover Designer:** Jack Davis; **Printer:** Braun-Brumfield

Printed in the United States of America   10 9 8 7 6

Human Kinetics
Web site: www.humankinetics.com

United States: Human Kinetics, P.O. Box 5076, Champaign, IL 61825-5076
1-800-747-4457
e-mail: humank@hkusa.com

Canada: Human Kinetics, 475 Devonshire Road, Unit 100, Windsor, ON N8Y 2L5
1-800-465-7301 (in Canada only)
e-mail: humank@hkcanada.com

Europe: Human Kinetics, P.O. Box IW14, Leeds LS16 6TR, United Kingdom
+44 (0)113-278 1708
e-mail: humank@hkeurope.com

Australia: Human Kinetics, 57A Price Avenue, Lower Mitcham, South Australia 5062
(08) 82771555
e-mail: liahka@senet.com.au

New Zealand: Human Kinetics, P.O. Box 105-231, Auckland Central
09-523-3462
e-mail: humank@hknewz.com

CONTENTS

CONTRIBUTORS

Senior Editor

J. Larry Durstine, PhD, FACSM
University of South Carolina

Section Editors

Lorraine E. Bloomquist, EdD, FACSM
University of Rhode Island

Stephen F. Figoni, PhD, RKT, FACSM
University of Kansas Medical Center

Geoffrey E. Moore, MD, FACSM
University of Pittsburgh

Patricia L. Painter, PhD, FACSM
University of California at San Francisco

Kenneth H. Pitetti, PhD, FACSM
Wichita State University

Scott O. Roberts, PhD, FAACVPR
Texas Tech University

Carol J. Pope, PhD
Texas Christian University
Consulting Editor

Contributors

Ann L. Albright, PhD
UCSF/California Department of Health Services

Oded Bar-Or, MD, FACSM
McMaster University
Chedoke Hospital
Children's Exercise Nutrition Center

Connie Bayles, PhD, FACSM
Mercy Hospital, Pittsburgh, PA

Thomas J. Birk, PhD, FACSM
Medical College of Ohio

Susan A. Bloomfield, PhD
Texas A & M University

Clinton Brawner, BS
Henry Ford Hospital

Christopher B. Cooper, MD, FACSM
UCLA School of Medicine

Bo Fernhall, PhD, FACSM
George Washington University

Michael Ferrara, PhD, ATC
Ball State University

Barry A. Franklin, PhD, FACSM
Wayne State University School of Medicine

Daniel Friedman, MD, FACSM
New Mexico Heart Institute

Andrew W. Gardner, PhD
Baltimore VA Medical Center

John R. Gates, MD
The University Epilepsy Group, P.A.

Neil F. Gordon, MD, PhD, MPH, FACSM
The Heart and Lung Group of Savannah

Joseph Jankovic, MD
Baylor College of Medicine

Tim Johnson, MD
Lovelace Medical Center

Donald R. Kay, MD, FACP, FACR
University of Missouri Health Sciences Center

Steven J. Keteyian, PhD, FACSM
Henry Ford Hospital

Nancy Klimas, MD
University of Miami School of Medicine

James Laskin, PhD, PT
University of Oklahoma Health Science Center

Arthur LaPerriere, PhD, FACSM
University of Miami School of Medicine

Patricia Major, MD
University of Miami School of Medicine

Marian A. Minor, PT, PhD
Missouri Arthritis Rehabilitation Research and
    Training Center

Janet A. Mulcare, PhD, FACSM
Andrews University

Jonathan N. Myers, PhD, FACSM
Palo Alto VA Medical Center

Karen L. Nau, PhD, PT
University of Kansas Medical Center

Patricia A. Nixon, PhD, FACSM
University of Pittsburgh

N.B. Oldridge, PhD, FACSM
University of Wisconsin

Karen Palmer-McLean, PhD, PT
University of Wisconsin, LaCrosse

Arlette Perry, PhD, FACSM
University of Miami School of Medicine

Elizabeth J. Protas, PT, PhD, FACSM
Texas Woman's University

Reed E. Pyeritz, MD, PhD
Medical College of Pennsylvania and Hahnemann
    University

James Rimmer, PhD
Northern Illinois University

George Selby, MD
University of Oklahoma Health Science Center

Kathy E. Sietsema, MD
Harbor - UCLA Medical Center

Gary S. Skrinar, PhD, FACSM
Sargent College of Allied Health Professions

Ronald H. Spiegel, MD
The University Epilepsy Group, P.A.

Rhonda K. Stanley, PT, PhD
University of Evansville

J.E. Stoll, MD
University of Wisconsin

Janet P. Wallace, PhD, FACSM
Indiana University

Michael West, MD
Lovelace Medical Center

Jack E. Wilberger, MD
Tri-State Neurosurgical Assoc., Inc.

REVIEWERS

James Agre, MD, FACSM
University of Wisconsin

Ed Balaban, DO
Geisinger Medical Group

Frank J. Cerny, PhD, FACSM
SUNY at Buffalo

Chuck Cortes, PhD
Philadelphia Geriatrics Center

Barbara Culatta, PhD
University of Rhode Island

J. Mark Davis, PhD, FACSM
University of South Carolina

Paul Davis, MS
University of South Carolina

Ted Dreisinger, PhD
Columbia Spine Center

James M. Hagberg, PhD, FACSM
University of Maryland

Martin Hoffman, MD, FACSM
Clement J. Zablocki VA Medical Center

Don Hoover, MS, PT
University of Kansas Medical Center

Linda Hughes, MA, CRC
Rhode Island Department of Human Services

James John, MD
University of Kansas Medical Center

Terrence Kavanagh, MD

Mark P. Kelly, MS

Fred Kusumoto, MD
Lovelace Medical Center

Barry Maron, MD
Minneapolis Heart Institute Foundation

Linda McClain, PhD, OTR
University of Kansas Medical Center

Brian McKiernan, ABD, PT
University of Kansas Medical Center

Carolee Moncour, PT, PhD
University of Utah

Mark S. Nash, PhD
University of Miami

Claire Peel, PhD

Scott Powers, PhD, FACSM
University of Florida

John B. Redford, MD
Kansas City VA Medical Center

Carlos Roldan, MD
Albuquerque Veterans Medical Center

Robert Rondinelli, MD, PhD
University of Kansas Medical Center

Jeffrey C. Rupp, PhD
Georgia State University

Mark Senn, PhD
South Carolina Heart Center

Martin Sullivan, MD
Duke University Medical Center

Catherine Thompson, MS, PT

Walter Rolph Thompson, PhD, FACSM
Georgia State University

George Varghese, MD
University of Kansas Medical Center

Ann Ward, PhD, FACSM
University of Wisconsin

Billy Webster, PhD, FACSM
HeartLife

PREFACE

J. Larry Durstine, PhD, FACSM

Lorraine E. Bloomquist, EdD, FACSM

Stephen F. Figoni, PhD, RKT, FACSM

Geoffrey E. Moore, MD, FACSM

Patricia L. Painter, PhD, FACSM

Kenneth H. Pitetti, PhD, FACSM

Carol J. Pope, PhD

Scott O. Roberts, PhD, FAACVPR

The fifth edition of *ACSM's Guidelines for Exercise Testing and Prescription* provides the basic principles of testing and training for normal healthy individuals and for those with cardiovascular disease. There is growing interest in the use of exercise for clients with other chronic diseases and disabilities. The purpose of this book is to provide a framework for determining functional capacity and developing appropriate exercise programming for optimizing functional capacity in persons with chronic diseases and/or disabilities. The basic principles for exercise testing and training stated in *ACSM's Guidelines for Exercise Testing and Prescription* provide the foundation for this book. When not otherwise stated, these principles are assumed to apply. However, some special situations created by a disease pathology, disability, or treatment alter these basic principles. For example, exercise testing is an important aspect of the approach used in this book, but some people will not have completed an exercise test before starting an exercise program. Participation in regular physical activity can enhance functional capacity, and a primary goal of this book is to get more individuals physically active. Thus, for many people exercise testing may not be absolutely necessary before starting a low-level physical activity program.

Exercise management for persons with a chronic disease and/or disability is now provided by a wide variety of health care and exercise professionals. Presently, management techniques depend on the provider's experience and are loosely, if at all, coordinated with other providers. A second goal of this book is to develop an integrated model of care so that everyone can work together in a program in which exercise is coordinated with other aspects of health care.

This is not an all-encompassing book on exercise testing and prescription for the populations of interest. Rather, it is a reference manual to use as a guide for managing people with a condition outside the exercise professional's primary expertise. The editorial board and authors were chosen by virtue of their clinical and research experience in exercise programming for persons with chronic diseases and disabilities. The editors established a format for the book and then worked with the authors in writing the text. During the writing process each chapter was peer-reviewed and revised accordingly. Before printing, the entire book was reviewed by individuals with a broad expertise in the use of exercise. The authors have suggested reading materials for more in-depth information; these are listed at the end of each chapter and are strongly recommended. If the reader is unable to solve a clinical problem using this manual and the suggested readings, we recommend contacting the chapter author or section editor for advice.

Many who have a chronic disease or disability enter a spiral downward toward exercise intolerance, so exercise intervention programs should be designed to resist this spiral and optimize functional capacity. Within any given population, there is a wide range of abilities, determined by several factors: progression of the disease, response to treatment, and presence of other concomitant illnesses. Expected outcomes of exercise training are not always known. Realistically, optimal exercise and medical programming may yield improvements or may merely prevent further deterioration. This book at times may recommend tests or programs that have not been validated, but that experience has shown to be successful. It is hoped that optimal management will bring the individual greater independence and improved quality of life.

Exercise programming must be regularly updated and adapted to the individual's clinical state. The prescription may change depending on the needs of the person, the progression/stabilization of the condition, or the therapy. As a result of disease progression, exercise programming may need to be discontinued—exercise at all costs is not our intent. Rather, we desire appropriate exercise management, including the astute clinical judgment of the exercise professional, leading to successful exercise programs.

We hope that this book will help improve the quality of life for individuals with chronic diseases or disabilities.

SECTION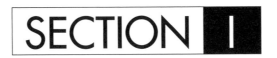

Introduction

Section Editor:

J. Larry Durstine, PhD, FACSM
University of South Carolina

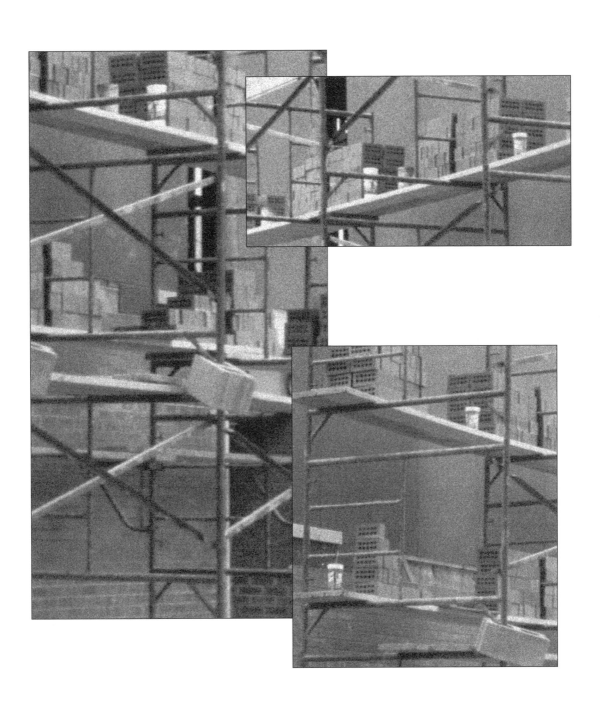

CHAPTER 1

Introduction

Geoffrey E. Moore, MD, FACSM
University of Pittsburgh

In general, our society has a bias toward curative rather than palliative medicine, toward making the disease go away rather than finding ways to cope with disease. An unfortunate consequence of this perspective is that for persons with chronic disease or disability, we devalue the palliative benefits of preserving functionality and well-being. Recent improvements in societal awareness of persons with disabilities, of the elderly, and of persons with terminal or end-stage disease have brought attention to medical issues surrounding individual rights of autonomy and self-determination. Since the 1960s, exercise has been promoted as a method of extending life, largely through prevention and moderation of cardiovascular disease. But in the 1980s, research and clinical applications for exercise expanded to populations with a variety of chronic diseases and disabilities, for whom exercise is perhaps more fundamentally related to *quality* of life than to *quantity* of life. Perhaps the greatest potential benefit of exercise is its ability to preserve functional capacity, freedom, and independence.

The exercise or health professional looking for guidance in managing exercise programs for people with chronic disease or disability will soon discover that most textbook chapters are grouped by diagnosis. Most chapters are written by specialists who discuss precautions and caveats for the performance of exercise in the context of a specific disease or disability. Since many diseases and disabilities have not been sufficiently studied to yield exact dose-response information, recommendations are vague, coming not from controlled trials but from empiricism and anecdote. While this approach is valid, one must recognize that its origins lie not in physiology, but in the structure of academia and the perception that exercise is an adjuvant therapy.

One major shortcoming of *diagnosis-oriented* management is that many people have multiple concomitant problems and do not fit neatly into a single special population. Furthermore, many diseases involve multiple organ systems. Exercise professionals need a paradigm useful for *anyone:* a paradigm based on the effects of disease or disability on the acute response to exercise, on the adaptations to training, on the interaction of exercise with medicines, and on the expected dose-response relationship. *Problem-oriented* exercise management provides a fundamental framework through which to approach any client with any combination of diseases and/or disabilities. Problem-oriented exercise management yields many advantages: it uses exercise testing to reveal physiologic dysfunction; it directs exercise therapy toward problems that might be improved by training; it integrates exercise into medical management; it assigns responsibility to the individual, thereby reinforcing the individual's sense of self-determination and autonomy; and, perhaps most importantly, it transforms problems of overwhelming complexity into components that are more manageable.

How to Use This Book

This manual provides an outline of how to effectively manage exercise for someone with chronic disease or disability. To use this manual, the reader should have extensive knowledge about exercise testing and training. Successful exercise management should also involve close teamwork between physicians, nurses, and allied health care providers. The editors assume that the reader is appropriately skilled in these matters and can adapt to individual circumstances. *ACSM's Resource Manual for Guidelines for Exercise Testing and Prescription* (second edition) and *ACSM's Guidelines for Exercise Testing and Prescription* (fifth edition) contain information on various exercise protocols, although some specific protocols or exercise devices may be described here. This manual does *not* provide detailed instruction on exercise physiology or disease, so the reader must do supplementary reading as needed in order to fully understand exercise management. For detailed information on diseases and disabilities, the reader should refer to standard physiology, medical, and adapted physical activity texts.

Each chapter deals with a common chronic disorder or disability that might limit functional capacity. Each chapter briefly lists the physiologic nature of the disease or disability, its effects on exercise response and adaptation, the effects of commonly used medicines, and any unique circumstances that should be considered. Recommendations for testing and programming are presented in tables for easy reference. The reader should refer to the chapter(s) relevant for each individual and use the information in those chapters as guidelines to develop an individualized exercise program.

In order to develop an integrated model, we have aggregated and consolidated old conventions and tried to create a comprehensive system. The first two chapters introduce these new conventions; all the remaining chapters follow this model. Some concepts are used interchangeably, such as "exercise prescription" and "exercise programming." Other concepts are new, such as "families of exercise tests." These conventions were not chosen to imply correctness, but to simplify. Some concepts remain unsimplified, for there seemed no easy approach and no substantial benefit to simplifying. For example, aerobic exercise intensity is expressed in a variety of ways: percentage $\dot{V}O_2$max, percentage peak heart rate, percentage heart rate reserve, and so on. These choices were largely left to each author's preference. One important convention in this book is the use of the words "clients" and "individuals" instead of "patients." This convention was chosen because not all exercise managers are health care professionals in a patient-caregiver relationship.

Problem-Oriented Management

A method of exercise management that uses problem-oriented techniques is presented here and is recommended by the editors. This technique uses the "SOAP" notes commonly employed by health care professionals. For those unfamiliar with this technique, the problem-oriented system is just an organizational tool. In brief, SOAP is an acronym that stands for *Subjective data, Objective data, Assessment, and Plan of action.* Notes, to oneself and others, are written in the SOAP style to clarify the thinking process and the rationale for a course of evaluation, therapy, or both. Problems and unique needs are identified and the intervention is documented, largely so that follow-up evaluations can be compared to earlier visits and success or failure can be fairly judged. The key benefit of problem-oriented management is that several problems can be independently tracked in their own time course but within the context of the overall situation. In healthy able-bodied persons, there is little need for this system, and there may not be much need even in persons with a single chronic disease or disability that doesn't alter the physiologic response to activity (e.g., sensory disorders such as deafness and visual impairment). But for persons in whom multiple chronic disease or disability circumstances affect exercise performance, there can be a real need for such a system. *The key to problem-oriented management is identifying all the problems and needs and then following each problem in its own appropriate time frame.*

How to Use the Tables

Each chapter contains tables describing appropriate exercise tests and programs for the chronic disease or disability addressed in that chapter. The table columns and rows are separated by lines. Columns contain categories of recommendations; rows are defined by family of exercise as described in chapter 2.

Each row contains recommendations regarding that family of exercise. For testing tables, the categories are **Methods** (to use), **Measures** (to take), **Endpoints** (and way-points to specifically note), and general **Comments**. For programming tables, the categories are **Modes** (of training), **Goals** (of the program), **Intensity/Frequency/Duration** (in the prescription), and **Time to Goal**. Both testing and programming tables have sections describing appropriate **Medications** and **Special Considerations**.

How to Read the Tables

To determine what exercise test to conduct, look under the testing table for the relevant chapter. In the first column, labeled Methods, find the family of exercise test you would like to perform. Then read across to the second column, Measures, to find out which physiologic measurements are recommended during the test. Continuing to read across within the family of exercise test, look for Endpoints in the third column. Endpoints are usually indications to terminate the test, though some "endpoints" are relevant way-points, or measurements taken during the test (e.g., ventilatory threshold). The fourth column contains Comments about relevant issues. In addition, special attention should be given to the sections in each table regarding appropriate Medications and Special Considerations.

Similarly, in developing an exercise program for an individual, look under the programming table. In the first column, labeled Modes, find the family of exercise you would like to prescribe. Within each family of exercise are recommended generic modes of training. Then read across to the second column, Goals, to find appropriate program objectives. Continuing to read across within the family of exercise, you will find appropriate Intensity/Frequency/Duration recommendations in the third column. The fourth column contains Time to Goal, which provides an idea of how long it will take to reach an established goal. As with exercise testing, special note should be taken of the sections in each table on appropriate Medications and Special Considerations.

What's in the Tables

The tables contain material summarized from the chapter as well as recommendations about exercise testing and programming. Protocols and programs are usually listed generically, rather than in specific terms, because detailed listing of all known protocols would be overly cumbersome. It is *assumed* that readers know how to conduct tests and design programs. If not, the reader should refer to the chapter's selected readings or to reference texts listed at the end of this chapter (e.g., *ACSM's Guidelines for Exercise Testing and Prescription*, fifth edition) or seek other guidance.

What's Not in the Tables

Although many tables are complete and comprehensive, many are not. Some tables contain areas that are left blank, or omit mention of a particular family of exercise, usually because the author, section editor, and reviewer felt that insufficient data were available to justify a recommendation. Sometimes recommendations for the corresponding testing and programming don't match; again, the reason is usually that research on exercise testing and training procedures is incomplete. Also, testing and programming tables in some sections are combined because the disability doesn't alter the normal response to exercise or adaptations to exercise training (e.g., visual impairment). In such cases, the reader is referred to *ACSM's Guidelines for Exercise Testing and Prescription*, fifth edition.

Suggested Readings

Exercise Physiology

American College of Sports Medicine. 1993. *ACSM's resource manual for guidelines for exercise testing and prescription.* Ed. J.L. Durstine, A.C. King, P.L. Painter, J.L. Roitman, L.D. Zwiren, and W.L. Kenney. 2nd ed. Philadelphia: Lea & Febiger.

American College of Sports Medicine. 1995. *ACSM's guidelines for exercise testing and prescription.* Ed. W.L. Kenney, R.H. Humphrey, C.X. Bryant, D.A. Mahler, V. Froehlicher, N.H. Miller, and T.D. York. 5th ed. Baltimore: Williams & Wilkins.

Astrand, P.O., and K. Rodahl. 1986. *Textbook of work physiology: Physiological bases of exercise.* 3rd ed. New York: McGraw-Hill.

Exercise in Chronic Disease and Disability

Shephard, R.J. 1990. *Fitness in special populations.* Champaign, IL: Human Kinetics.

Sherrill, C. 1993. *Adapted physical activity, recreation and sport: Cross-disciplinary and lifespan.* 4th ed. Madison, WI: Brown & Benchmark.

Skinner, J.B., ed. 1993. *Exercise in special populations: Theoretical basis and clinical application.* 2nd ed. Philadelphia: Lea & Febiger.

Medicine

Berlow, R., and A.J. Fletcher, eds. 1992. *Merck manual of diagnosis and therapy.* Rahway, NJ: Merck & Co.

Harvey, A.M., R.J. Johns, V.A. McKusick, A.H. Owens, Jr., and R.S. Ross, eds. 1988. *Principles and practice of medicine.* 2nd ed. Norwalk, CT: Appleton & Lange.

Pharmacology

American Medical Association. 1995. *Drug evaluations.* Chicago: American Medical Association.

Olin, B.R., S.K. Hebel, and J.L. Gremp, eds. 1995. *Drug facts and comparisons.* St. Louis: Wolters Kluwer.

CHAPTER 2

Framework

Geoffrey E. Moore, MD, FACSM
University of Pittsburgh

J. Larry Durstine, PhD, FACSM
University of South Carolina

This chapter introduces a method to manage exercise in persons with chronic disease or disability. The first section provides an overview of this model. Subsequent sections offer greater detail about factors to consider.

An exercise history should be taken from the individual to provide *subjective* data on aerobic ability, anaerobic ability (for athletes), endurance, strength, flexibility, neuromuscular skill, and overall functional performance. This information defines the person's problem(s), and these aspects of physical activity are easily tested in the laboratory to provide *objective* data. The objective data quantify the person's limitations in physiologic terms, and this information is used to *assess* the cause(s) of exercise intolerance. From this assessment, an exercise training *plan* is developed. Formulation of a plan is complex, and includes (1) medication effects; (2) exercise dose-response (desired goal; type of exercise; intensity, duration, and frequency of training; adaptability to training as well as exhaustion/overtraining limits); (3) risks of training; (4) the cost/benefit ratio; and (5) any necessary coordination among members of the health care team.

Problem-Oriented Exercise Management

Problem-oriented exercise management is the cornerstone of our approach to exercise in persons with chronic disease and disability. Problem-oriented medical management was developed in the late 1960s and has been beneficial to health care professionals. The major benefit is that this approach organizes extremely complex problems into simpler parts that are more easily tracked and solved. Given the enormous complexity of exercise in chronic disease and disability, it may not be possible to manage some persons without this technique.

Problem-oriented management consists of five steps, commonly documented in the SOAP format: (1) collection of subjective data, (2) collection of objective data, (3) assessment and generation of a problem list, (4) formulation of a diagnostic or therapeutic plan, or both, and (5) periodic reassessment (follow-up). Since the SOAP note provides a quick conceptual reminder of the situation and of any progress that has been made, SOAP notes are useful not only to the manager, but also to any colleagues who may be assisting.

Getting Subjective Data

Before testing someone with a chronic disease or disability, characterize his or her problem. Take a history of physical activity and medical problems to obtain the person's complaints and symptoms. With regard to exercise intolerance, symptoms might include shortness of breath, exertional chest pain, weakness, ease of fatigability, back pain, and so forth. Find out why the person is coming to you, what exercises have been done in the past, what the limitations are now, what injuries have occurred, and what medical problems (heart, lung, circulatory, gastrointestinal, metabolic, and neurological disorders) and musculoskeletal problems are present now. Determine present medicines that are being taken. Obtain results of any recent medical and exercise tests. Even if you are not highly skilled in physical examination, a simple physical examination is valuable in establishing the extent of obvious musculoskeletal limitations.

Learning these facts will guide you toward the exercise measures that are probably subnormal. These are the problems that limit functional capacity, and they should be characterized by an exercise test. If a person cannot go to the store because he or she becomes winded or worn out, aerobic and endurance exercise tests are indicated. If the person can't go to the store because he or she is too weak to carry the bags home, strength tests are indicated. For someone who is too clumsy to walk to the store, neuromuscular and functional performance tests are indicated. It is not helpful or cost-effective to use every exercise test on everyone, nor is it wise to use only certain tests for persons with a specific disease or disability. Subjective data help you figure out what tests to use.

Getting Objective Data

Objective data include information collected during physical examination and laboratory studies. Having discovered the client's problem(s), perform tests that best characterize the exercise capacity. Appropriate medical and laboratory tests may provide measurements that confirm or refute possible causes of the symptoms. Since there are many kinds of exercise tests you could use, recommending a specific test is difficult. Furthermore, it is often not clear which test protocol is the best method. This is the main reason tests have been grouped into seven families based on what they are designed to quantify (see discussion of families of exercise test measures later in this chapter). These are the families:

- *Aerobic tests* - measure the ability to do exercise using high rate of oxygen consumption.
- *Anaerobic tests* - measure the ability to do unsustained very high intensity exercise.
- *Endurance tests* - measure the ability to sustain submaximal aerobic exercise for an extended time.
- *Strength tests* - measure the ability to do unsustained exercise against a high resistance.
- *Flexibility tests* - measure the ability to move joints through their range of motion.
- *Neuromuscular tests* - measure the ability to do activities that require coordination and skill.
- *Functional performance tests* - measure the ability to do specific physical activities of daily living.

Exercise testing protocols should be individualized to suit each person and, as a result, provide the best possible information for developing the management plan. In order to complete this task, the exercise professional may need to develop an opinion regarding the individual's potential exercise capacity. That opinion, along with professional knowledge and the information presented in this book, may then be used to attain optimal test results.

Making the Assessment

Using information from the subjective and objective steps, you should generate a list of specific problems. For example, an individual's problems may include (1) low aerobic capacity, (2) low ventilatory threshold, (3) low endurance at 75% of aerobic capacity, (4) weak hip and knee extensors, and so on. This assessment may explain the person's problem(s) or lead to further testing for problems that aren't fully explained or evident. Complete assessment may take several rounds of testing and reassessment before you have enough information to clearly identify the problem(s). Organize the assessment either by family of exercise test or by physiologic problem, and number each problem in sequence. Doing so will help you keep track of all the problems in a systematic fashion. For most people, obtaining subjective and objective data and making an assessment will not be difficult.

Formulating a Plan

The plan of action is the path that will lead to diagnosis of the problem(s), treatment, or both. Making this plan is usually far more difficult than the first three steps, because exercise prescription for persons with chronic disease or disability is often complex. The initial plan for some people will require performing further assessment and obtaining additional data, but sooner or later, an overall management plan including exercise programming must be formulated. Executing this plan is difficult because part of the plan will include following a problem for a period of time. This period can be a few days, a few weeks, or a few months. When numerous problems are present, it is possible to lose track of some of them during this time, making sequential numbering of the problems important.

First, establish an exercise prescription that has realistically achievable long-term goals. Then establish shorter-term intermediate goals that are easily achieved. This helps to develop a feeling of success. Make the goals something meaningful to the person—a specific activity such as yard work, for example. Use the exercise test measures only for your own records. Telling someone that he or she has achieved a 25% increase in aerobic capacity may mean little, but celebrating a renewed ability to mow the lawn is something most can understand.

Second, consider any unique circumstances such as prosthetics, medicines, exercise facilities, and other conditions that may require modification of a more typical program. Also evaluate the risks, benefits, and costs of the program. Remember that anyone who exercises has some *activity-dependent* risks such as injuries. But persons with a chronic disease or disability have risks related to their disease or disability. The risks of exercise are commonly conceived in terms of heart attacks and sudden death, but these are really *disease-dependent* risks for persons with heart disease. Heart attacks and sudden death are distinctly uncommon in people who don't have heart disease, so other disease-dependent risks may prove more important. The relative risks of any activity are determined by the severity of the disease and the inherent danger of the activity. Benefits of the program will usually be an increase in physical activity, quality of life, or both, but may well be a reduction in medicines or a moderation of disease severity. Costs will generally be time and energy, particularly for people who can do unsupervised exercise, although equipment and facility costs must also be considered. Be aware that for some, exercise training will be more bother than benefit.

Third, design an exercise program incorporating each of the considerations identified. Start from the person's current fitness and choose practical levels of intensity, duration, and frequency of exercise sessions. Do not be unnecessarily bound to standard programs (e.g., 20-40 minutes, three to four times a week). Such programs typically have the goal of decreasing cardiac morbidity and mortality, but these are often not the best goals for the purposes of persons with chronic disease or disability. Be careful not to exhaust the individual with work sessions that are too difficult. Choose a realistic time frame for achieving the goals, and pay attention to the necessary rate of improvement. Be careful not to overtrain the individual; there is no real purpose in overexercising a person with limited reserve who is not competing in sports. However, some persons with chronic diseases and/or disabilities can participate in athletic competition. The risk, cost, and benefit of exercise training will be discussed later in this chapter.

Lastly, a schedule for follow-up reassessment should be developed. Sometimes it is easy to make an assessment and a logical plan is readily apparent. More often, the assessment and plan are iterative processes—assessment, data collection, reassessment, more data collection, more reassessment, and so on, until the problem is solved. A *therapeutic trial* is a way to obtain objective data by seeing how well empiric therapy solves the problem. Once a solution has been settled upon, the appropriate time between reassessments is determined by individual circumstances. Following up too soon is a poor use of time and resources, but following up too late risks letting an old problem get out of control or a new problem go unnoticed. During follow-up, evaluate the progress and reassess the appropriateness of the prescription. Do this for each problem that is not stable and needs more attention. Problems that are not relevant may be skipped.

Organizing problems by exercise family has the advantages of maintaining the context of the exercise test and prescription, focusing strategy, and helping track the minor problems. In many cases, the person in fact has several problems but really only one major problem. However, one must not lose sight of the fact that secondary problems and sedentary lifestyle compound the situation. It is easiest to keep it all straight if these problems are organized by exercise family. Organizing by physiologic problem is a good alternative. Note that the tables for recommended testing and programming found in each chapter of this book are organized by family of exercise.

Tips on SOAP Notes

To make writing SOAP notes quick and easy, follow these guidelines:

- Be concise.
- Avoid sentences; use key phrases.
- Leave out irrelevant information.
- Discuss only currently relevant problems.
- Organize the problems by exercise family (i.e., aerobic, strength, flexibility, and the like).
- Assign a number to each problem, and *always* refer to that problem by its number.
- *Always* follow up unresolved problems.

Families of Exercise Test Measures

All forms of exercise involve most of the systems found in the body, whereas different types of exercises have different physiologic effects. In this manual, exercises are grouped into seven families of laboratory measurements that characterize the capacity to perform specific activities: (1) aerobic, (2) anaerobic, (3) endurance, (4) strength, (5) flexibility,

(6) neuromuscular skill, and (7) functional performance. These generic groupings provide a rationale for selecting an appropriate laboratory test and prescribing a training program. From a physiologic perspective these groupings do overlap to an extent, but in a problem-oriented system these families of exercises are nonetheless useful for organizational purposes. Exercise measures that characterize each family are as follows:

- *Aerobic* exercise tests measure ability to do exercise requiring use of high rates of oxygen consumption. Examples of aerobic test measures include maximal oxygen consumption ($\dot{V}O_2$max), peak oxygen consumption ($\dot{V}O_2$peak), maximal steady state oxygen consumption ($\dot{V}O_{2MSS}$), ventilation (spirometry, $_T$, etc.), 12-lead electrocardiogram (ECG), heart rate, blood pressure, perceived exertion, metabolic equivalents (METs), time to exhaustion, and lactate threshold.

- *Anaerobic* exercise tests measure the ability to exercise at an intensity that exceeds maximal (peak) oxygen consumption. Examples of anaerobic test measures include capacity for oxygen debt, 30-second peak power output, time trial performance, and peak lactate. This type of test is useful mostly for athletes.

- *Endurance* exercise tests measure ability to sustain submaximal aerobic exercise for an extended time. Examples of endurance test measures include time trial performance, 6- and 12-minute walk, 1-mile walk, time to exhaustion or rate of perceived exertion at a constant work rate, and maximal number of repetitions.

- *Strength* exercise tests measure ability to do unsustained work against a high resistance. Examples of strength test measures include maximal number of repetitions, isokinetic work and peak torque, maximal voluntary contraction, and peak power output.

- *Flexibility* tests measure ability to move joints through a prescribed range of motion. Examples of flexibility test measures include sit-and-reach distances and goniometry (range of motion).

- *Neuromuscular* tests measure ability to do activities that require coordination and skill. Examples of neuromuscular test measures include gait analysis, balance times, hand-eye coordination scores, and reaction time.

- *Functional performance* tests measure ability to do specific physical activities of daily living. Examples of functional performance test mea-

sures include sit-and-stand scores, lifting, timed walk, and gait.

The redundancy that is found among the families reflects the integrated nature of physical activity and a means of characterizing specific aspects of exercise. Note that this manual usually does *not* recommend the mode of exercise (i.e., in the *aerobic family:* walking, jogging, cycling, rowing, combined arm/leg cycling, stair climbing, swimming, aerobic dance, and so on).

Speed of fatigability is a common complaint in people who are severely challenged by activities we commonly consider routine, such as grocery shopping. Daily activities are complex physical activities that require integrated function between many of the organ systems and use all seven families of exercise. In this way, factors such as endurance and neuromuscular skill can determine daily activities and quality of life more than measures of $\dot{V}O_2$, strength, flexibility, or combinations of these measures.

Aerobic Exercise Tests

The ability to do aerobic exercise is very important for completing activities of daily living, and is commonly tested in the laboratory setting through use of graded exercise tests. Maximal oxygen consumption is an important physiologic measurement, and several criteria are used to determine whether or not oxygen consumption has truly reached a physiologic maximum (see *ACSM's Resource Manual for Guidelines for Exercise Testing and Prescription,* second edition). However, even though oxygen consumption may be increasing, most persons with a chronic disease or disability do not achieve a "true" $\dot{V}O_2$max, but do reach a point at which they cannot continue. Such individuals are said to reach symptom-limited exhaustion, which is referred to as peak $\dot{V}O_2$.

Another critical point that can be revealed during exercise testing is the point at which the person experiences a transition from an exercise intensity that can be sustained more or less indefinitely to an intensity that can be sustained for only a short time. A variety of methods are used to measure this transition, including lactate threshold, onset of blood lactate accumulation, ventilatory threshold, and Conconi heart rate threshold. Several protocols designed to detect this transition are available. For our purposes, the transition from sustainable to unsustainable exercise is the common aspect and will be referred to as the oxygen consumption at maximal steady state ($\dot{V}O_{2MSS}$).

Measurement of $\dot{V}O_{2MSS}$ is important in persons with chronic disease or disability. Many such people have a very low peak $\dot{V}O_2$, usually less than 25 ml·kg^{-1}·min^{-1} and often less than 20 ml·kg^{-1}·min^{-1}. The usual range for $\dot{V}O_{2MSS}$ is 40% to 70% of the $\dot{V}O_2$max. Many common activities of daily living, usually taken for granted by those who are healthy and able-bodied, require oxygen consumption in the range of 12 to 30 ml·kg^{-1}·min^{-1}. Many people with a chronic disease or disability have a $\dot{V}O_2$max *below* that required for activities of daily living, employment, and maintenance of individual independence, resulting in a lower quality of life. For this reason, $\dot{V}O_2$max is a critically important measurement.

In general, constant increment or continuously increasing (or *ramp)* work rate protocols are preferred over some standard protocols (e.g., Bruce protocol). Many standard protocols increase work rate in relatively large, often nonlinear increments and are effective in screening for ischemic heart disease. In exercise management, however, we are more interested in characterizing the exercise response in the submaximal range. Ramp protocols are far superior in this regard because they indicate submaximal exercise responses while still detecting coronary artery disease.

A disadvantage with use of a ramp protocol is that one cannot individualize exercise tests so that each subject can complete the test in 8 to 10 minutes. Many deconditioned persons have low endurance exercise capacity and will not be able to exercise for this length of time. At the same time, tests lasting for 12 to 15 minutes or longer can give falsely low results. Therefore, one must know the client's approximate ability, estimate his or her peak exercise capacity, and design a test to yield four to eight changes in work rates during an 8- to 10-minute test period. Low-level ramp protocols may require special programming and manual operation, and may be difficult to reproduce on equipment that is imprecise at low exercise levels. For example, some persons can generate only 10 watts and will not be able to pedal a standard stationary cycle against any measurable resistance. Therefore, the subject must be tested by freewheel pedaling, in which only the pedaling rate is increased. With careful consideration and planning, successful exercise testing can be accomplished in nearly everyone.

Anaerobic Tests

Anaerobic tests usually consist of short-term exercise that supplements strength test data or offers data on ability to do brief periods of high-intensity exercise. In several chronic diseases, this type of test correlates closely with a variety of measures of functional capacity, including $\dot{V}O_2$max. Anaerobic tests may also be of value for athletes preparing for competition.

Endurance Tests

Endurance tests are potentially useful because many inactive persons cannot exercise longer than five minutes but can sustain exercise for one hour or more after training (even without an increase in peak $\dot{V}O_2$). Unfortunately, endurance tests have not been well developed and often lack test-retest reliability, well-defined endpoints, and clear physiologic meaning. Claudication tests (e.g., walk distance to onset of pain, maximal walk distance) are useful in arterial insufficiency because they satisfy these criteria.

Strength Tests

Muscular strength is a critical component of exercise capacity, particularly in persons with chronic disease or disability. Resistance testing is essential because skeletal muscle weakness can limit functional capacity. Like aerobic exercise response, skeletal muscle function can be evaluated in myriad ways: for example, maximal repetitions for a given weight (using either free weights or a machine); isokinetic force, work, and power; and isometric force. Each of these forms of testing has its own advantages and disadvantages, and the method chosen should be carefully matched to the problems being addressed and to the person's situation. Resistance testing can reveal several important aspects of strength, including maximal force, the smoothness of contraction and relaxation (lack of spasticity), balance of strength between extensor and flexor muscle groups, symmetry between left and right sides, and resistance to fatigue. Resistance training is also an excellent addition to a rehabilitation program and is often overlooked in cardiovascular rehabilitation programs. Strength training may well belong in virtually every program for persons with a chronic disease or disability.

Flexibility Tests

Flexibility is also a critical aspect of exercise programming. Range of motion is important because muscle force, in order to be useful, must be applied through a full range of movement for the proper performance of physical work. Normal joint and spine movement can maintain symmetry of function and protects muscles, joints, and bones from strain and injury. Like other forms of exercise testing, assessment of flexibility can be performed in a variety of ways, but the easiest, most versatile, and least expensive is use of a simple goniometer. For our purposes, goniometry is probably most worthwhile in people with neuro-musculoskeletal disability, such as those with extreme scar tissue in joints, contractures, spasticity, and so on. Many exercise programs complete flexibility training (i.e., stretching) during the warm-up and cool-down segments of an exercise training session. Some people may require more extensive stretching, perhaps in combination with specific programs, in order to regain and maintain flexibility.

Neuromuscular Tests

Neuromuscular tests, which assess coordination and skill, are most useful in persons with a neuromuscular disability or those who are severely debilitated from chronic disease or are frail. As a result, these types of tests are more commonly used by physical, occupational, and kinesiotherapists than by exercise physiologists. Examples include reaction time, hand-eye coordination tests, and gait analysis. These kinds of tests should be used for the most part in persons with neuromuscular deficits that need specific assessment and programming.

Functional Performance Tests

Functional performance tests are advantageous in that they present real-life challenges in a laboratory setting where performance can be quantified. While there are a large number of neuromuscular and functional tests that are scientifically accepted, it may be possible to create a measurement that is particularly well suited to a given individual's clinical situation.

No Exercise Tests

One predicament that exercise professionals encounter is the need to design a program without having any exercise test data. It isn't necessary to have an exercise test to begin a program. By using two or more techniques to measure relative intensity (such as heart rate and perceived exertion), you can compare them against each other as well as prior experience. Err on having your client exercise

on the low side; you'll soon discover that it's too easy and can then increase the work rates to a more appropriate level. Within a week or two, your client will be on the right track.

On the other hand, you may wish to improvise a test. It is possible to use age- and gender-predicted values as "test results," but this can lead to inappropriate prescriptions in persons who aren't close to the average values. One common example is peak heart rate in persons on beta-antagonist drugs. Many authors have attempted to refine methods to yield more accurate predictions, and if these methods work successfully for you, use them. A more pragmatic approach, however, is to improvise an informal submaximal exercise study in the form of an exercise session, or several studies over the course of a week. The simple rules recommended in this chapter, and the protocols in each chapter's table on exercise testing, provide useful information. For example, you can perform a submaximal bicycle ergometer study by using a ramped protocol and recording heart rates and rating of perceived exertion up to a level of 17 on a 20-point scale. You would then prescribe a range of exercising heart rates based on perceived exertion.

Summary

The exercise specialist working with persons with a chronic disease or disability must be able to employ techniques from each of the seven families of exercise tests. In the past, much of the emphasis has been on aerobic exercise testing, largely because of the prevalence of cardiovascular disease and the popularity of aerobic exercise. However, many exercise professionals have long used measures of strength, flexibility, neuromuscular skill, and functional performance. Since activities of daily living are integrated functions that require some element from each family of exercise, exercise specialists working with persons having a chronic disease or disability should incorporate the various test results in developing a comprehensive exercise management plan. In addition, many of the new exercise machines are useful as tools in obtaining these measurements, but exercise specialists at facilities without these specialized machines can still assess exercise intolerance by using simple tools and a little ingenuity. A thorough knowledge of testing and test devices and an ability to improvise will be required. For some exercise specialists, this success may be enhanced by collaborating with other specialists who have complementary expertise and skills.

Exercise and Medicines

Most persons with a chronic disease or disability take medicines to treat their medical problems. Unfortunately, little is known about the side effects that most medicines have as they relate to exercise capacity and quality of life. Some medicines improve exercise performance in general, whereas some improve exercise performance when used for specific chronic diseases. However, some medicines reduce exercise performance and thereby can have an adverse impact on quality of life. The development of an exercise management plan includes consideration of drug-induced changes in exercise performance, as well as optimal dosing of medicines to achieve a desired exercise response. Very little is known about the effects of most medicines on adaptations to exercise training, but drug effects on exercise adaptability should be a consideration in exercise management.

It is easier to understand the effects of medicines on exercise performance if one thinks of exercise itself as a medicine. Exercise, in one sense, is an idealized "intensive care unit" in which neural, hormonal, and local factors alter heart rate and redirect blood flow to deliver oxygen and nutrients. Metabolic control of energy resources is profoundly affected while thermal, acid-base, and electrolyte regulation are altered to support exercise activity. Myriad changes constitute what we call the *exercise response,* but these physiologic changes reflect biochemical alterations in the body's control of metabolism. No modern intensive care unit can match the body's extraordinary and sophisticated system for delivery of biochemical compounds during exercise, despite the fact that some natural compounds (including hormones) are often used as prescription drugs. In this way exercise is a medicine.

Part of the difficulty in prescribing exercise as a drug is that exercise doesn't allow independent control over each biochemical process. During exercise, many biochemical reactions take place and we are unable to alter the sophistication of the whole process completely to our liking. However, we can take advantage of the interactions between exercise and medicines. *First*, different kinds of physical activity (e.g., aerobic, strength, flexibility) stimulate biochemical and physiologic processes in slightly different ways. *Second*, most medicines work by *blocking* or *enhancing* specific processes and as a result cause the desired (and undesired) effects. Drug-exercise interactions are determined by the blocked or stimulated processes common to both medicine and exercise. Thus, to understand the effect of a medicine on exercise, one must know both the biochemistry and the physiology of both exercise and the medicine. The challenge is to use these differing effects to the person's advantage.

The study of drug-exercise interactions has generally centered on high blood pressure, angina pectoris (chest pain), congestive heart failure, and ergogenic aids (drugs that improve performance). Most drug-exercise studies compare exercise response on and off medication or on different medications. This is largely for two reasons: (a) these studies are easier than longitudinal drug-training studies, and (b) these kinds of studies are part of FDA approval and pharmaceutical marketing programs. As a result, the effects of drugs on aerobic exercise response are better known than are the effects of drugs on training adaptations. Most drug-exercise studies have investigated drugs that alter cardiovascular function: alpha- and beta-adrenergic antagonists (alpha and beta blockers), calcium channel antagonists (calcium channel blockers), angiotensin-converting enzyme (ACE) inhibitors, vasoactive nitrates, and diuretics. Many neuromuscular drugs, such as antiparkinsonian drugs, have also been studied in relation to functional performance.

Paradoxical Effects

One paradox of drug-exercise interactions is that disease can alter physiologic action so that a drug can have opposite effects on exercise capacity when used in some combinations or in different disease states. Beta blockers are the most thoroughly studied drug with regard to exercise and provide a good example of paradoxical effects. In persons with high blood pressure, beta blockers typically reduce exercise capacity. However, in persons with mild to moderate congestive heart failure, beta blockers can increase exercise capacity. In severe congestive heart failure, beta blockers typically worsen exercise capacity, although careful prolonged use sometimes increases exercise capacity. The ACE inhibitors provide another example of paradoxical effects. In persons with high blood pressure, ACE inhibitors have no effect on exercise capacity, but in those with congestive heart failure, ACE inhibitors usually increase exercise capacity. The beta blocker example shows that drug therapy can help the person's disease but reduce exercise capacity. The mechanisms of these effects are complex and will not be discussed here, but these examples show that the effect on exercise capacity is not inherent in the drug, but rather in how the drug interacts with the biochemistry of exercise.

Adverse Effects

Sometimes drugs are recommended as preferred therapy even though they reduce exercise capacity. Beta blockers and diuretics are examples. Recommended as drugs of first choice for high blood pressure, beta blockers and diuretics are proven to prevent strokes and heart attacks and to increase longevity. Furthermore, they are inexpensive in comparison to newer medicines such as calcium channel blockers, ACE inhibitors, vasodilators, and alpha blockers. However, beta blockers and diuretics often impair exercise response, aerobic capacity, and quality of life, while the newer drugs generally do not have these particular side effects. Unfortunately, there are little data on efficacy in preventing strokes or heart attacks and prolonging life for most of these newer drugs. Thus, beta blockers and diuretics are recommended for high blood pressure even though newer (more expensive) drugs may make it possible to control blood pressure with fewer side effects on exercise capacity and quality of life.

Effects on Muscle

Medicines without cardiovascular action can alter exercise response through effects on skeletal muscle. Corticosteroids, beta blockers, and ACE inhibitors are examples. Corticosteroids are used for suppression of inflammatory and autoimmune diseases, as well as for immunosuppression in transplant recipients. In the absence of exercise, corticosteroids cause peripheral muscle wasting. In contrast, corticosteroids have no effect on the usual muscle adaptations to exercise training. Beta blockers also act on skeletal muscle and may attenuate skeletal muscle adaptations to training. On the other hand, long-term ACE inhibitor therapy appears to increase muscle blood flow, although this might be a result of increased physical activity. These examples suggest that the poorly understood effects of medicines on skeletal muscle may be critically important in people who are weak and lacking in endurance.

Drugs That Affect Metabolism

Use of hormones that regulate metabolism can alter functional capacity and response to training. Thyroid hormone and insulin are examples. *Hyperthyroidism* and *hypothyroidism* reduce exercise performance, and overreplacement or underreplacement of thyroid hormone can reduce exercise capacity. However, persons on adequate thyroid replacement have normal exercise performance. In one remarkable example, sprinter Gail Devers suffered from severe hyperthyroidism, but recovered after therapy to win gold medals in both the Olympic Games and World Championships. Insulin is used to control blood sugar in persons with diabetes, but insulin dosing usually should be reduced (or a snack eaten before exercise) in order to prevent life-threatening lowering of blood sugar during exercise.

Ergogenic Aids

Medicines that improve the ability to exercise are called ergogenic aids, and competitors are not allowed to use them because they provide an unfair advantage. However, it might be reasonable to make judicious use of ergogenic aids in some persons with a chronic disease or disability. For example, use of growth hormone or anabolic steroids may someday reveal the potential for improving exercise capacity in people who are weak and frail. Other ergogenic aids, such as stimulants, might also be helpful in carefully selected circumstances. For example, caffeinated beverages should be avoided by people with coronary artery disease, but might provide benefit to other people with exercise intolerance.

Other Medications

Little is known about the effects of most other drugs on exercise performance. Notable among these are drugs with antiparkinsonian and anticholinergic activity. Almost nothing is known about the effects of polypharmacy (use of multiple drugs). Many people take several medications several times a day. Under these circumstances, it is well known that people forget to take their medicines. Furthermore, when adherence or timing of a medication dose varies, the exercise response may be affected. Finally, while the effects of exercise on medicines are generally unexplored, it is worth noting that even less is known about the effects of exercise on the metabolism of medicines (i.e., whether a drug's metabolism is increased or decreased).

The examples in this section provide no details about the interactions between medicines and exercise. Nonetheless, exercise professionals must know (or learn) about the medications their clients are taking and must be able to assess how the medicine may alter each person's physiology. A pharmacology textbook should be a standard reference for anyone attempting to manage exercise for someone who takes medicines. Exercise professionals should establish a working relationship with the individual's physician so that suggestions about changing medications or dosing schedules can be smoothly integrated into overall medical management. The reader is referred to appendix A for a table on the effects of selected medications.

Exercise Dose-Response

Prescribing exercise for persons with chronic disease or disability is a very complex art. The objective is to decrease physiologic limitations and improve physical capacity through specific therapies. The biggest dilemmas are not in determining which therapies to use, but in defining the goals and choosing the appropriate training intensity, duration, and frequency. The key question is: What is the dose-response relationship of exercise training for each disease and disability?

In considering exercise programming for persons with chronic disease or disability, one often has little data on which to base decisions. Recommendations for preventing death from heart disease are based on large studies, but since these studies generally have not included persons with chronic disease or disability, present data may not be applicable. Furthermore, restoring and maintaining functional capacity and independence are very different goals from preventing cardiovascular disease. Unfortunately, exercise training to optimize functional capacity has not been well studied in the context of most chronic diseases or disabilities. As a result, many exercise professionals have used clinical experience to develop their own methods for prescribing exercise. Many of the recommendations in this manual were derived in this manner.

Experience is an acceptable way to guide exercise management, but a systematic approach would be better. One logical alternative would be to model exercise in the same way that pharmacologists model medications—through the use of exercise principles for dose response. Exercise prescriptions are similar to medical prescriptions. Medicines are prescribed by action (type of chemical), bioavailability (which determines the dose), therapeutic level (the goal of therapy), and half-life (metabolism of the medicine). Prescription of exercise is quite similar. The family of exercise specifies the action (e.g., aerobic training increases $\dot{V}O_2$max; strength training increases muscle strength and mass); exercise dose is a function of intensity and duration (hard workouts at high intensity or long duration yield a higher

number of total MET-minutes); exercise frequency is determined by the desired fitness level (therapeutic goal) and the length of time for recovery from an exercise session (half-life).

These principles explain some common practices in exercise science and sport. Athletes who desire to be very fit exercise daily or even twice daily, whereas wellness enthusiasts exercise three or four times a week. People who recover quickly can exercise on the day after a big workout, whereas other people may need an intervening day of rest, particularly after a very high-dose session. Like people who are sensitive to medicines and require lower doses, those with low functional capacity are easily exhausted, and it is common to prescribe short, low-intensity workouts with long rest periods (low-dose exercise). Just as a therapeutic drug level in the blood can be achieved with use of a lower dose more frequently, conditioning can be achieved through use of lower-intensity exercise two or three times a day. Just as slowly metabolized drugs must be given less often, persons who are slow to recover and adapt need more rest between exercise sessions.

Prescribing the right dose of exercise is important, because one can experience an acute "overdose" of exercise. Like marathoners "hitting the wall," persons with chronic disease or disability can suddenly become worn out, often by small amounts of exercise. Common sense suggests that one should probably avoid exhaustion (an exercise overdose), but there are few data to support or refute this notion. In comparison, overtraining is essentially a chronic overdose of exercise, and is associated with psychologic and physiologic decompensation as well as musculoskeletal injury. Acute exercise overdoses and chronic overtraining must be avoided in persons who have limited reserve because of chronic disease or disability.

One area in which pharmacologists are ahead of exercise specialists is in following the therapeutic effect of medicines. Pharmacologists can do this by measuring drug levels in the blood. This information can then be used to help guide dose frequency. Exercise specialists can try using exercise tests to assess progress, but this information is not as helpful as data on drug level in the blood are to pharmacologists. A systematic way to guide frequency of exercise training has not been developed, largely because we do not fully understand fatigue and adaptation.

The person's starting level, resistance to fatigue, and adaptability to training are probably what determine the total dose of exercise required to achieve a given fitness level. Perceived fatigue is not like perceived exertion, which is proportional to exercise intensity (e.g., the 20-point Borg scale). Fatigue seems to have a threshold; after this threshold is reached, exhaustion occurs quite rapidly. Adaptability is also poorly understood. It is possible to increase the adaptation rate by training harder (increasing the intensity or frequency of exercise sessions), but training too hard leads to decompensation or injury. Thus, all we can say at present is that high doses of exercise increase the risk of exhaustion; high frequency of exercise superimposes more training on incomplete recovery and risks overtraining.

Risk, Cost, and Benefit

It is common to think of musculoskeletal injury, heart attack, and sudden death as the risks of exercise. In fact, persons who are healthy and able-bodied are at risk largely for musculoskeletal injuries. For example, despite highly publicized cases of sudden death, basketball players are at greater risk for spraining their ankles. Only the basketball players with heart disease are at risk for sudden death. So exercise involves two kinds of risks: *disease-dependent* and *activity-dependent*. Disease-dependent risks are the adverse effects of exercise that are a consequence of disease. Activity-dependent risks are the adverse effects of exercise that are a consequence of accidents occurring during an activity. Activity- and disease-dependent risks must be considered for each person with a chronic disease or disability.

In general, the most important risks are disease-dependent: arthritic joints can become more inflamed, diabetics can lose control of their blood sugar, people with high blood pressure can have a stroke or heart attack, patients with heart failure can have abnormal heart rhythms, patients with poor balance can fall, prosthetics can cause skin trauma and irritation, and so on. The most common activity-dependent complications are probably musculoskeletal injury and exhaustion, while the most feared risks of heart attack and sudden death occur largely in people with heart disease. Accurate estimates of these risks are not available. Although few clinical exercise trials in persons with a chronic disease or disability have reported life-threatening complications, virtually all studies have used small, selected populations that precluded high-risk subjects. Some data suggest a high incidence of musculoskeletal injury with the use of intense exercise in weak and frail individuals, although this has not been a universal finding. Although the data on risk are generally not clear, it is prudent to monitor vigilantly for potential complications.

The costs of exercise training include time, energy, and money put into the program. Fortunately, exercise can be inexpensive compared to other modern medical therapies (particularly so for unsupervised exercise). Even so, exercise is far from cost-free. Membership in a YMCA/YWCA, health club, or fitness center can cost several hundred dollars per year. Some individuals may need to choose a center that caters to persons who have special medical circumstances and need medical supervision. Investment in the appropriate clothing, shoes, and assorted equipment can also be substantial. This can be particularly true for those who must invest in prosthetic equipment or sport/racing wheelchairs. Protective equipment such as pads, gloves, skin protection materials, and helmets must not be overlooked. Since very few people can participate in a lifetime of exercise and be totally free from medical complications (especially activity-dependent problems), it may be reasonable to assume that there will be at least some associated medical costs. Lastly, personal time and energy are major costs of any program, but these are difficult to quantify in monetary terms.

The various investments in an exercise program must be weighed against the probable benefits. Benefits from exercise training are usually related to functional capacity and quality of life, although some populations also benefit from decreased morbidity and mortality. Furthermore, it is sometimes possible to decrease the doses of medications and reap a direct financial return on investment. There has been some success in predicting outcome for cardiac rehabilitation patients, and this technique may be useful for other populations. Until then, an exercise trial is probably worthwhile in any person with a chronic disease or disability. In contrast, a person who has several diseases and/or disabilities may gain little or may even be adversely affected by exercise training. Thus, it is difficult to know who is too sick to benefit from exercise. In people who are too sick to improve, it usually becomes apparent that exercise is of little benefit. Unfortunately, it is not currently possible to know how much someone will benefit from a given exercise program, and in many cases it is impossible to compare the benefits to costs in monetary terms. Better methods of predicting adaptation would improve goal setting and improve risk/benefit as well as cost/benefit analyses.

Putting It All Together

Now comes the point of putting it all together. Some of the techniques suggested in this manual will be new to exercise specialists, who will require some time to learn them and become proficient in their use. Successful exercise management does not require use of these principles, but thinking about exercise in the contexts presented here can help determine what exercise tests to use, how to accommodate medicines, how to develop goals, how to estimate the dose response, and how to assess the risk/benefit and cost/benefit relationships. These considerations may be particularly complicated in persons with a low exhaustion threshold, frequent intercurrent illness, multiple chronic diseases, and poor adherence. In someone with only one relatively minor medical problem or disability, these tasks may be simple and straightforward. In someone with a severe chronic disease or disability or multiple chronic diseases and/or disabilities, these tasks are very complex. Problem-oriented exercise management using SOAP notes is one mechanism that can be employed to solve these problems. When using this approach, be sure to follow some key steps.

When taking subjective data:

- Uncover the nature of the problem as it relates to exercise.
- Ask about old and new musculoskeletal injuries.
- Look at the person for obvious problems.

When choosing exercise tests (objective data):

- Select the families of exercise tests that provide insight into the problem.
- Use modes and protocols that can be individualized.
- Use tests that provide specific measures that either will further define the problem or will determine specific aspects of the exercise program.
- Be aware of medications that may affect the test results, and know the times they are taken.
- Be aware of concomitant conditions and any special circumstances.

When making an assessment:

- Organize the assessment either by family of exercise or by physiologic problem.
- Consider possible need for additional tests.

- Be flexible in assessing multiple problems, and attack each one independently (but watch for interactions).
- Be aware that each problem may follow its own time course.
- If unsure, consider a therapeutic trial.

When developing an exercise program:

- Choose the families and modes of exercise that best treat the problem.
- Choose goals that are realistically attainable to increase the chance of success.
- Adjust exercise doses on the basis of exercise test measures, perceived exercise intensity, and the "fatigue threshold."
- Recommend frequency of training based on the total exercise dose and the person's adaptability.
- Accommodate any need for prosthetic, orthotic, or assistive devices.
- Consider the potential interactions of exercise and medications.
- Consider the disease-dependent and activity-dependent risks.
- Be aware that most of the benefits are probably related to quality of life.

When monitoring:

- Beware the sudden onset of exhaustion, as well as insufficient recovery and overtraining.
- Monitor stability of the underlying medical problems and changes in medications.
- When in doubt about safety, or if an activity causes pain, don't do it.
- When in doubt about progression, increase in small increments.
- Don't allow people to push themselves hard unless they are well warmed up.

When following up:

- Report progress in terms that have meaning to the individual, not in exercise jargon.
- Estimate dose response and be willing to consider failure to benefit.
- Always follow up on unresolved problems.
- Use the numbers you assign to the problems to help keep track of everything.
- Most interventions take weeks (if not months) to achieve a benefit—so be patient.

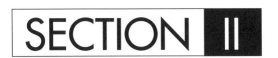

SECTION II

Cardiovascular and Pulmonary Diseases

Section Editors:

Geoffrey E. Moore, MD, FACSM

University of Pittsburgh

Scott O. Roberts, PhD, FAACVPR

Texas Tech University

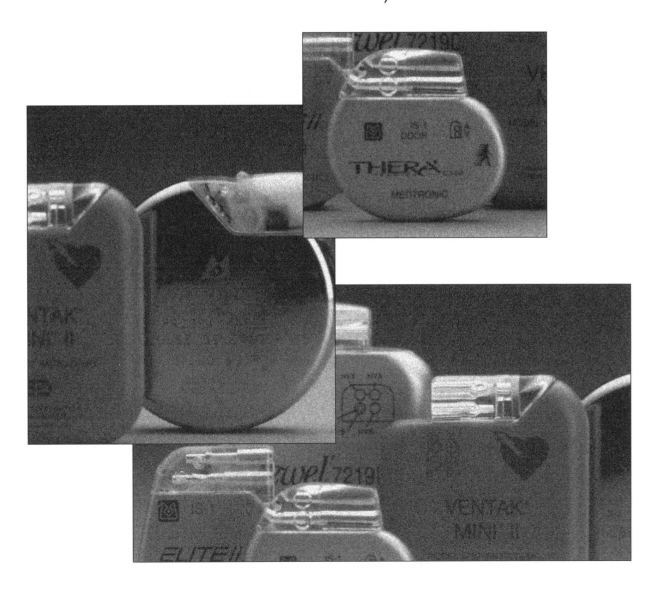

CHAPTER 3

Myocardial Infarction

Barry A. Franklin, PhD, FACSM

William Beaumont Hospital,
Wayne State University
School of Medicine

Overview of the Pathophysiology

Coronary atherosclerosis involves a localized accumulation of lipid and fibrous tissue within the coronary artery, progressively narrowing the lumen of the vessel. Fatty streaks may progress over time (generally 20 to 40+ years) to fibrous plaques and eventually to atheromata. Clinically significant lesions (> 75% of the vessel's cross-sectional area) that produce myocardial ischemia and left ventricular dysfunction often develop in the proximal, epicardial segments of coronary arteries at sites of abrupt curvature or branching. Atherosclerotic plaques may be complicated by hemorrhage, ulceration, calcification, or thrombosis (a clot). Prolonged ischemia (> 60 minutes) of cardiac tissue causes irreversible cellular damage and cell death, leading to acute myocardial infarction (MI). More than 1.5 million Americans have an MI each year; of these, approximately 500,000, or one-third, will die.

Myocardial infarction is classically characterized by a diagnostic triad of signs and symptoms:

- Severe, prolonged chest discomfort or pressure that may radiate to the arms, back, or neck, frequently associated with sweating, nausea, or vomiting.

- Increased serum levels of cardiac enzymes released by dying myocardial cells (aspartate transaminase, also called serum glutamic oxaloacetic transaminase; creatine phosphokinase or creatine kinase; or lactic dehydrogenase).

- Electrocardiographic changes in the leads overlying the area of infarction, consisting of ST-segment elevation and T-wave inversion; these changes result from ischemic injury and disappear over time. Finally, pronounced Q waves indicate myocardial necrosis and become a permanent change in the person's ECG.

Myocardial infarction usually affects the left ventricle and is associated with permanent loss of contractile function in the area of dead muscle cells, as well as impaired contractility in the surrounding muscle. Two types of infarctions are generally described, depending upon the amount of myocardial tissue involved:

- A **transmural infarction** (**Q-wave infarction**) involves the full thickness of the ventricular wall.

- A **subendocardial infarction** (**non-Q-wave infarction**) is limited to the inner half of the myocardium.

Thus, not everyone who has an MI gets the Q waves described above.

Infarctions are further described according to the involvement of the coronary arteries and location on the ventricle. For example, anterior infarctions result from lesions in the left anterior descending coronary artery and involve the anterior wall of the left ventricle, whereas inferior wall infarctions are generally the result of right coronary artery lesions. Other common infarct sites are lateral, posterior, and septal. Extensive infarctions involving large portions of the ventricle are referred to by combining the adjacent locations into one word (e.g., anteroseptal, inferolateral).

After an acute MI, the risk of future cardiovascular morbidity and mortality is largely determined by two variables:

- The extent of left ventricular damage or dysfunction

- The degree of residual myocardial ischemia

Ventricular dysfunction is characterized by a parameter called *ejection fraction*, which is the portion of blood pumped out with each beat. Normal ejection fraction is about $62 \pm 6\%$, measured at rest. Residual myocardial ischemia, as manifest by exertional chest discomfort and/or ECG changes in the ST segment, suggests that there is an open but narrowed artery, which could become occluded in the future and cause a second MI.

Effects on the Exercise Response

Acute MI may alter the individual's cardiorespiratory and hemodynamic responses to submaximal and maximal exercise. People who have suffered a previous MI often have a subnormal aerobic capacity (50-70% of age, gender predicted). The reduced oxygen transport capacity is attributable primarily to diminished cardiac output (stroke volume, heart rate, or both) rather than to a reduction in peripheral extraction of oxygen. In some individuals, a primary limitation appears to be the decreased contractile force of the left ventricle because of residual ischemia or scarring, causing a progressive decrease in ejection fraction and stroke volume. This decreased ejection fraction and stroke volume is often manifested as a blunted or decreasing systolic blood pressure response to progressive exercise (exertional hypotension). In other people, cardiac output may be limited by the restriction in the rise of the heart rate due to intrinsic disease of the sinoatrial node or atrioventricular node (chronotropic impairment) or by the appearance of anginal symptoms, with or without ischemic ST-segment depression; these preclude exercising to a higher level. Life-threatening exercise-induced ventricular dysrhythmias also occur more commonly in persons with previous MI than in individuals without heart disease. In addition, since these persons are often taking medications to decrease heart rate and blood pressure (to lower myocardial oxygen demands), the type and dose of these medications should be noted before the individual undergoes exercise testing or training.

Effects of Exercise Training

Common rationales for exercise training of persons with previous MI include

- increased maximal oxygen consumption ($\dot{V}O_2$peak; mean about 20%), which generally varies inversely with the pretraining $\dot{V}O_2$peak;

- relief of anginal symptoms, since training will lower the heart rate and/or blood pressure (and thus myocardial oxygen demand) at any given submaximal work rate;

- modest decreases in body fat, blood pressure (particularly in hypertensive patients), total blood cholesterol, serum triglycerides, and low-density lipoprotein (LDL) cholesterol;

- increases in the "antiatherogenic" high-density lipoprotein (HDL) cholesterol;

- improved well-being and self-efficacy; and

- protection against the triggering of MI by strenuous physical exertion (6 MET s).

On the other hand, conventional exercise training, as an isolated intervention, does little to improve left ventricular ejection fraction or myocardial perfusion. Numerous training studies have now demonstrated increased exercise tolerance in persons with impaired left ventricular function, despite the lack of improvement in resting hemodynamics or ejection fraction. However, those who have *both* left ventricular dysfunction and exercise-induced myocardial ischemia show little or no increase in $\dot{V}O_2$max after early outpatient cardiac rehabilitation.

Meta-analyses of previous randomized, controlled clinical trials of rehabilitation with exercise after MI have shown a 20% to 25% reduction in total and cardiovascular-related mortality, with no difference in the rate of nonfatal recurrent events. However, current thrombolytic and revascularization procedures, which markedly decrease postinfarction mortality, would be likely to diminish these benefits of adjunctive contemporary cardiac rehabilitation programs.

The advisability of vigorous exercise training for two client subsets has been recently questioned:

- Individuals with exertional ST-segment depression without symptoms (silent ischemia; see chapter 5, "Angina and Silent Ischemia")

- Persons recovering from MI involving a large portion of the anterior wall

Although isolated reports have suggested that vigorous exercise training in these individuals may actually worsen cardiac function, others suggest that increased fibrosis, infarct expansion, and a deterioration in left ventricular function are unlikely outcomes of exercise training.

Management and Medications

Medical management of the individual is essentially undertaken to minimize the severity of clinical sequelae and to potentially slow, halt, or even reverse the progression of atherosclerosis. Persons at moderate-to-high risk of dying might live longer if they have successful percutaneous transluminal coronary angioplasty or coronary artery bypass graft surgery. Risk factor interventions aimed at smoking cessation, lipid/lipoprotein modification, hypertension control, and increasing physical activity, as well as beneficial drugs (including beta blockers and aspirin) have produced significant reductions in cardiovascular-related morbidity and mortality.

Appropriate drug therapy decreases mortality after acute MI, reduces complications in unstable angina, improves symptoms in stable angina and heart failure, suppresses worrisome atrial and ventricular dysrhythmias, and inhibits clot formation. Accordingly, many persons take one or more medications after acute MI, including anti-ischemic drugs (beta blockers, calcium channel-blocking agents, nitroglycerin, and longer-acting nitrate drugs—see chapter 5, "Angina and Silent Ischemia"), platelet inhibitors, anticoagulants, drugs for the treatment of heart failure (digitalis, diuretics, angiotensin-converting enzyme inhibitors—see chapter 8, "Congestive Heart Failure"), vasodilators, antiarrhythmic drugs, and lipid-altering drugs (see chapter 17, "Hyperlipidemia"). Several of the cardiovascular medications, however, may influence the responses to exercise testing and training.

- **Diuretics** do not alter chronotropic reserve or aerobic capacity. Thus, the prescribed exercise heart rate can be determined in the standard fashion.

- **Beta blockers** decrease submaximal and maximal heart rate and sometimes exercise capacity, especially with nonselective agents. Nevertheless, exercise trainability appears to be uncompromised, despite a reduced training heart rate. Because beta blockers do not alter the remarkably consistent relationship between %HRpeak and % $\dot{V}O_2$peak, the generally prescribed metabolic work rate for training (60-80% $\dot{V}O_2$peak) may be achieved at the conventional relative heart rate recommendation for training (70-85% HRpeak).

- **Central nervous system–active drugs** have varying effects on the heart rate and blood pressure during exercise. Thus, the potential hypotension, dizziness, and syncope should be carefully monitored.

- **Vasodilators and angiotensin-converting enzyme inhibitors** generally do not affect the heart rate response to exercise. Consequently, exercise training intensity can be prescribed in the usual manner. Persons on these medications may be subject to hypotensive episodes in the postexercise period unless an adequate cooldown is performed.

- **Calcium channel blockers** do not generally impair functional capacity or exercise trainability. However, certain calcium channel blockers may alter the heart rate response to exercise (e.g., verapamil). Consequently, the prescribed training heart rate should be based on the medicated person's response to an exercise test.

- **Alpha-receptor blockers** significantly lower systolic (SBP) and diastolic blood pressure (DBP) but appear to have minimal effects on the heart rate and on metabolic responses to exercise. Therefore, training heart rates may be prescribed in the usual manner.

Recommendations for Exercise Testing

The test protocol should be selected to accommodate the person's ability to perform lower-extremity exercise (see table on exercise testing at the end of this chapter). People unable to perform treadmill or cycle ergometer exercise may, alternatively, be evaluated by arm crank ergometry or pharmacologic stress testing at rest.

The exercise test should begin at an intensity level considerably below the anticipated peak or symptom-limited capacity and should increase gradually in 2- or 3-minute stages, with cardiorespiratory measures made at each progressive stage. A target test duration of 10 ± 2 minutes has been suggested. Contraindications to testing and indications for terminating exercise should be closely observed.

The primary objectives of exercise testing of these persons are to evaluate quantitatively and accurately the following functions:

- Chronotropic capacity

- Aerobic capacity of the body ($\dot{V}O_2$peak)

- Myocardial aerobic capacity, estimated by the peak rate-pressure product

- Exertional symptoms (e.g., increasing chest pain or light-headedness)

- Associated changes in electrical functions of the heart (e.g., dysrhythmias, ST-T-wave changes)

These data are critical to establish a safe and effective metabolic load for aerobic exercise training.

Because ST-segment abnormalities that develop during exercise are difficult to interpret or uninterpretable in some circumstances (presence of digitalis, substantial ST-segment depression at rest, left ventricular hypertrophy, or left bundle-branch block), exercise testing with myocardial perfusion imaging (e.g., thallium-201 chloride or Technetium Tc 99m Sestamibi [Cardiolite] scintigraphy) is often recommended to screen for myocardial ischemia in persons with these conditions.

Recommendations for Exercise Programming

Simple exposure to orthostatic or gravitational stress (e.g., intermittent sitting or standing during the bed rest stage of hospital convalescence [Phase I]) can obviate much of the deterioration in exercise performance that normally follows acute MI. Large muscle group exercise that is rhythmic—for example, walking, cycle ergometry, rowing, or stair climbing—is appropriate for outpatient (Phase II-IV) physical conditioning. Because the training benefits do not substantially cross over from the legs to the arms and vice versa, both sets of limbs should be exercised. Mild-to-moderate resistance training can also provide a safe and effective method for improving muscular strength and endurance in selected cardiac individuals.

Recommendations for exercise programming are found in the table at the end of this chapter. They can be summarized as follows:

- **Intensity** generally corresponds to 40% to 85% of maximal heart rate reserve, with rate of perceived exertion (RPE; 11 to 16 [6-20 scale]) used as an adjunct to heart rate as an intensity guide.

- **Frequency** of exercise is at least three days per week.

- **Duration** of training involves 20 to 40 minutes of continuous or interval exercise, preceded and followed by warm-up and cool-down periods of about 10 minutes.

Suggested Readings

American College of Sports Medicine. 1994. Position stand. Exercise for patients with coronary artery disease. *Med. Sci. Sports Exerc.* 26: i-v.

Arvan, S. 1988. Exercise performance of the high risk acute myocardial infarction patient after cardiac rehabilitation. *Am. J. Cardiol.* 62: 197-201.

Fletcher, G.F., G. Balady, V.F. Froelicher, L.H. Hartley, W.L. Haskell, and M.L. Pollock. 1995. Exercise standards: A statement for healthcare professionals from the American Heart Association. *Circulation* 91: 580-615.

Franklin, B.A. 1989. Aerobic exercise training programs for the upper body. *Med. Sci. Sports Exerc.* 21: S141-S148.

Franklin, B.A., K. Bonzheim, S. Gordon, and G.C. Timmis. 1991. Resistance training in cardiac rehabilitation. *J. Cardiopulmonary Rehabil.* 11: 99-106.

Franklin, B.A., S. Gordon, and G.C. Timmis. 1992. Amount of exercise necessary for the patient with coronary artery disease. *Am. J. Cardiol.* 69: 1426-32.

Franklin, B.A., H.K. Hellerstein, S. Gordon, and G.C. Timmis. 1989. Cardiac patients. In *Exercise in modern medicine*, ed. B.A. Franklin, S. Gordon, and G.C. Timmis, 44-80. Baltimore: Williams & Wilkins.

Froelicher, V.F., D. Jensen, F. Genter, M. Sullivan, M. McKirnan, K. Witztum, J. Scharf, M. Strong, and W. Ashburn. 1984. A randomized trial of exercise training in patients with coronary heart disease. *JAMA* 252: 1291-97.

Giannuzzi, P., L. Tavazzi, P.L. Temporelli, U. Corra, A. Imparato, M. Gattone, A. Giordano, L. Sala, C. Schweiger, and C. Malinverni. 1993. Long-term physical training and left ventricular remodeling after anterior myocardial infarction: Results of the exercise in anterior myocardial infarction (EAMI) trial. *J. Am. Coll. Cardiol.* 22: 1821-29.

Giannuzzi, P., P.L. Temporelli, L. Tavazzi, U. Corrá, M. Gattone, A. Imparato, A. Giordano, C. Schweiger, L. Sola, C. Molinverni, and the EAMI Study Group. 1992. EAMI-Exercise training in anterior myocardial infarction: An ongoing multicenter randomized study: preliminary results of left ventricular function and remodeling. *Chest* 101: 315S-321S.

Jugdutt, B.I., B.L. Michorowski, and C.T. Kappagoda. 1988. Exercise training after anterior Q wave myocardial infarction: Importance of regional left ventricular function and topography. *J. Am. Coll. Cardiol.* 12: 362-72.

Lau, J., E.M. Antman, J. Jimenez-Salva, B. Kupelnick, F. Mosteller, and T.C. Chalmers. 1992. Cumulative meta-analysis of therapeutic trials for myocardial infarction. *N. Engl. J. Med.* 327: 248-54.

Mark, D.B., M.A. Hlatky, R.M. Califf, J.J. Morris, Jr., S.D. Sisson, C.B. McCants, K.L. Lee, F.E. Harrell, Jr., D.B. Pryor. 1989. Painless exercise ST deviation on the treadmill: long-term prognosis. *J. Am. Coll. Cardiol.* 14: 885-892.

Mittleman, M.A., M. Maclure, G.H. Tofler, J.B. Sherwood, R.J. Goldberg, and J.E. Muller. 1993. Triggering of acute myocardial infarction by heavy physical exertion: Protection against triggering by regular exertion. *N. Engl. J. Med.* 329: 1677-83.

Pashkow, F.J. 1993. Issues in contemporary cardiac rehabilitation: A historical perspective. *J. Am. Coll. Cardiol.* 21: 822-34.

Schuler, G., G. Shlierf, A. Wirth, H. Mautner, H. Scheurlen, M. Thumm, H. Roth, F. Schwarz, M. Kohlmeier, H. Mehmel, W. Kübler. 1988. Low fat diet and regular, supervised physical exercise in pateients with symptomatic coronary artery disease: reduction of stress-induced myocardial ischemia. *Circulation* 77: 172-81.

Sullivan, M.J., M.B. Higginbotham, and F.R. Cobb. 1988. Exercise training in patients with severe left ventricular dysfunction: hemodynamic and metabolic effects. *Circulation* 78: 506-15.

MYOCARDIAL INFARCTION: EXERCISE TESTING

METHODS	MEASURES	ENDPOINTS*	COMMENTS
Aerobic power **Cycle** (17 watts/min) ramp protocol (25-50 watts/3 min stage) **Treadmill** (1-2 METs/3 min stage)	• 12-lead ECG, heart rate	• Serious dysrhythmias • > 2 mm ST-segment depression or elevation • Ischemic threshold • T-wave inversion with significant ST change	• Use low-level treadmill protocol for acute MI clients. • Important in establishing a safe training intensity. • Chronotropic impairment results in poor prognosis. • Minimal treadmill speed should be $\leq$ 1.0 mph.
	• Blood pressure	• SBP > 260 mmHg or DBP > 115 mmHg	• Exertional hypotension (drop of $\geq$ 20 mmHg or failure to rise) suggests poor prognosis.
	• RPE (Borg 6-20 or 0-10 scale)		• May be useful, but approximately 10% of clients use scale inappropriately.
	• Angina scale	• +3 or earlier on +1 to +4 scale (see table on testing in chapter 5)	
	• Gas analysis (peak $\dot{V}O_2$)		• Only if exact measures are indicated, ventilatory threshold is often useful.
	• Radionuclide testing		• Is more sensitive and specific than exercise ECG in assessing ischemic heart disease.
Strength **Isokinetic/isotonic**	• 90% maximal voluntary contraction (MVC) greatest load lifted 2-3 times	• 3 consecutive repetitions	• Useful in planning resistance exercise program. • Meant to improve muscle strength/ endurance and reverse or delay the deleterious effects of bed rest. • Use 1 repetition maximum (estimated from 90% MV) to establish training load.

*Measurements of particular significance; do not *always* indicate test termination.

(continued)

MYOCARDIAL INFARCTION: EXERCISE TESTING (continued)

MEDICATIONS	SPECIAL CONSIDERATIONS
• See appendix A. • Beta blockers: Decrease submaximal and maximal HR and blood pressure (BP) response and sometimes exercise capacity, especially with nonselective medications. • Vasodilators and ACE inhibitors: Do not generally affect exercise HR response. However, clients may be more susceptible to postexercise hypotension. • Calcium channel blockers: May alter exercise HR response (e.g., verapamil). • Central nervous system–active drugs: Have varied effects on HR and BP during exercise. Caution for hypotension, dizziness, and syncope. • Alpha blockers: Decrease systolic and diastolic BP response, but have minimal effects on HR and $\dot{V}O_2$ responses to exercise. • Digitalis: May promote spurious ST-T–wave changes (interpret with caution). Sometimes used to control atrial dysrhythmias. • Nitroglycerin: May mask or attenuate ischemic responses.	• Clients with concomitant orthopedic limitations may require cycle or arm ergometer testing, or alternatively, pharmacologic stress testing to assess cardiac function. • Clients with coronary artery disease are more likely to demonstrate limiting signs or symptoms including angina, ischemic ST depression, BP abnormalities, and serious ventricular dysrhythmias. • Clients with high-grade peripheral vascular disease may not be able to achieve cardiac stress ($\geq$ 85% maximal age-predicted heart rate) with conventional treadmill testing. • Maximal stress testing should not be performed immediately prior to hematologic screening. • Some cardiac medications can influence temperature regulation. • 12-hour fast or light meal is recommended prior to testing.

MYOCARDIAL INFARCTION: EXERCISE PROGRAMMING

MODES	GOALS	INTENSITY/ FREQUENCY/DURATION	TIME TO GOAL
Aerobic • Large muscle activities • Arm/leg ergometry	• Increase aerobic capacity. • Decrease BP and HR response to submaximal exercise. • Decrease myocardial $\dot{V}O_2$ demand. • Decrease coronary artery disease risk factors.	• Borg RPE of 11-16. • 40-85% $\dot{V}O_2$ max or HR reserve. • 3-4 days/week. • 20-40 minutes/session. • 5-10 minutes of warm-up and cool-down activities.	• 4-6 months
Strength • Circuit training	• Increase ability to perform leisure, occupational, and daily living activities. • Increase muscle strength and endurance.	• 40-50% maximal voluntary contraction (avoid Valsalva). • 2-3 days/week. • 1-3 sets, 10-15 repetitions. • Resistance should be gradually increased over time.	• 4-6 months
Flexibility • Upper and lower body range-of-motion activities	• Decrease risk of injury.	• 2-3 days/week.	• 4-6 months

MEDICATIONS	SPECIAL CONSIDERATIONS
• See appendix A. • Beta blockers: No major effect on exercise trainability in cardiac patients. • Calcium channel blockers: No major effect on exercise trainability in cardiac patients.	• Low-fit clients (functional capacity 5 MET s) can often train at 40-50% $\dot{V}O_2$ peak; 70% is appropriate for most clients. • Monitor for abnormal signs and symptoms, i.e., chest pain or pressure, dizziness, and dysrhythmias. • High-intensity exercise may precipitate cardiovascular complications in post-MI patients. • Supervision is suggested for moderate-to high-risk patients, e.g., those with exercise-induced myocardial ischemia manifested as ST-segment depression and/or angina pectoris and those with poor left ventricular function (ejection fraction < 30%). • Many post-MI patients have peripheral arterial disease and/ or diabetes mellitus (see tables in chapters 11 and 16 for additional guidelines). • When possible, select exercise equipment that can be adjusted in 1 MET increments. • Increasing muscular strength is an important component of an exercise program for post-MI clients, as it will decrease heart rate, blood pressure, and myocardial $\dot{V}O_2$ demand at any given resistance.

CHAPTER 4

Coronary Artery Bypass Grafting and Angioplasty

Barry A. Franklin, PhD, FACSM

William Beaumont Hospital,
Wayne State University
School of Medicine

Overview of the Pathophysiology

Coronary atherosclerosis involves a localized accumulation of lipid and fibrous tissue within the coronary artery, causing progressive narrowing of the lumen of the vessel. Clinically significant lesions, producing myocardial ischemia and ventricular dysfunction, usually obstruct over 75% of the vessel lumen. The aims of *revascularization* are

- to increase blood flow and oxygen delivery to ischemic myocardium beyond an obstructive arterial lesion and
- to potentially reduce cardiovascular-related morbidity and mortality.

Two basic revascularization techniques are widely used: coronary artery bypass grafting (CABG) and percutaneous transluminal coronary angioplasty (PTCA). The surgical technique involves bypassing the obstruction with either a saphenous vein removed from the person's leg, or with an internal mammary artery (one of the major arteries carrying blood to the chest wall). In PTCA, a balloon catheter is directed to the site of an atherosclerotic lesion until the balloon lies within the vascular stenosis. Inflation of the balloon produces

- plaque compression and redistribution and
- stretching of the vessel wall with an increase in the vessel diameter.

Today, more than half of all persons diagnosed with ischemic heart disease who are referred for revascularization (> 600,000 patients per year) undergo PTCA.

Coronary Artery Bypass Grafting

Current indications for CABG, after definition of coronary anatomy and left ventricular function by cardiac catheterization, are

- to relieve anginal symptoms that are refractory to pharmacologic therapy;
- when PTCA is contraindicated;
- to prolong life in persons with left main coronary artery disease, triple-vessel disease, or double-vessel disease and left ventricular dysfunction and/or proximal left anterior descending coronary artery disease; and
- to preserve left ventricular function in persons with diffuse or compelling coronary artery disease and significant additional myocardium in jeopardy, particularly when previous myocardial infarction has already compromised left ventricular function.

People who undergo CABG today are generally older and are more likely to have three-vessel disease and intrinsically poor ventricular pump function. The left ventricular ejection fraction in persons who undergo CABG averages 38%; the ejection fraction for those undergoing PTCA averages 55%. Complications of CABG, such as perioperative infarction, occur more frequently in older individuals, women, obese persons, individuals with left ventricular dysfunction (ejection fraction < 30%), and persons undergoing emergency bypass surgery. Current graft patency (an open lumen) rates for saphenous vein grafts are 90%, 80%, and 60% after 1, 5, and 11 years, respectively. Unfortunately, nearly half of these grafts become severely atherosclerotic within a decade. In contrast, internal mammary grafts have a 93% 10-year graft patency and appear to be resistant to atherosclerosis. This fact may partially explain the impressive 10-year actuarial survival advantage in persons undergoing CABG who received internal mammary grafts as compared to those who received vein bypass grafts. Total relief of angina pectoris typically occurs in 70% of persons who had CABG 5 years earlier; approximately 50% are asymptomatic at 10 years.

Percutaneous Transluminal Coronary Angioplasty

Although the use of PTCA was initially restricted to elective cases of low-risk individuals who had discrete, proximal, single-vessel lesions, indications for the procedure have since broadened to include persons with

- two-vessel or three-vessel disease,

- impaired left ventricular function, or

- acute occlusion during myocardial infarction.

However, people undergoing PTCA must be willing to undergo emergency CABG if dilation fails or complications occur. Compared to CABG, which historically requires a hospital stay of 6 to 9 days, the recovery period after elective PTCA is much shorter (1 to 2 days) and the initial cost is considerably less. However, failure remains the biggest limitation of PTCA. Approximately 30% to 40% of individuals undergoing PTCA will develop restenosis of the treated vessel within six months of the procedure.

Effects on the Exercise Response

Successful revascularization may alter the exercise response to a single session of exercise in several ways. By increasing the blood flow and oxygen supply to myocardial regions beyond an obstructive coronary arterial lesion, CABG or PTCA may reduce or eliminate electrocardiographic changes resulting from ischemia—that is, T-wave inversion, ST-segment depression, or both—as well as anginal symptoms on exertion. The latter may serve to increase physical work capacity in persons who are symptomatic at low levels of exercise. Correcting the imbalance between myocardial oxygen supply and demand may also improve ventricular contractility and wall motion, favorably altering the hemodynamic response to exercise. Chronotropic impairment and/or exertional hypotension may normalize after revascularization. Ischemia-related ventricular dysrhythmias may also be abolished by successful PTCA or CABG. Indeed, recent studies suggest that silent ischemia may increase risk of cardiac arrest in persons who don't have symptoms during exercise.

Effects of Exercise Training

The benefits and limitations of exercise training for persons undergoing PTCA or CABG are similar to those for survivors of acute myocardial infarction (see chapter 3). The average improvement in physical work capacity and maximal oxygen uptake is about 20%. Moreover, training-induced reductions in heart rate and blood pressure serve to decrease myocardial O_2 demands at rest and at any given submaximal work rate.

Although results from several meta-analyses have demonstrated a 20% to 25% reduction in fatal cardiovascular events and total mortality after myocardial infarction, the contribution of exercise training to survival of persons after CABG and PTCA has not been evaluated. It is also unclear what role physical conditioning plays in maintaining graft patency, preventing restenosis, or retarding atherosclerotic coronary disease after successful revascularization. Unfortunately, studies to date generally suggest that exercise training is largely ineffective in achieving these outcomes.

Management and Medications

The treatment of revascularization clients has progressed from the use of nitrate drugs and beta-blocking agents to an aggressive multi-modality approach using coronary risk factor modification, pharmacologic therapy (e.g., calcium channel-blocking drugs, new antiarrhythmic and lipid-lowering drugs), thrombolytic enzymes, PTCA, surgical interventions, and, when necessary, the implantable cardioverter defibrillator. The exact roles of these modalities in clients undergoing PTCA or CABG are uncertain today. Nevertheless, lifestyle interventions designed to slow, halt, or even reverse the underlying atherosclerotic disease process remain the mainstay of treatment; these include

- regular aerobic exercise,
- blood pressure control,
- smoking cessation,
- stress management, and
- cholesterol lowering.

Smoking cessation, for example, is associated with a higher prevalence of disease-free bypass grafts over time.

Empiric experience has shown that close observation and monitoring of revascularization clients during exercise-based cardiac rehabilitation can often detect a deterioration in clinical status. Exercise-related signs or symptoms that may indicate restenosis of a treated vessel, occlusion of vein grafts, or progression of atherosclerotic disease include

- recurring anginal pain (chest pain or pressure, an ache in the jaw or neck, pain across the shoulders or back),
- dizziness or light-headedness, and
- threatening forms of ventricular ectopy (frequent paired or multiform ventricular premature beats, couplets, or ventricular tachycardia).

Cardiac and lipid-lowering medications commonly used to treat revascularization clients are summarized elsewhere (in chapter 3 and appendix A), with specific reference to their hemodynamic and electrocardiographic effects. Unfortunately, interventions to prevent restenosis using aspirin (alone or in combination with dipyridamole), anticoagulants (e.g., warfarin, heparin), N-3 omega fatty acids, corticosteroid hormone therapy, and calcium channel-blocking drugs have been largely ineffective. Repeat PTCA is the usual treatment for restenosis, and most persons experience sustained improvement after the procedure.

Recommendations for Exercise Testing

Exercise testing can follow the general protocols and procedures outlined for individuals after myo-cardial infarction. Treadmill or cycle ergometer testing three to five weeks after CABG is valuable in assessing exercise tolerance and in prescribing levels of physical activity. In contrast, arm ergometer testing at this time may be uncomfortable because of midsternal incisional pain. Follow-up testing procedures are similar to those after acute myocardial infarction, that is, after an additional three to six months of exercise training and yearly thereafter. A functional capacity of 9 METs or more indicates a favorable prognosis, regardless of other responses.

The exercise test soon after PTCA may be more intense than that typically recommended after myocardial infarction or CABG. However, among asymptomatic subjects with single-vessel disease, the detection of restenosis and the utility of the exercise test to predict cardiovascular morbidity or mortality after PTCA is generally low. Preliminary signs or symptoms of restenosis, manifested as significant ST-segment depression, the provocation of angina pectoris, or both, may be apparent with exercise testing as early as two to three days after PTCA. A more accepted time period for initial evaluation of PTCA persons is two to five weeks, followed by another exercise test at six months. Thereafter, exercise testing once a year is generally considered adequate.

Recommendations for Exercise Programming

Walking is recommended as the major mode of exercise soon after coronary revascularization. General recommendations for exercise training are found in the table at the end of this chapter. Compared with persons with myocardial infarction, individuals after CABG typically

- begin inpatient exercise rehabilitation sooner,
- progress at a more accelerated rate, and
- devote more attention to upper extremity range-of-motion exercises.

However, upper-body ergometry or resistive exercises should be avoided until healing of the sternal incision is complete (generally four to eight weeks after CABG).

Subjects may begin to resume normal activities, including light to moderate exercise such as brisk walking, within 24 to 48 hours after PTCA. Exercise-based cardiac rehabilitation (Phase II) provides close monitoring and supervision in which failures (restenosis) can be detected early.

Suggested Readings

Acinapura, A.J., I.J. Jacobowitz, M.D. Kramer, M.S. Adkins, Z. Zisbrod, and J.N. Cunningham, Jr. 1990. Demographic changes in coronary artery bypass surgery and its effect on mortality and morbidity. *Eur. J. Cardiothorac. Surg.* 4: 175-81.

Balady, G.J., M.L. Leitschuh, A.K. Jacobs, D. Merrell, D.A. Weiner, and T.J. Ryan. 1992. Safety and clinical use of exercise testing one to three days after percutaneous transluminal coronary angioplasty. *Am. J. Cardiol.* 69: 1259-64.

Connolly, M.W., and R.A. Guyton. 1992. Surgical intervention in coronary heart disease. In *Rehabilitation of the coronary patient*, ed. N.K. Wenger and H.K. Hellerstein, 323-47. 3rd ed. New York: Churchill Livingstone.

Deligonul, U., M.G. Vandormael, Y. Shah, K. Galan, M.J. Kern, and B.R. Chaitman. 1989. Prognostic value of early exercise stress testing after successful coronary angioplasty: Importance of the degree of revascularization. *Am. Heart J.* 117: 509-14.

Dubach, P., V. Froelicher, J. Klein, and R. Detrano. 1989. Use of the exercise test to predict prognosis after coronary artery bypass grafting. *Am. J. Cardiol.* 65: 530-33.

Fitz Gibbon, G.M., A.J. Leach, and H.P. Kafka. 1987. Atherosclerosis of coronary artery bypass grafts and smoking. *Can. Med. Assoc. J.* 136: 45-47.

Fletcher, G.F., G. Balady, V.F. Froelicher, L.H. Hartley, W.L. Haskell, and M.L. Pollock. 1995. Exercise standards: A statement for healthcare professionals from the American Heart Association. *Circulation* 91: 580-615.

Hoberg, E., G. Schuler, B. Kunze, A.L. Obermoser, K. Hauer, H.P. Mautner, G. Schlierf, W. Kubler. 1990. Silent myocardial ischemia as a potential link between lack of premonitoring symptoms and increased risk of cardiac arrest during physical stress. *Am. J. Cardiol.* 65: 583-89.

Laarman, G., H.E. Luijten, L.G. van Zeyl, K.J. Beatt, J.G. Tijssen, P.W. Serruys, and J. de Feyter. 1990. Assessment of silent restenosis and long-term follow-up after successful angioplasty in single vessel coronary artery disease: The value of quantitative exercise electrocardiography and quantitative coronary angiography. *J. Am. Coll. Cardiol.* 16: 578-85.

Lytle, B.W., D. Cosgrove, and F.D. Loop. 1991. Future implications of current trends in bypass surgery. *Cardiovasc. Clin.* 21: 265-78.

Sabri, M.N., and M.J. Cowley. 1992. Coronary angioplasty and coronary atherectomy. In *Rehabilitation of the coronary patient*, ed. N.K. Wenger and H.K. Hellerstein, 303-22. 3rd ed. New York: Churchill Livingstone.

Schelkum, P.H. 1992. Exercise after angioplasty: How much? How soon? *Physician Sportsmed.* 20 (3): 199-212.

CABG/PTCA: EXERCISE TESTING

METHODS	MEASURES	ENDPOINTS*	COMMENTS
Aerobic power **Cycle** (17 watts/min) ramp protocol (25-50 watts/3 min stage) **Treadmill** (1-2 METs/3 min stage)	• 12-lead ECG, heart rate	• Serious dysrhythmias • > 2 mm ST-segment depression or elevation • Ischemic threshold • T-wave inversion with significant ST change	• ST-segment displacement can occur with restenosis or partial occlusion. • Important in establishing a safe training intensity. • Chronotropic impairment sug- gests poor prognosis. • Minimal treadmill speed should be 1.0 mph.
	• Blood pressure	• SBP > 260 mmHg or DBP > 115 mmHg	• Exertional hypotension (drop of $\geq$ 20 mmHg or failure to rise) suggests poor prognosis.
	• RPE (Borg 6-20 or scale)		• Useful as an adjunct to HR as an exercise intensity guide.
	• Gas analysis ($\dot{V}O_2$ peak)		• Only if exact measures are indi- cated. • For CABG clients, a peak work rate of 9 METs or more suggests a good prognosis.
Strength **Isokinetic/isotonic**	• 90% maximal voluntary contraction (MVC) greatest load lifted 2-3 times	• 3 consecutive repetitions	• Useful in planning resistance exercise program. • Use 1 repetition maximum (esti- mated from 90% MVC) to estab- lish training load. • Meant to improve muscle strength/endurance and reverse or delay the harmful effects of bed rest. • Should not be performed until sternum has healed.

*Measurements of particular significance; do not *always* indicate test termination.

MEDICATIONS	SPECIAL CONSIDERATIONS
• See testing table in chapter 3 and appendix A.	• See testing table in chapter 3. • Chest and leg wounds usually require 4 to 8 weeks for complete healing. Upper-body arm crank ergometer testing that may cause sternal tension should be avoided until healing is complete. • An extended active cool-down after peak or symptom-limited exercise testing has been suggested to reduce the risk of cardiovascular complications that commonly occur in the postexercise period. • Prolonged convalescence after CABG may further serve to decrease $\dot{V}O_2$ max. • After CABG, exercise testing often increases self-confidence and self-efficacy. • Clients often resume normal or near-normal activities soon after PTCA (i.e., within 24-48 hours).

CABG/PTCA: EXERCISE PROGRAMMING

MODES	GOALS	INTENSITY/ FREQUENCY/DURATION	TIME TO GOAL
Aerobic • Large muscle activities • Arm/leg ergometry	• Increase aerobic capacity. • Decrease blood pressure and heart rate response to submaximal exercise. • Decrease myocardial O_2 demand. • Decrease CAD risk factors.	• Borg RPE of 12-14. • 40-85% $\dot{V}O_2$ max or HR reserve. • Intensity must be kept below ischemic threshold. • 3-7 days/week. • 20-60 minutes/session. • 5-10 minutes of warm-up and cool-down activities.	• 4-6 months
Strength • Circuit training	• Increase ability to perform leisure, occupational, and daily living activities. • Increase muscle strength and endurance.	• 40-50% maximal voluntary contraction (avoid Valsalva). • 2-3 days/week. • 1-3 sets of 10-15 repetitions. • Start with 1-2 lb. Wait 6 weeks postoperation before using heavier weights. • Resistance can be progressively increased over time.	• 4-6 months
Flexibility • Upper and lower body range-of-motion activities	• Decrease risk of injury • Improve range of motion in CABG patients.	• 2-3 days/week.	• 4-6 months

MEDICATIONS	SPECIAL CONSIDERATIONS
• See chapter 3 programming table and appendix A. • Beta blockers: No major effect on exercise trainability in cardiac patients. • Calcium channel blockers: No major effect on exercise trainability in cardiac patients.	• See programming table in chapter 3. • CABG patients typically begin inpatient rehabilitation sooner and progress at a more accelerated rate. • CABG patients generally devote more time to upper extremity range-of-motion exercises. • Carefully monitor for signs and symptoms (e.g., angina) of graft occlusion (CABG) or restenosis (PTCA). Periodic intermittent or continuous ECG monitoring may be helpful in this regard. • The upper limits of early exercise prescription (i.e., inpatient) for CABG clients include RPE of 11-13 and HR at rest + 30 beats/min.

CHAPTER 5

Angina and Silent Ischemia

Daniel Friedman, MD, FACSM

New Mexico Heart Institute

Overview of the Pathophysiology

Angina is classically described as a discomfort in the chest that has a heavy, vise-like, and/or squeezing effect. It is usually retrosternal and often radiates to the shoulders, arms, neck, or jaw. Some people experience shortness of breath, nausea, or diaphoresis (sweating). Some patients have these symptoms without chest discomfort. Symptoms generally last from 10 to 20 seconds at a time, but occasionally for as long as 30 minutes or more. Clinicians sometimes refer to angina that predictably occurs with exercise as *stable angina*. Some individuals have atypical angina that is difficult to distinguish from gastrointestinal, musculoskeletal, or pulmonary symptoms.

Silent ischemia does not demonstrate classical symptoms of ischemia, but is generally demonstrated by some type of cardiac stress test. It is more common in individuals with diabetes; why some persons with coronary artery disease do not have symptoms is still unclear. Silent ischemia during exercise testing (ST-segment depression without angina) generally indicates milder forms of coronary artery disease (CAD) and has a lower risk than ST-segment depression accompanied by angina. In general, silent ischemia responds to measures similar to those used to treat persons with angina.

Ischemia occurs when the obstruction of the artery reaches a magnitude that results in blood flow inadequate to meet myocardial oxygen demand.

Ischemia may be symptomatic or silent. Initially ischemia occurs only during intense exertion or stress; however, as size of the plaque increases, symptoms may occur with minimal activity or even at rest. Any change in the status of a person's angina (i.e., increased episodes, increased pain, increase in episodes at rest or during mild exercise) must be reported to his/her physician immediately.

In contrast to stable angina, *unstable angina* occurs when an individual experiences a noticeable increase in the frequency of angina or begins to experience angina at rest. This acceleration of symptoms is thought to be a precursor to an acute myocardial infarction. The pathogenesis of unstable angina is most likely multifactorial, and may include

- transient periods of vasospasm at the atherosclerotic plaque,

- platelet aggregation or thrombosis at a site of coronary artery narrowing, and

- rupture and hemorrhage into an atherosclerotic plaque.

Since unstable angina has the potential to progress to an acute myocardial infarction, unstable angina is a medical emergency; these persons should not exercise and generally need immediate medical attention.

Effect on the Exercise Response

In people with CAD, exercise is important as a diagnostic tool and as a therapeutic modality. Angina is a common cardiac symptom during exercise. Angina is graded on a scale of +1 to +4: +1 = light, barely noticeable; +2 = moderate, bothersome;

+3 = severe, very uncomfortable; +4 = most severe ever experienced.

Angina that develops during exercise can be a predictor of CAD, but only 50% of individuals with CAD experience angina during a maximal exercise test. ST-segment depression during an exercise test in persons with CAD increases the probability of subsequent cardiac events, regardless of whether angina occurs during the test. ST-segment depression with angina symptoms during exercise significantly increases the probability of future cardiac events.

Effects of Exercise Training

Persons with stable angina generally benefit from exercise training, and for these people the risks associated with exercise are minimal. Individuals with unstable angina should not exercise until their clinical symptoms improve. Exercise alone, or in combination with other lifestyle behavior changes, helps to reduce overall cardiac risk and can help prevent, retard growth of, or reverse atherosclerotic plaques. The overall goal for persons with angina is to raise their ischemic threshold, or the point during physical stress at which angina symptoms occur. Optimal pharmacologic therapy will help enhance exercise performance. After exercise training, individuals should be able to perform more leisure- and exercise-related physical activity without signs and symptoms of angina.

Management and Medications

Many medications exist that can help reduce the symptoms in persons with angina. Antiplatelet therapy (aspirin) has been shown to reduce platelet aggregation and thrombosis (clotting) and is thus commonly prescribed to angina patients. Aspirin, in a dose as low as 81 milligrams per day, reduces the likelihood of heart attacks. Beta blockers block the effect of adrenaline in the heart and thus reduce angina while improving exercise capacity. They also decrease myocardial oxygen demand by decreasing contractility and heart rate, but beta blockers may also reduce the sensitivity of exercise testing. They may also prolong life in many persons after a heart attack. Nitrates (both short- and long-acting nitroglycerin) are commonly prescribed to individuals suffering from angina. Nitrates decrease myocardial oxygen demand by decreasing preload while at the same time increasing oxygen supply by

way of an increase in coronary perfusion and decrease in coronary vasospasm. Calcium channel blockers have also been found to be useful at controlling symptoms of angina (for specific drug effects see chapters 3 and 4 and appendix A).

Individuals with known or suspected CAD should strongly consider modifying those lifestyle behaviors that contributed to their disease (i.e., stop smoking, eat a diet that is low in fat and cholesterol, participate regularly in an exercise program, and learn to control stress through appropriate psychological intervention). Such acquired "healthy" behaviors have been demonstrated to slow the progression of CAD and in some cases reverse it. If pharmacologic therapy or lifestyle behavior change is unsuccessful in relieving angina, other invasive procedures such as angioplasty or coronary artery bypass grafting are most likely necessary (see chapter 4).

Recommendations for Exercise Testing

Exercise testing is most commonly used to evaluate persons suspected of having CAD that causes ischemia. Exercise testing is contraindicated in persons with unstable angina, or who are within three to seven days of having had an acute myocardial infarction. After this time, a standard exercise test should monitor heart rate, blood pressure, and 12-lead ECG. In addition to ECG changes such as ST-segment alterations, blood pressure, and provokable ventricular ectopy, important information comes from the aerobic capacity of the individual. The duration of the exercise test also has important prognostic implications. Even in persons with confirmed significant CAD, the capacity to exercise into stage IV of a Bruce protocol is associated with a 93% eight-year survival rate. In contrast, persons who can complete only stage I have a 45% eight-year survival rate. A hypotensive response to exercise is associated with an 80% predictive value for significant CAD. A low work capacity and early onset of angina combined with marked ST-segment depression, especially continuing into recovery, are associated with very significant CAD including left main and three-vessel diseases.

A complete description of angina symptoms, the rating of angina, and the exact onset and duration of angina should be carefully documented. Indications for terminating exercise testing include a fall in systolic pressure, increasing angina pain, signs of poor perfusion, dysrhythmias, marked ECG changes, and the subject's desire to stop. Added sensitivity and, in some cases, specificity in diagnosing CAD can be obtained by combining cardiac imaging with the test. Echocardiography and nuclear imaging are particularly useful when the resting ECG is abnormal, making interpretation of ECG changes during exercise difficult.

In persons unable to exercise adequately to perform the test, other modalities may be employed. Dobutamine is often used to increase myocardial oxygen consumption mostly by an increase in heart rate and contractility. This procedure is often performed in conjunction with echocardiography, with which the physician looks for wall motion abnormalities. Persantine (dipyridamole) and adenosine may be used during nuclear imaging of the heart; these agents dilate normal coronary arteries more than diseased ones. Blood flow to the heart is assessed at rest and during infusion of either compound, along with simultaneous nuclear imaging with thallium or technetium.

Recommendations for Exercise Programming

Comprehensive exercise programming (cardiac rehabilitation) is now considered a vital component in the effort to prevent, retard, and reverse CAD. Before entry into a cardiac rehabilitation program, all people who have experienced angina symptoms should have a diagnostic exercise test to establish functional capacity and the severity of their disease. In addition, if angina occurs during the exercise test, the work rate and heart rate at which angina occurred are useful for determining the initial upper training limits for that person. Before clients are allowed to exercise, they must be able to

- define angina,
- identify angina symptoms,
- identify their own angina symptoms, and
- describe the immediate treatment for it.

Such education generally occurs during cardiac rehabilitation. In addition, persons with angina should understand and be able to verbalize the protocol for taking nitroglycerin in the event of an angina attack.

Upper limits of heart rate, rate of perceived exertion (RPE), and angina scale ratings should be clearly established before the first exercise training session. Clients can begin with an exercise intensity, duration, and frequency that allows them to exercise without any signs and symptoms of angina. A safe heart rate range for clients with angina is 10 to 15 beats below their ischemic threshold (the heart rate/blood pressure where they have angina). The exercise prescription will periodically need to be re-evaluated so new upper limits may be set. A prolonged warm-up and cool-down (approximately 10 minutes or longer) may be indicated for persons with angina. Clients with angina may also benefit from more frequent, shorter duration-type exercise (five to six days per week with 5 to 10 minutes per session and two to three sessions per day). Individuals with angina should generally be counseled against exercising in the cold.

Any change in angina symptoms before, during, or after exercise needs to be recorded and a physician notified. If angina occurs during an exercise session, exercise should be terminated and standard nitroglycerin protocol administration followed. Blood pressure should be checked routinely after the administration of nitroglycerin to monitor for hypotensive responses. It is important to know the exercise-related side effects of all cardiac medications a person is currently taking. Lastly, any change in cardiac medications needs to be reported to the cardiac rehabilitation staff before the next exercise session.

Suggested Readings

Bogaty, P., G.R. Dagenais, B. Cantin, P. Alain, and J.R. Rouleau. 1989. Prognosis in patients with a strongly positive electrocardiogram. *Am. J. Cardiol.* 64: 1284-88.

Boran, K., R.A. Oliveros, C.A. Boucher, C.H. Beckmann, and J.F. Seaworth. 1983. Ischemia-associated intraventricular conduction disturbances during exercise testing as a predictor of proximal left anterior descending coronary artery disease. *Am. J. Cardiol.* 51: 1098-1102.

Chaitman, B. 1992. Exercise stress testing. In *Heart disease*, ed. E. Braunwald, 161-79. 4th ed. Philadelphia: Saunders.

Dubach, P., V.F. Froelicher, J. Klein, D. Oakes, M. Grover-McKay, and R. Friis. 1988. Exercise-induced hypotension in a male population. Criteria, causes and prognosis. *Circulation* 78: 1380-87.

Ho, S.W.C., M.J. McComish, and R.R. Taylor. 1985. Effect of beta-adrenergic blockade on the results of exercise testing related to the extent of coronary artery disease. *Am. J. Cardiol.* 55: 258-62.

Stuart, R.J., and M.H. Ellestad. 1980. National survey of exercise stress testing facilities. *Chest* 77: 94-97.

ANGINA AND SILENT ISCHEMIA: EXERCISE TESTING

METHODS	MEASURES	ENDPOINTS*	COMMENTS
Aerobic power **Cycle** (17 watts/min) ramp protocol (25-50 watts/3 min stage) **Treadmill** (1-2 METs/3 min stage)	• 12-lead ECG, heart rate	• Serious dysrhythmias • > 2 mm ST-segment depression or elevation • Ischemic threshold • T-wave inversion with significant ST change	
	• Blood pressure	• Plateau or drop in SBP with increased work rate • SBP > 260 mmHg or DBP > 115 mmHg	• Drop in BP with exercise is associated with increased prognosis of ischemic heart disease.
	• RPE (Borg 6-20 scale)		• May be useful for setting exercise intensity.
	• Angina scale	• +3 or earlier on +1 to +4 scale	• Onset of angina at low work rates is predictive of ischemic heart disease.

*Measurements of particular significance; do not *always* indicate test termination.

MEDICATIONS	SPECIAL CONSIDERATIONS
• See appendix A. • Most cardiac medications can alter the hemodynamic responses to exercise and possibly reduce the sensitivity of the test.	• Clarify symptoms of angina with client before testing. • Unstable angina is a contraindication to exercise testing. • Poor left ventricular function may lead to dyspnea.

ANGINA AND SILENT ISCHEMIA: EXERCISE PROGRAMMING

MODES	GOALS	INTENSITY/ FREQUENCY/DURATION	TIME TO GOAL
Aerobic	• Improve functional capacity. • Decrease CAD risk factors. • Decrease blood pressure and heart rate response to submaximal exercise. • Decrease myocardial O_2 demand.	• HR 10-25 contractions/minute below ischemic threshold. • 3-7 days/week. • 20-60 minutes/session. • 5-10 minutes of warm-up and cool-down activities.	• 4-6 months
Strength	• Improve functional capacity.	• Light resistance/40-50% maximal voluntary contraction (avoid Valsalva). • 2-3 days/week. • 15-20 minutes/session. • Avoid isometric exercises.	• 4-6 months
Flexibility • Upper and lower body range-of-motion activities	• Decrease risk of injury.	• 2-3 days/week.	• 4-6 months

MEDICATIONS	SPECIAL CONSIDERATIONS
• See appendix A. • Most cardiac medications can alter hemodynamics during exercise.	• See table on exercise programming in chapter 3. • Clients need to be encouraged to stay below their ischemic threshold. • If signs or symptoms change, the client should be referred to his/her physician. • Clients should always carry nitroglycerin if diagnosed with CAD. • Lower-intensity walking is useful. • Patients with low ejection fraction, poor exercise capacity, or frequent dysrhythmias should be closely monitored. • Home-based cardiac rehabilitation may be appropriate for many low-risk patients (see Home Exercise Guidelines in the fifth edition of *ACSM's Guidelines for Exercise Testing and Prescription*). • Prolonged warm-up and cool-down (> 10 min) have an antianginal effect.

CHAPTER 6

Pacemakers and Implantable Cardioverter Defibrillators

Michael West, MD and Tim Johnson, MD
Department of Cardiology
Lovelace Medical Center

Scott O. Roberts, PhD, FAACVPR
Texas Tech University

Overview of the Pathophysiology

Several factors contribute to optimal cardiac function, including atrioventricular synchronization and the responsiveness of heart rate and contractility to the neurohumoral control. Loss of the normal sequence of atrial and ventricular filling and contraction can result in deterioration of hemodynamics and significant symptoms at rest and during exercise. Pacing techniques are sometimes used in such persons to improve symptoms and exercise performance. Individuals who cannot increase heart rate in response to increased metabolic demand have sinus node dysfunction and may also be highly symptomatic and require some form of cardiac pacing. Other individuals who have worrisome life-threatening ventricular dysrhythmias are sometimes candidates for an *implantable cardioverter defibrillator (ICD)*.

Review of Pacing Terminology

• *Chronotropic incompetence*—The inability to increase the heart rate above 100 contractions per minute or reach 85% of maximal predicted heart rate despite maximal exertion.

• *Symptomatic bradycardia*—Symptoms directly attributable to a slow heart rate: transient dizziness, light-headedness, and complete or near loss of consciousness (syncope).

• *Rate-adaptive pacemakers*—Pacemakers equipped with sensors that allow adaptation of the pacemaker's rate commensurate with increases in demand (i.e., exercise). These units utilize various types of sensors including those that respond to physiological, mechanical, or electrical signals. This facilitates pacing in a more "physiologic" manner.

• *Pacemaker syndrome*—Constellation of clinical signs and symptoms that usually occur as a consequence of single-chamber (i.e., ventricular) pacing. Generally, symptoms result from a reduced cardiac output, "negative" atrial contribution to stroke volume, or both. Symptoms include lethargy, fatigue, hypotension, shortness of breath, syncope, neck pulsations, and impaired exercise capacity.

• *Hypertrophic cardiomyopathy*—A group of ventricular disorders that cause an impediment to filling, outflow, or both. This includes clients with muscular subaortic stenosis, concentric left ventricular hypertrophy, valvular aortic stenosis, and combinations of these. These persons typically have symptoms of low cardiac output and heart failure despite normal left ventricular performance during systole.

• *Tiered therapy*—Latest generation of implanted defibrillators that utilize anti-tachycardia pacing, shock therapies, and bradycardia safety pacing in a step-wise approach to the treatment of life-threatening ventricular dysrhythmias.

• *Sudden cardiac death syndrome*—A clinical scenario during which the person experiences loss of consciousness due to a ventricular tachydysrhythmia, usually ventricular tachycardia (VT) or ventricular fibrillation (VF). Unless there is prompt restoration to normal rhythm, death ensues. Severe bradycardia and asystole can also account for sudden death in a minority of cases.

Pacemakers

The use of permanent cardiac pacemakers increases survival, decreases symptoms, and improves quality of life. Commonly accepted indications for pacemaker implantation include

- acquired atrioventricular (A-V) block,
- persistent advanced A-V block after myocardial infarction, and
- sick sinus syndrome with symptomatic bradycardia.

Other less common indications for use of a pacemaker are in

- individuals with hypertrophic cardiomyopathies,
- those with dilated cardiomyopathies with symptoms of low cardiac output, and
- those in whom A-V block is intentionally created by ablative procedures.

A typical pacemaker system consists of two basic components: one or two leads and a pulse generator. Leads are insulated and are implanted transvenously into the right atrium, right ventricle, or both. The leads are connected to the pulse generator, which is typically implanted near the clavicle. The two main functions of the leads are sensing and pacing. Sensing involves receiving electrical signals from the heart (P waves and R waves). In the absence of such sensed signals, the pacemaker generator will fire, causing the atria or ventricles to contract. Optimally, the pacing system utilizes an atrial and ventricular lead to maintain A-V synchrony, which in turn facilitates cardiac output and exercise capacity.

Pacemakers are categorized by a standardized code. For example, VVIR is an abbreviation for V—ventricle chamber being paced, V—ventricle chamber being sensed, I—sensing response being inhib-

iting, and R—rate-responsive programming. A common pacemaker system is a VVIR, or a single-chamber rate-adaptive pacing system. A DDD system both senses and paces the atrium and ventricle, providing rate-responsiveness for persons with chronotropic incompetence from sinus node dysfunction. The simpler DDD system is widely regarded as the optimal pacing mode in individuals who have normal sinoatrial node function because it provides atrioventricular synchrony and utilizes sinus rhythm for the sensor-driven heart rate.

Implantable Cardioverter Defibrillators

Persons with coronary artery disease, prior infarction, congestive heart failure, as well as those with various forms of cardiomyopathy, are at increased risk of sudden cardiac death. Implantable cardioverter defibrillators are used to electrically terminate life-threatening ventricular tachyarrhythmias. They consist of two basic parts—the lead system and the cardioverter defibrillator. The newest generation of ICDs have lead systems that are placed transvenously, typically by way of the subclavian and cephalic vein. The ICD leads track the cardiac rhythm and transmit the information to the pulse generator, which is usually implanted subcutaneously in the abdominal or pectoral region. When a tachydysrhythmia is detected, preprogrammed therapies are sent back to terminate the dysrhythmia. The units can pace-terminate a dysrhythmia and/or deliver small and large electric cardioversion shocks. In order to terminate a dysrhythmia, the pulse generator must be programmed to recognize specific tachydysrhythmias. Ventricular tachycardia and fibrillation are typically recognized by their rapid rates. If either is sensed, the pulse generator will deliver the appropriate preprogrammed therapy to the heart through the lead system.

Effects on the Exercise Response

Because of abnormalities in sinus node function, cardiac conduction, and neurohormonal systems, many persons benefit from an improved heart rate response to exercise. Inadequate heart rate responses to exercise, with attendant symptoms, can be markedly improved with current pacemaker technologies.

Persons with ICDs are at risk of receiving inappropriate shocks during exercise. This can occur if the sinus heart rate exceeds the programmed threshold rate or if the person develops an exercise-induced supraventricular tachycardia. For this reason, people with ICDs should be closely monitored during exercise to ensure that their heart rate does not approach the activation rate for the device.

Effects of Exercise Training

During exercise, cardiac output must increase to support the increased tissue oxygen demand. This increase is accomplished primarily through an increase in the heart rate via sympathetic stimulation and activation of neurochemical and hormonal systems. Recent technologic advances have dramatically advanced pacemaker function to the point where pacemakers can nearly mimic normal cardiac function at rest and during exercise. It is important that the exercise training "upper" heart rate limit in DDD and VVIR pacemakers be set below the person's ischemic threshold. At least a 10% safety margin between exercise heart rate and rate cutoff for the device is advised.

An inappropriately delivered shock can be proarrhythmic and itself induce a life-threatening ventricular dysrhythmia. Despite a high level of caution, however, inappropriate shocks are common and have many causes. Therefore, full knowledge of the person's ICD programming is essential before exercise, and close consultation with the client's electrophysiologist is advised.

Management and Medications

Individuals with pacemakers or ICDs may be taking cardiac medications such as antihypertensives or beta blockers. Persons receiving a pacemaker or ICD may have left ventricular dysfunction, necessitating vasodilator therapy. In addition to the precautions associated with a pacemaker or ICD, precautions for possible side effects during exercise or exercise training should be followed on the basis of the type of medications the person is currently taking (see appendix A).

Recommendations for Exercise Testing

Exercise testing can be used as a diagnostic tool as well as a therapeutic tool in the adjustment of rate-responsive pacemakers. Once a permanent pace-maker with rate-responsive pacing capabilities has been implanted, exercise testing is sometimes useful in the evaluation of pacemaker behavior as well as for optimization of the pacemaker activity response. As for all people, those with pacemakers and ICDs require an exercise protocol suited to their age, health/medical status, and present functional capacity. Exercise protocols such as the modified Bruce, Balke, or Naughton protocol can often be helpful in this population. It is important to remember that in persons with a pacemaker, induced heartbeat ST-segment changes may not reflect ischemic changes and thus other diagnostic tests should be considered. Stress imaging with echo or thallium is often useful in these circumstances.

Recommendations for Exercise Programming

Persons with ICDs and pacemakers can benefit from exercise training. In addition to improving functional capacity, exercise training can also help reduce cardiac risk factors (e.g., through cholesterol modification, hypertension reduction) and improve psychosocial outcomes. Activities should be selected so that the intensity can be carefully regulated during exercise. Because some upper body movement may dislodge implanted leads, upper-body exercises are not advised initially for people with pacemakers. Before exercise training, full knowledge of the individual's ICD programming is essential, and close consultation with the client's electrophysiologist is advised. The upper exercise training intensity must be set below the person's ischemic threshold and must not approach a heart rate causing activation of the ICD.

Suggested Readings

Pashkow, F.J. 1992. Patients with implanted pacemakers or implanted cardioverter defibrillators. In *Rehabilitation of the coronary patient*, ed. N. Wenger and H. Hellerstein, 431-38. 3rd ed. New York: Churchill Livingstone.

Pashkow, F.J., C. Walters, G. Blackburn, and P. McCarthy. 1993. Exercise training with an implantable ventricular assist device. *J. Am. Coll. Cardiol.* 21 (2): 188A.

Podrid, P.J., and Kowey, P.R., eds. 1995. *Cardiac dysrhythmia: Mechanisms, diagnosis, and management.* Baltimore: Williams & Wilkins.

Smith, L.K. 1991. Exercise training in patients with impaired left ventricular function. *Med. Sci. Sports Exerc.* 23 (6): 654-60.

Wilkoff, B.L., and R.E. Miller. 1992. Exercise testing for chronotropic assessment. *Cardiol. Clinics* 10 (4): 705-17.

PACEMAKER AND ICD: EXERCISE TESTING

METHODS	MEASURES	ENDPOINTS*	COMMENTS
Aerobic power **Cycle** (10-25 watts/3 min stage) **Treadmill** (1-2 METs/3 min stage)	• 12-lead ECG, heart rate	• Peak HR must be below activation rate for ICD • Serious dysrhythmias • > 2 mm ST-segment depression or elevation • Ischemic threshold • T-wave inversion with significant ST change	• Peak HR may be blunted. • ECG sensitivity low for detecting ischemia. • Know HR activation rate for ICD before testing.
	• Blood pressure	• SBP > 260 mmHg or DBP > 115 mmHg • Watch for drop or no increase in SBP with increased work rate	• Peak SBP may be blunted. SBP may decrease or not increase with left ventricular dysfunction.
	• RPE (Borg 6-20 scale)		• Better guide of intensity because of possible inability of HR to increase with exercise.
	• Radionuclide or stress echocardiogram testing		• May be more useful in assessing ischemic heart disease.
Strength **Isokinetic**			• Not recommended following pacemaker or ICD implantation. May later be useful in planning exercise program.

*Measurements of particular significance; do not *always* indicate test termination.

MEDICATIONS	SPECIAL CONSIDERATIONS
• See table on exercise testing in chapter 3.	• Individuals with ICDs are at risk for receiving inappropriate shocks. • HR should not approach the activation rate of the ICD. • Some individuals with pacemakers and ICDs have moderate to severe left ventricular dysfunction. Therefore, appropriate precautions for this population may need to be followed as well (see chapter 8).

PACEMAKER AND ICD: EXERCISE PROGRAMMING

MODES	GOALS	INTENSITY/ FREQUENCY/DURATION	TIME TO GOAL
Aerobic • Large muscle activities	• Increase functional capacity and ability to perform daily living activities. • Increase self-efficacy.	• 50-85% $\dot{V}O_2$ peak or HR reserve. • Target HR should be kept below ischemic threshold and ICD activation threshold. • 4-7 days/week. • 20-60 minutes/session.	• 4-6 months
Strength • Circuit training	• Increase ability to perform leisure, occupational, and daily living activities. • Increase muscle strength and endurance.	• Low to moderate intensity. • 2 days/week. • 15-20 minutes/session. • Should be avoided initially after implantation.	
Flexibility • Upper and lower body range-of-motion activities		• 2-3 days/week	

MEDICATIONS	SPECIAL CONSIDERATIONS
• See table on exercise programming in chapter 3.	• Upper-extremity range of motion may be limited due to pacemaker and ICD incision. • Important to know the type and function of pacemaker. • RPE should be used in conjunction with HR to monitor intensity. • Know ICD activation rate. • Ventricular tachyarrhythmias should be anticipated. • Guidelines for left ventricular dysfunction may be indicated (see chapter 8).

CHAPTER 7

Valvular Heart Disease

Daniel Friedman, MD, FACSM

New Mexico Heart Institute

Overview of the Pathophysiology

The symptoms, limitations, and recommendations with respect to physical activity in patients with valvular heart disease depend on

- the valve(s) involved,
- whether the valve(s) is stenotic (does not open adequately) or regurgitant,
- the severity of the valve lesions, and
- the presence of coronary artery disease, myocardial dysfunction, or other organ system disease.

Mitral Stenosis

The predominant cause of mitral stenosis is rheumatic fever (approximately 60%). Other causes include a congenital etiology, systemic lupus erythematosus, carcinoid, and amyloid disease. A congenital membrane (cor triatriatum) or a tumor in the left atrium can cause identical symptoms. Mitral annular calcification generally causes mitral regurgitation, but mild stenosis can occur (rarely). Table 7.1 shows the classifications of mitral valve disease.

Exercise capacity is related to the severity of vascular disease. Patients with mild vascular disease may have normal exercise capacity. As mitral valve stenosis progresses, however, exercise intolerance worsens. As the mitral valve area decreases, the pressure gradient between the left atrium and ventricle increases. As left atrial pressure rises, pulmonary vascular pressure also rises and eventually results in dyspnea. Since the rate of flow through the mitral valve also affects the pressure gradient, dyspnea is initially present only during high levels of exertion. As mitral stenosis worsens, dyspnea occurs at progressively lesser levels of activity. Dyspnea, including orthopnea and even frank pulmonary edema, are the most common symptoms in mitral valve disease. Other symptoms include hemoptysis, chest pain, thromboembolism, infective endocarditis, and hoarseness. Neck veins often demonstrate an elevated pressure and a prominent A wave. On auscultation, a loud S_1, an opening snap, and a low pitched diastolic murmur is present. Echocardiography is helpful in evaluating the left atrial size to determine the mitral valve area, assess the presence and severity of mitral regurgitation and pulmonary hypertension. Echocardiography also helps define the feasibility of balloon valvuloplasty.

Table 7.1 MITRAL VALVE DISEASE CLASSIFICATION		
	MITRAL VALVE AREA	**SYMPTOMS**
Normal	4-6 cm^2	None
Mild mitral stenosis	1.5-2.0 cm^2	Minimal dyspnea on exertion
Moderate mitral stenosis	1.0-1.5 cm^2	Dyspnea, orthopnea, paroxysmal nocturnal dyspnea
Critical mitral stenosis	< 1.0 cm^2	Dyspnea at rest

Mitral Regurgitation

The causes of mitral regurgitation include rheumatic heart disease, myxomatous degeneration of mitral valve leaflets, mitral valve prolapse, and age-related degenerative disease. Other causes include Marfan syndrome, infectious endocarditis, a ruptured valve chordae or papillary muscle, mitral annular dilation (most often in congestive heart failure), various congenital lesions, and cardiac tumors. There are many other causes both in native and in prosthetic mitral valves. During the early stages of the disease, patients will have normal exercise capacity. The symptoms of mitral regurgitation will depend on the severity and the rate of development of the regurgitation. Often symptoms do not develop until the left ventricle begins to fail. In fact, many persons never develop symptoms. In others, by the time symptoms such as dyspnea and fatigue appear, irreversible ventricular dysfunction has developed. A holosystolic murmur is the most prominent feature during physical exam. Echocardiography is useful to determine the etiology and the severity of mitral regurgitation. It can also help to determine whether or not left ventricular dysfunction or pulmonary hypertension has developed. Although the superiority of angiography is questioned, it remains the gold standard for determining the severity of mitral regurgitation.

Aortic Stenosis

Aortic stenosis in older persons is most often caused by calcification and probably results from years of the normal stress on the valve. Other causes include congenital aortic stenosis, a bicuspid valve, and rheumatic heart disease. Aortic stenosis accompanied by heart failure symptoms (dyspnea), angina, and/or syncope is the most common presentation during the seventh decade of life. From the time of the development of symptoms, persons without surgery usually survive two to five years. On physical examination, carotid upstrokes are diminished, the second heart sound is single and may be soft, and a harsh murmur at the upper left sternal border (often radiating to the neck) is present. Echocardiography can noninvasively determine the severity of aortic stenosis. Along with watching symptoms, it is a good practice to follow persons with mild or moderate disease in anticipation of a future requirement for surgery. Angiography is performed before surgery in order to determine whether coronary bypass is necessary.

Aortic Regurgitation

Aortic regurgitation may be caused by disease of the aortic root or valve leaflets. Valvular disease may develop in the setting of rheumatic disease, infective endocarditis, trauma, or congenital lesions, or in connective tissue-related diseases including Marfan syndrome and Ehlers-Danlos syndrome. Aortic root disease occurs in a wide range of conditions that cause dilation of the ascending aorta. In general these persons maintain normal exercise capacity. Individuals who have aortic regurgitation often present in their fourth or fifth decades with exertional dyspnea. When symptoms develop, irreversible left ventricular dysfunction may have occurred. Thus it is important to diagnose and follow these individuals appropriately. Exaggerated arterial pulses are noted, as are a systolic ejection murmur and an early diastolic murmur. Echocardiography can both diagnose this lesion and help one to follow patients so as to determine the appropriate time for surgical intervention.

Tricuspid Stenosis

Tricuspid stenosis is almost always secondary to rheumatic heart disease, and some mitral valve disease is usually present as well. Tumors and infection are among other causes. Persons most often complain of fatigue and lower-extremity and abdominal swelling. Upon physical examination, neck veins are distended and significant edema is present. The lungs are often clear, and the murmur may be difficult to auscultate. Echocardiography is a noninvasive method to determine the presence, cause, and severity of this lesion.

Tricuspid Regurgitation

Tricuspid regurgitation is often caused by dilation of the right ventricle and tricuspid annulus. Most common causes are left-sided myocardial or valvular disease and pulmonary lung disease leading to pulmonary hypertension and right ventricular enlargement. Often, less common but more specific causes include Ebstein's anomaly, carcinoid syndrome, rheumatic heart disease, and infection. If pulmonary hypertension is absent, tricuspid regurgitation is generally well tolerated. If pulmonary arterial pressure is elevated, fatigue and peripheral edema develop. A holosystolic murmur that leads to increase with inspiration is heard at the lower left sternal border. With use of Doppler echocardiography, the presence and severity of this lesion can be determined and the right ventricular pressure estimated.

Pulmonic Valve Disease

Pulmonic stenosis is often congenital. Other causes include rheumatic heart disease and carcinoid plaques. Pulmonic regurgitation is caused by dilation of the pulmonary artery or valve ring due to pulmonary hypertension. Persons with a mild pulmonic stenosis are usually asymptomatic. In more significant cases, patients experience heart failure, exertional dyspnea, syncope, or chest pain because they cannot increase pulmonary blood flow during exercise. The major symptoms of pulmonic regurgitation usually relate to the underlying cause. Persons with pulmonic stenosis often have a harsh, rapidly louder then softer, systolic murmur at the upper left sternal border. In the setting of significant pulmonic regurgitation, an early diastolic murmur in the same region can be heard. Echocardiography can generally determine the presence and possible cause and at least estimate the significance of each of these lesions.

Effects on the Exercise Response

Exercise testing is not important in the specific diagnosis of most valvular diseases but can help quantify functional capacity. ST changes may be nonspecific in aortic stenosis. In general, exercise testing is contraindicated in persons with critical aortic stenosis because of the risk of dysrhythmia and death. This is probably caused by some combination of carotid hyperactivity, baroreceptor stimulation, left ventricular failure, and dysrhythmia. It is important to follow blood pressure carefully and watch for dysrhythmias or slowing of heart rate. For individuals with significant pulmonic stenosis, exercise testing should be performed carefully because of the risk of syncope. In mitral stenosis, ST depression may represent reduced coronary perfusion or pulmonary hypertension. In mitral valve prolapse, ST depression has been seen with normal coronary arteries. These changes can be medicated with beta blockade.

Effects of Exercise Training

Persons with clinically significant mitral stenosis will have marked limitation to exercise because their cardiac output does not meet demands of the exercising muscle. In general, if this substantially limits activity, surgical correction is indicated. There is no specific therapeutic role for exercise training in mitral stenosis. Of course, improved skeletal muscle efficiency will allow such a person to do more activity at a given cardiovascular work rate. In addition, exercise may help reduce other cardiovascular risk factors.

There is no specific therapeutic role for exercise training in mitral regurgitation. People with severe aortic stenosis should avoid vigorous physical activity because of the added risk of sudden death. Persons with cardiac dysfunction or limited cardiac reserve secondary to aortic insufficiency should refrain from vigorous exertion or sports. Those with significant pulmonic stenosis should refrain from vigorous physical activity because of the risk of syncope.

Management and Medications

In individuals with diagnosed mitral valve disease, antibiotic prophylaxis is used prior to dental work or minor surgery because such persons are at high risk for infective endocarditis as a result of these procedures. Diuretics, beta blockers, and digoxin are useful in controlling symptoms. Anticoagulation therapy (see chapter 22) is used to prevent blood clots. Surgery is indicated once severe symptoms develop, particularly when the mitral valve area is < 1.0 cm². Afterload reduction, digitalis, appropriate antibiotic prophylaxis, and perhaps diuretics are common treatments for mitral regurgitation. The ideal timing of surgical treatment is difficult to determine for mitral regurgitation. One would like to intervene before irreversible left ventricular dysfunction develops without subjecting individuals unnecessarily to the risk of surgery. Although some valves can be repaired, many have to be replaced.

Antibiotic prophylaxis is considered prior to dental procedures or minor surgery in persons with aortic stenosis. In general, individuals with aortic stenosis do not respond to medical therapy. Once symptoms develop, aortic valve replacement is generally necessary. Although balloon valvuloplasty can increase the valve area, it is not highly effective in this condition. Treatment for people with aortic regurgitation who are minimally symptomatic or asymptomatic with normal or minimally increased cardiac size can be managed medically. Antibiotic prophylaxis is extremely important prior to dental procedures or minor surgery to prevent endocarditis. Afterload reduction is helpful, and there is a specific improvement in outcome with nifedipine therapy. Digoxin has an important role as well.

When significant symptoms or left ventricular dilation develops as a result of aortic regurgitation, surgery with aortic valve replacement is indicated.

For persons with tricuspid stenosis, salt restriction and diuretics can help lessen the volume overload. Surgical repair of the tricuspid valve is the treatment of choice and is usually done at the time of mitral valve surgery. For individuals with isolated tricuspid regurgitation, no intervention is generally required. These people generally respond best to an improvement or correction of the underlying cause when possible. Narrowing the tricuspid annulus with a prosthesis called a *Carpentier ring* can improve tricuspid regurgitation. If pulmonic valve disease is significant, it can usually be repaired with a balloon or through surgery. Pulmonic regurgitation responds best to treatment of the underlying cause. Antibiotic prophylaxis should be considered prior to dental work or minor surgeries.

Recommendations for Exercise Testing

Although not important for the diagnosis of mitral valve disease, exercise testing can provide important information about a person's functional capacity. Exercise testing can be utilized to quantify the extent of hemodynamic impairment consequent to valvular heart disease. The results can be used to follow individuals and determine the appropriate time for intervention. At least a brief cardiac examination should be performed before exercise testing to rule out aortic stenosis and determine whether exercise testing is contraindicated. Atrial dysrhythmias may occur in persons with mitral valve disease, and in particular, atrial fibrillation will eliminate the effective atrial contraction and worsen symptoms. Exercise testing is not important in the diagnosis of tricuspid stenosis or regurgitation. Because of the risk of syncope, exercise testing should be performed carefully in persons with pulmonic valve disease if significant pulmonic stenosis is considered.

Recommendations for Exercise Programming

With mitral valve disease, including mitral regurgitation, physical activity is mostly limited by the individual's symptoms. Before an exercise program begins, the upper training rate and description of any symptoms should be documented from a diagnostic exercise test. The extent of the stenosis should be known. When symptoms of aortic stenosis including angina, congestive heart failure, or syncope occur, valve replacement is generally pursued. There is no specific role of exercise training in aortic regurgitation. Persons with significant pulmonic stenosis should refrain from vigorous physical activity because of the risk of syncope. In the setting of mild disease, no limitation is necessary.

Suggested Readings

Atwood, J.E., S. Kawanishi, J. Myers, and V.F. Froelicher. 1988. Exercise testing in patients with aortic stenosis. *Chest* 93: 1083-87.

Braunwald, E. 1992. Valvular heart disease. In *Heart Disease*, ed. E. Braunwald, 1007-77. 4th ed. Philadelphia: Saunders.

Broustet, J.P., H. Douard, and B. Mora. 1987. Exercise testing in dysrhythmias of idiopathic mitral valve prolapse. *Eur. Heart J.* 8 (suppl. D): 37-42.

Fletcher, G.F., G. Balady, V.F. Froelicher, L.H. Hartley, W.L. Haskell, and M.L. Pollock. 1995. Exercise standards: A statement for healthcare professionals from the American Heart Association. *Circulation* 91 (2): 580-615.

VALVULAR HEART DISEASE: EXERCISE TESTING

METHODS	MEASURES	ENDPOINTS*	COMMENTS
Aerobic power **Cycle** (17 watts/min) ramp protocol (25-30 watts/3 min stage) **Treadmill** (1-2 METs/3 min stage)	• 12-lead ECG, heart rate • Blood pressure • RPE (Borg 6-20 scale) • Stress echocardiogram	• Serious dysrhythmias • > 2 mm ST-segment depression or elevation • Ischemic threshold • T-wave inversion with significant ST change • SBP > 260 mmHg or DBP > 115 mmHg	• Useful in developing exercise prescription and determining need for surgery. • Useful in determining degree of stenosis, regurgitation, left ventricular function, and proper time for surgery. • ST changes may lose specificity with mitral and aortic valve stenosis and mitral valve prolapse in terms of the diagnosis of CAD.
Strength **Isokinetic/isotonic**			

*Measurements of particular significance; do not *always* indicate test termination.

MEDICATIONS	SPECIAL CONSIDERATIONS
• Most cardiac medications can alter hemodynamic responses to exercise (see appendix A).	• Follow the guidelines for exercise testing individuals at risk in the fifth edition of *ACSM's Guidelines for Exercise Testing and Prescription.* • Watch for new symptoms of fatigue, chest pain, shortness of breath, and syncope. • Beware of critical aortic stenosis.

VALVULAR HEART DISEASE: EXERCISE PROGRAMMING

MODES	GOALS	INTENSITY/ FREQUENCY/DURATION	TIME TO GOAL
Aerobic • Large muscle activities	• Increase functional capacity.	• Borg RPE of 11-14 • 60-85% peak HR • 3-7 days/week • 20-60 minutes/session • Resting HR + 30 beats/minute after surgery.	• 4-6 months
Strength • Isokinetic/isotonic	• Improve muscle function.		
Flexibility • Upper and lower body range-of-motion activities • Shoulder wheel	• Improve range of motion.		

MEDICATIONS	SPECIAL CONSIDERATIONS
• Coumadin: No effect on HR or BP.	• See precautions for exercise after CABG if client has had prosthetic valve replacement (programming table in chapter 4). • Monitor high-risk patients closely.

CHAPTER 8

Congestive Heart Failure

Jonathan N. Myers, PhD, FACSM
Palo Alto VA Medical Center

Overview of the Pathophysiology

Chronic congestive heart failure (CHF) is characterized by the inability of the heart to adequately deliver oxygen to the metabolizing tissues. The underlying pathophysiology in most persons with CHF is depressed systolic function of the left ventricle, due to either loss of muscle (i.e., myocardial infarction) or reduced contractility. Nearly all persons who have systolic dysfunction also have some degree of diastolic dysfunction, which implies abnormal filling characteristics related to poor ventricular compliance. Several central hemodynamic changes are associated with CHF:

- Decreased cardiac output during exercise, or in severe cases, at rest
- Elevated left ventricular filling pressures
- Compensatory ventricular volume overload
- Elevated pulmonary and central venous pressures

In addition to these abnormalities in central hemodynamics, CHF is associated with secondary organ changes, including major derangements in skeletal muscle metabolism, impaired vasodilation, and renal insufficiency leading to sodium and water retention. These changes underlie the hallmark signs and symptoms of CHF, namely, fatigue, dyspnea, and reduced exercise tolerance.

Effects on the Exercise Response

A number of central, peripheral, and ventilatory abnormalities influence the acute response to exercise among persons with CHF:

- Central factors
  1. Systolic dysfunction
  2. Pulmonary hemodynamics
  3. Diastolic dysfunction
  4. Neurohumoral mechanisms
- Peripheral factors
  1. Blood flow abnormalities
  2. Vasodilatory capacity
  3. Skeletal muscle biochemistry
- Ventilatory factors
  1. Pulmonary pressure
  2. Physiologic dead space
  3. Ventilation-perfusion mismatch
  4. Respiratory control
  5. Breathing pattern

The major pathophysiologic feature of the client with CHF is a reduction in cardiac output relative to the demands of the work; this leads to a number of characteristic responses to exercise. Poor cardiac output underlies a mismatching of ventilation to perfusion in the lung, causing an elevation in physiologic dead space and leading to shortness of breath.

Interestingly, although dyspnea on exertion is a hallmark of CHF, most individuals (roughly two-thirds) are limited by leg fatigue during exercise testing. Early fatigue is related to the heart's inability to supply adequate blood flow and oxygen to the working muscles. Lactate accumulates in the blood at low work rates relative to those for healthy individuals. This contributes to the hyperventilatory response to exercise and early fatigue.

Abnormal neurohumoral mechanisms contribute to reduced cardiac performance during exercise in persons with CHF. Catecholamine levels are usually elevated among these persons, and abnormalities in beta-receptor density probably contribute to reduced contractile function. This is so because beta-adrenergic receptors play an important inotropic regulatory role in the myocardium and are less sensitive to endogenous and exogenous beta-agonist stimulation in CHF. Altered baroreceptor reflexes have been observed in animals with heart failure, and may also contribute to diminished chronotropic responses or to reduced systolic pressure during exercise, the latter perhaps contributing to peripheral perfusion abnormalities.

There are significant peripheral abnormalities in response to exercise in persons with CHF. These include not only reductions in blood flow, but also abnormal redistribution of blood, vasodilatory capacity, and skeletal muscle biochemistry. Abnormalities in skeletal muscle metabolism include reduced mitochondrial enzyme activities and histologic changes (reduced type I aerobic fibers and increased type II fibers). The cumulative effect of these skeletal muscle abnormalities is reduced exercise tolerance as a result of

- greater glycolysis,
- reduced oxidative phosphorylation, and
- greater metabolic acidosis.

Effects of Exercise Training

Before the 1980s, persons with CHF were generally discouraged from participating in formal programs of exercise training. This was a result of concerns over safety and questions about whether or not exercise training caused harm to a weak heart. But in the last decade, several notable studies have documented increases in exercise capacity after exercise training in persons with heart failure. These studies suggest that improvements in exercise capacity after training result more from peripheral adaptations (i.e., skeletal muscle metabolism) than

from cardiac changes (i.e., central hemodynamics including volumes, ejection fraction, and pulmonary pressures at rest and during exercise).

A recent controversy has arisen regarding the possibility that exercise training in patients with heart failure could cause abnormal ventricular remodeling and infarct expansion, particularly for exercise performed early after a heart attack. This concern arose because a group of individuals who had ventricular asynergy were found to have worsening of asynergy, myocardial expansion, peak shape distortion, and decreased ejection fraction. However, two more recent reports have allayed these concerns. Although some people with ejection fractions of less than 40% may develop global and regional left ventricular deterioration, exercise training appears to have no effect on ventricular function.

Management and Medications

Initial management of CHF involves identifying the underlying cause. For example, a stenotic valve may need to be replaced, hypertension or myocardial ischemia controlled, or alcohol use discontinued. In some persons, these measures alone may restore cardiac function to normal. A major manifestation of CHF is increased ventricular volume and pressure; therefore, the second goal is to reduce these manifestations with medications. Therapy generally reduces symptoms; often, however, a period of time on therapy is required before exercise capacity improves. Since excessive salt and water retention is a hallmark of CHF, many persons will need to use a diuretic. Also, agents such as nitroglycerin or nitroprusside dilate the venous capacitance system; this permits a shift of blood volume from the central to peripheral venous beds, resulting in a reduction of central cardiac and pulmonary pressures. Afterload reduction by angiotensin-converting enzyme (ACE) inhibition or other arterial vasodilators tends to reduce left ventricular end-diastolic pressures and improve stroke volume and cardiac output, and this reduces symptoms. ACE inhibition may lower mortality, while digoxin or other inotropic agents increase myocardial contractility.

Recommendations for Exercise Testing

Exercise testing can be a valuable tool to objectively characterize the severity of CHF and to evaluate the efficacy of therapeutic interventions. In general, the standard exercise electrocardiogram offers little insight into the nature of the person's symptoms. It is frequently more appropriate to characterize the cardiopulmonary (ventilatory gas exchange) response to exercise, quantify exercise tolerance, and identify the pathophysiologic abnormalities responsible for the limitation in exercise capacity. Exercise capacity measured by gas exchange techniques enhances risk stratification in persons with CHF. The normal central and peripheral responses to the exercise test may not be present in these persons. For example, relative to what is seen in healthy individuals, cardiac output is reduced, blood is redistributed poorly, and peripheral vascular resistance is high. Exercise can cause a drop in ejection fraction, stroke volume, or both, and exertional hypotension may occur. Although exercise testing in these individuals has the potential for more complications, the safety of exercise testing in CHF is similar to that observed among persons with coronary artery disease. The following considerations relate to exercise testing with this population:

- Symptoms are frequently observed under 5 METs, so lower-level, moderately incremented, individualized protocols are recommended (Naughton or ramp).

- Symptoms indicative of unstable or decompensated CHF are a contraindication.

- Respired gas measurements increase precision and permit assessment of breathing efficiency and patterns; these are particularly useful in patients with CHF.

- Six-minute walk tests are an effective supplement to the graded exercise tests.

- Be prepared for exertional hypotension, significant dysrhythmias, and chronotropic incompetence.

- Test endpoints should focus on symptoms, hemodynamic response, and indications for stopping (and not target heart rate).

Recommendations for Exercise Programming

Because of improvements in therapeutic and surgical techniques, persons with CHF compose one of the fastest-growing cardiac rehabilitation populations. Formal exercise training programs are effective in lessening their symptoms and improving their exercise capacity. An improvement in the ability to sustain low-level activities can mean that a person can live independently and continue to work instead of being disabled. For these reasons, exercise programs may significantly enhance the quality of these individuals' lives.

However, the potential complications and outcomes differ from those of the standard cardiac rehabilitation client. For example, many clients with CHF will deteriorate irrespective of exercise or medical therapy. In these persons, the exercise regimen needs to be reassessed. Persons with CHF are at higher risk of sudden death, and they frequently experience psychosocial and vocational problems brought on by their disease. Some may experience prolonged fatigue after a single exercise session. Careful consideration should be given to absolute contraindications (particularly obstruction to left ventricular outflow, decompensated CHF, or unstable dysrhythmias). Relative contraindications to exercise are the same for persons with CHF as for persons with normal left ventricular function. These considerations necessitate that programs be designed carefully and that the staff be trained to recognize specific needs of this population and specific precautions that should be taken:

- Status can change quickly, and patients should be reevaluated frequently (for signs of decompensation, rapid changes in weight or blood pressure, worse-than-usual dyspnea or angina on exertion, or increases in dysrhythmias).

- Warm-up and cool-down sessions should be prolonged.

- Patients may tolerate only limited workloads; use low-intensity/long-duration sessions.

- Perceived exertion and dyspnea scales should take precedence over heart rate and workload targets.

- Avoid isometric exercise.

- ECG monitoring is required for persons with a history of ventricular tachycardia, cardiac arrest (sudden death), or exertional hypotension.

- Consider ancillary study data (exercise echocardiogram, radionuclide studies, hemodynamic studies, respired gas analysis) when developing the exercise program. In general, do not exceed a work rate that produces wall motion abnormalities, a drop in ejection fraction, a pulmonary wedge pressure greater than 20 mmHg, or the ventilatory threshold.

Suggested Readings

Adamopoulos, S., A.J.S. Coats, F. Brunotte, L. Arnolda, T. Meyer, C.H. Thompson, J.F. Dunn, J. Stratton, G.J. Kemp, G.K. Radda, and B. Rajagopalan. 1993. Physical training improves skeletal muscle metabolism in patients with chronic heart failure. *J. Am. Coll. Cardiol.* 21: 1101-06.

Bristow, M.R., R. Ginsburg, W. Minobe, R.S. Cubiccitti, W.S. Sageman, K. Lurie, M. R. Billingham, D. C. Harrison, and E. B. Stinson. 1982. Decreased catecholamine sensitivity and beta-adrenergic receptor density in failing human hearts. *N. Engl. J. Med.* 307: 205-11.

Giannuzzi, P., L. Tavazzi, P.L. Temporelli, U. Corra, A. Imparato, M. Gattone, A. Giordano, L. Sala, C. Schweiger, and C. Malinverni. 1993. Long-term physical training and left ventricular remodeling after anterior myocardial infarction: Results of the exercise in anterior myocardial infarction (EAMI) trial. *J. Am. Coll. Cardiol.* 22: 1821-29.

Jette, M., R. Heller, F. Landry, and G. Blümchen. 1991. Randomized 4-week exercise program in patients with impaired left ventricular function. *Circulation* 84: 1561-67.

Jugdutt, B.I., B.L. Michorowski, and C.T. Kappagoda. 1988. Exercise training after anterior Q-wave myocardial infarction: Importance of regional left ventricular function and topography. *J. Am. Coll. Cardiol.* 12: 362-72.

Myers, J., and V.F. Froelicher. 1991. Hemodynamic determinants of exercise capacity in chronic heart failure. *Ann. Intern. Med.* 115: 377-86.

Myers, J., A. Salleh, N. Buchanan, D. Smith, J. Neutel, E. Bowes, and V.F. Froelicher. 1992. Ventilatory mechanisms of exercise intolerance in chronic heart failure. *Am. Heart J.* 124: 710-19.

Sullivan, M.J., H.J. Green, and F.R. Cobb. 1988. Exercise training in patients with severe left ventricular dysfunction: Hemodynamic and metabolic effects. *Circulation* 78: 506-15.

Sullivan, M.J., H.J. Green, and F.R. Cobb. 1988. Increased exercise ventilation in patients with chronic heart failure: Intact ventilatory control despite hemodynamic and pulmonary abnormalities. *Circulation* 77: 552-59.

Sullivan, M.J., H.J. Green, and F.R. Cobb. 1989. Exercise training in patients with chronic heart failure delays ventilatory anaerobic threshold and improves submaximal exercise performance. *Circulation* 79: 324-29.

Sullivan, M.J., H.J. Green, and F.R. Cobb. 1991. Altered skeletal muscle metabolic response to exercise in chronic heart failure: Relation to skeletal muscle aerobic enzyme activity. *Circulation* 84: 1597-1607.

CONGESTIVE HEART FAILURE: EXERCISE TESTING

METHODS	MEASURES	ENDPOINTS*	COMMENTS
Aerobic power **Cycle** (10-15 watts/min) ramp protocol (25-50 watts/3 min stage) **Treadmill** (Naughton—see Special Considerations below)	• 12-lead ECG, heart rate • Blood pressure • Dyspnea/RPE scales • Respired gas analysis	• Serious dysrhythmias • T-wave inversion with significant ST change • Hypotensive response • Perceived shortness of breath and fatigue • $\dot{V}O_2$ peak and ventilatory threshold	• Peak performance is often < 5 METs, so a low-level ramp or Naughton protocol is preferred.
Endurance **6-minute walk**	• Distance	• Time	• Useful throughout training program.
Strength **Isokinetic/isotonic**			• Weakness due to sedentary lifestyle and/or to abnormal muscle energy metabolism may be improved with resistance training.
Functional capacity **Lifestyle-specific tests**	• Performance related to daily living activities		

*Measurements of particular significance; do not *always* indicate test termination.

MEDICATIONS	SPECIAL CONSIDERATIONS
• Digoxin: Diffuse ST effects. May increase performance. • Diuretics: May induce ectopy. May lower BP. • Vasodilators: May increase HR, lower BP, and increase performance. • ACE inhibitors: Lower blood pressure and may improve performance. • Antiarrhythmics: May increase HR, but have little or no effect on performance.	• Peak performance is often < 5 METs, so a low-level ramp or Naughton protocol is preferred. • Ventilation/perfusion inequalities cause increased dead space and hyperventilation/dyspnea. • Increased risk of dysrhythmias.

CONGESTIVE HEART FAILURE: EXERCISE PROGRAMMING

MODES	GOALS	INTENSITY/ FREQUENCY/DURATION	TIME TO GOAL
Aerobic • Large muscle activities	• Increase $\dot{V}O_2$ peak and ventilatory threshold. • Increase peak work and endurance.	• Borg RPE of 11-16. • 40-70% $\dot{V}O_2$ peak or HR reserve. • 3-7 days/week. • 20-40 minutes/session.	• 3 months
Strength • Circuit training	• Reduce atrophy.	• High repetitions, low resistance.	• 3 months
Flexibility • Upper and lower body range-of-motion activities	• Decrease risk of injury.	• 2-3 days/week.	• 4-6 months
Functional • Activity-specific exercise	• Increase daily living activities. • Return to work. • Improve quality of life and maintain independence.		• 3 months

MEDICATIONS	SPECIAL CONSIDERATIONS
• Beta blockers: Attenuate HR by about 10 to 30 contractions/min. Long-term effects may be beneficial. • ACE inhibitors and diuretics: Combining with a vasodilator may increase performance but cause postexertional hypotension.	• See table on exercise programming in chapter 3. • Tolerance of exercise intensity will most likely be lower in these patients. • Some patients have prolonged fatigue after exercise. • Weight gain and/or increased dyspnea may indicate decompensated heart failure.

CHAPTER 9

Cardiac Transplant

Steven J. Keteyian, PhD, FACSM
Clinton Brawner, BS
The Henry Ford Heart and Vascular Institute
Henry Ford Hospital

Overview of the Pathophysiology

Cardiac transplantation represents an effective therapeutic alternative for persons with end-stage heart failure. Approximately 2,800 such procedures are performed annually, with one- and three-year survival rates for adults of 83% and 77%, respectively. Presently, almost all cardiac transplant procedures are orthotopic, performed by anastomosis of the atria of the recipient's heart to the atria of the donor's heart.

After surgery, clients with cardiac transplant often continue to experience exercise intolerance. Causes for this may include the extended period of inactivity experienced by the individual before surgery, slow resolution of the skeletal muscle derangements that are characteristic of persons with heart failure, loss of skeletal muscle mass and strength, the absence of autonomic innervation in the transplanted heart, or combinations of these. People with cardiac transplant are unique in that their heart is *decentralized*, which means that except for the parasympathetic, postganglionic nerve fibers that are left intact, all other cardiac autonomic fibers are disrupted. Spontaneous reinnervation after surgery is felt to be uncommon, and if it occurs, it is likely to be a late phenomenon years after transplantation. Thus, decentralization is prolonged if not permanent.

Effects on the Exercise Response

As a consequence of the decentralized myocardium, many differences in the cardiopulmonary and neuroendocrine response are evident at rest and during exercise when comparing persons with cardiac transplant versus healthy individuals. Some of these differences are the following:

- Resting heart rate is increased (90-110 contractions per minute); chronotropic response to exercise is reduced; and peak heart rate is lower.

- Systolic and diastolic blood pressures are elevated at rest; this is likely to be attributable to (a) elevations in catecholamines and atrial natriuretic peptide, (b) the side effects of immunosuppressive medications (cyclosporine and prednisone), and (c) altered baroreceptor function. However, peak exercise systolic pressure is usually lower than in normal persons.

- There is less of an increase in cardiac output, with increases during light exercise predominantly due to stroke volume (muscle and respiratory pump actions augment venous return to maintain/increase preload) rather than heart rate. Increases in cardiac output during moderate- to high-intensity exercise are attributable to catecholamine-related increases in heart rate and further increases in stroke volume. Peak stroke volume is lower, and peak cardiac output is reduced by approximately 25%.

- Peak oxygen consumption and oxygen consumption at ventilatory threshold are reduced.

- Greater increase is seen in plasma norepinephrine during submaximal exercise.

- Because of the absence of efferent innervation to the sinoatrial node, the increased plasma catecholamines that develop during exercise exert a positive chronotropic effect in early recovery. As a result, the heart rate declines slowly while the systolic blood pressure recovers in a normal fashion (catecholamines disappear from the blood at a normal rate).

Effects of Exercise Training

The response to exercise training in persons with cardiac transplant is also influenced, to some extent, by the fact that the heart is decentralized. Although the specific response may differ from one person to another, common responses to exercise training are as follows:

- No change in resting heart rate associated with exercise training of less than 16 weeks. A small (4 beats per minute) decrease in resting heart rate, however, has been noted after 16 months of training. Mechanisms for this finding may include down-regulation of cardiac beta-receptor sensitivity, a decrease in resting plasma norepinephrine, or both.

- An increase in peak exercise heart rate.

- No change in resting stroke volume or cardiac dimensions.

Management and Medications

Controlling immune system rejection of the donor heart while avoiding the adverse side effects of immunosuppressive therapy (hyperlipidemia, hypertension, obesity, and diabetes) is the main issue soon after transplantation. One year after surgery, the likelihood for acute rejection lessens, but there is increased probability of developing accelerated atherosclerosis in the coronary arteries of the donor heart.

Acute graft rejection is common among all transplant individuals and is characterized by perivascular infiltration of killer T lymphocytes into the myocardium, including possible cellular necrosis. The severity of acute rejection is generally classified as mild early, moderate, or severe. Treatment for acute graft rejection includes medications (corticosteroids, antilymphocyte globulin) and, in rare cases, re-transplantation.

Two approaches are used to lessen the occurrence of acute rejection. First, since rejection can be silent, endomyocardial biopsy (by catheters) is performed both to detect preclinical cellular involvement and to assess the efficacy of therapy. Second, immunosuppressive agents (prednisone, cyclosporine, azathioprine) are used to prophylactically suppress killer T lymphocyte function. Doing so, however, renders individuals more susceptible to certain infections and cancers. Also, although confirmatory evidence is lacking, the calf discomfort experienced in approximately 15% of the individuals during walking may be due to cyclosporine therapy. Otherwise, the immunosuppressive medications mentioned do not necessarily affect exercise testing or training.

Recommendations for Exercise Testing

Considerations that relate to graded exercise testing in individuals with cardiac transplant are as follows:

- Conduct continuous incremental testing using a treadmill or stationary cycle ergometer. Arm ergometry testing can be used to assess the safety and capacity of these individuals to perform arm work.

- Exercise protocols can be either ramp or steady state (three minutes per stage). With the use of cycle ergometry, work rates should be increased by 17 watts per minute or 25 to 30 watts per stage for ramp or steady state protocols, respectively. Exercise tests conducted with use of a treadmill should increase work rates by 1 to 2 METs per stage.

- Because of the delayed and blunted response of heart rate to exercise, ratings of perceived exertion as well as oxygen consumption should be assessed. These assessments will be helpful for quantifying functional capacity, developing an appropriate exercise prescription, and determining whether a peak effort was attained. Peak oxygen consumption in untrained cardiac transplant individuals is generally between 12 and 22 ml·kg^{-1}·min^{-1}.

- Although isolated cases of chest pain associated with accelerated graft atherosclerosis have been observed, decentralization of the myocardium eliminates anginal symptoms. Exercise electrocardiography is also inadequate with respect to assessing ischemia, as evidenced by its low sensitivity (0% to 21%) for detecting true disease in these individuals. Thus, radionuclide testing may be more useful for assessing ischemic heart disease.

- To assess recovery following a bout of maximal or submaximal exercise, observation of systolic blood pressure is a better indicator than heart rate alone.

Recommendations for Exercise Programming

As in most other people with chronic disease, progressive exercise training in individuals with cardiac transplant is an effective means to improve cardiorespiratory fitness and reestablish self-efficacy. Less well established, however, is whether the modification of cardiovascular risk factors through exercise alters the progression of accelerated graft atherosclerosis, which is the major factor limiting long-term survival in these individuals. In this disorder a concentric fibrointimal hyperplasia occurs that affects the coronary arteries.

The current recommended methods to guide exercise intensity in persons with cardiac transplant are ratings of perceived exertion, fixed distance/fixed speed, percentage of peak oxygen consumption, and ventilatory threshold. When incorporated into training studies involving persons with cardiac transplant, these methods have resulted in increases in peak oxygen consumption of 15% to 27%. The minimal threshold of intensity (i.e., 40%, 50%, 60% of peak) needed to significantly improve $\dot{V}O_2$ peak is not known.

The use of heart rate alone to guide exercise intensity is not appropriate. In fact, it is not uncommon to find persons with cardiac transplant achieving an exercise heart rate that not only exceeds 85% of measured peak but is equal to or greater than peak. These persons should perform an aerobic activity four to six times per week while progressively increasing the duration from 15 to 60 minutes. Also, since a leg-strength deficit contributes, in part, to the reduced peak oxygen consumption observed in these individuals, many may need to include two sessions per week of progressive resistance training in their plan.

Suggested Readings

Albrecht, A.E., D. Lillis, M.D. Pease, P. Harrison, B.J. Morgan, J.E. Schairer, and W.H. Boganhagen. 1993. Heart rate and catecholamine responses during exercise and recovery in cardiac transplant recipients. *J. Cardiopulmonary Rehabil.* 13: 182-87.

Banner, N.R. 1992. Exercise physiology and rehabilitation after heart transplantation. *J. Heart Lung Transplant.* 11 (4): S237-S240.

Braith, R.W., M.C. Limacher, S.H. Leggett, and M.L. Pollock. 1993. Skeletal muscle strength in heart transplant recipients. *J. Heart Lung Transplant.* 12: 1018-23.

Ehrman, J.K., S.J. Keteyian, A.B. Levine, K.L. Rhoads, L.R. Elder, T.B. Levine, and P.D. Stein. 1993. Exercise stress tests after cardiac transplantation. *Am. J. Cardiol.* 71: 1372-73.

Kavanaugh, T. 1992. Exercise and therapy of the cardiac transplant patient. In *Exercise and the heart in health and disease*, ed. R.J. Shepard and H.S. Miller, Jr., 257-82. New York: Marcel Dekker.

Keteyian, S.J., J. Ehrman, F. Fedel, and K. Rhoads. 1989. Exercise following cardiac transplantation, recommendations for rehabilitation. *Sports Med.* 8 (5): 251-59.

Keteyian, S.J., C.R.C. Marks, A.B. Levine, F. Fedel, T. Kataoka, and T.B. Levine. 1994. Cardiovascular responses of cardiac transplant patients to arm and leg exercise. *Eur. J. Appl. Physiol.* 68: 441-44.

Keteyian, S.J., C.R.C. Marks, A.B. Levine, T. Kataoka, F. Fedel, and T.B. Levine. 1994. Cardiovascular responses to submaximal arm and leg exercise in cardiac transplant patients. *Med. Sci. Sports Exerc.* 26 (4): 420-24.

McGregor, C.G.A. 1992. Cardiac transplantation: Surgical considerations and early postoperative management. *Mayo Clin. Proc.* 67: 577-85.

Savin, W.M., J.S. Shroeder, and W.L. Haskell. 1981. Response of cardiac transplant recipients to static and dynamic exercise: A review. *Heart Transplantation* 1 (1): 72-79.

Shepard, R.J. 1992. Responses of the cardiac transplant patient to exercise and training. *Exerc. Sport Sci. Rev.* 7: 297-320.

Squires, R.W. 1991. Rehabilitation after cardiac transplantation: 1980 to 1990. *J. Cardiopulmonary Rehabil.* 11: 84-92.

Young, J.B., W.L. Winters, R. Bouge, and B.F. Uretsky. 1993. Task Force 4: Function of the heart transplant recipient. *J. Am. Coll. Cardiol.* 22: 31-41.

CARDIAC TRANSPLANT: EXERCISE TESTING

METHODS	MEASURES	ENDPOINTS*	COMMENTS
Aerobic power **Cycle** (17 watts/min) ramp protocol (25-30 watts/3 min stage) **Treadmill** (1-2 METs/3 min stage)	• 12-lead ECG, heart rate	• Serious dysrhythmias	• Exercise and peak HR may be blunted. • Delayed slowing of HR in recovery; thus SBP may be a better indicator of recovery from a test. • ECG sensitivity low for detecting ischemia.
	• Blood pressure	• SBP > 260 mmHg or DBP > 115 mmHg	• Increased resting and submaximal BP due to cyclosporine therapy. • Peak SBP may be blunted.
	• RPE (Borg 6-20 scale)		• Better guide of intensity because of delayed and/or blunted response to exercise.
	• Gas analysis for $\dot{V}O_2$ peak $\dot{V}O_2$ at ventilatory threshold		• $\dot{V}O_2$ peak and $\dot{V}O_2$ at ventilatory threshold blunted.
	• Radionuclide testing		• May be more sensitive in assessing ischemic heart disease.
Strength **Isokinetic/isotonic**	• 1-3 repetitions maximum		• Useful in planning exercise program. • Meant to improve muscle strength/endurance and reverse or delay the harmful effects of long-term corticosteroid therapy.

*Measurements of particular significance; do not *always* indicate test termination.

MEDICATIONS	SPECIAL CONSIDERATIONS
• See table on exercise programming in chapter 3. • Prednisone: Muscle atrophy and decreased leg strength. May cause myopathy. • Cyclosporine: Increase in resting and submaximal BP.	• Calf muscle cramps can occur in approximately 15% of patients. • Leg-strength deficits are common and result in decreased exercise time. • Obesity due to long-term corticosteroid use and increased appetite. • Increased HR and decreased stroke volume at rest; decreased HR, stroke volume, cardiac output during peak exercise; decreased HR reserve. • Be cautious in using high-resistance exercise in persons who have had long-term, high-dose corticosteroids, which thin bone and thus risk fracture.

CARDIAC TRANSPLANT: EXERCISE PROGRAMMING

MODES	GOALS	INTENSITY/ FREQUENCY/DURATION	TIME TO GOAL
Aerobic • Large muscle activities	• Weight management. • Increase self-efficacy. • Increase cardiorespiratory fitness.	• Borg RPE of 11-16. • 50-75% $\dot{V}O_2$ peak. • 4-6 days/week. • 15-60 minutes/session.	• 4-6 months
Strength • Circuit training	• Increase ability to perform leisure, occupational, and daily living activities. • Increase muscle strength and endurance.	• Low to moderate intensity. • 2 days/week. • 15-20 minutes/session.	
Flexibility • Upper and lower body range-of-motion activities		• 2-3 days/week.	

MEDICATIONS	SPECIAL CONSIDERATIONS
• Prednisone: Possible bone/joint-related disorders because of demineralization effects.	• Due to sternotomy, postoperative range of motion may be limited for up to 8 to 10 weeks. • RPE should be primary method of monitoring exercise intensity. • Cardiac symptoms such as angina are absent because of decentralized myocardium. • Calf muscle cramps can occur in approximately 15% of patients. • Within the first postoperative year, exercise training HR may approach or exceed the maximal HR achieved on a previous exercise test. • Delayed slowing of HR is common during recovery. • Exercise adherence is important in this population. • Be cautious in using high-resistance exercise in persons who have had long-term, high-dose corticosteroids, which thin bone and thus risk fracture.

CHAPTER 10

Hypertension

Neil F. Gordon, MD, PhD, MPH, FACSM

The Heart and Lung Group of Savannah

Overview of the Pathophysiology

Hypertension is a major public health problem in most Western industrialized countries. It is estimated that in the United States, as many as 50 million individuals have an elevated blood pressure (BP) or are taking antihypertensive medication. In these persons, the risk for nonfatal and fatal cardiovascular disease (especially coronary artery disease and stroke), renal disease, and all-cause mortality increases progressively with higher levels of both systolic and diastolic BP. At any level of high BP, risks of cardiovascular disease are increased several-fold for persons with target-organ disease. Cardiovascular risks are also related to the presence of other risk factors.

Table 10.1 shows how adult BP is classified in the 1993 report of the Joint National Committee on Detection, Evaluation, and Treatment of High Blood Pressure.

Among hypertensive adults between the ages of 18 and 65 years who are seen in typical clinical practice, 95% have no identifiable cause. Their hypertension is defined as either primary, essential, or idiopathic. Although their cardiac output may be high initially, hypertension usually persists in these patients because of an increased peripheral resistance.

Secondary (and possibly reversible) forms of hypertension include renal parenchymal disease, renal vascular hypertension, adrenal hyperfunction (pheochromocytoma, Cushing's syndrome, primary

Table 10.1 CLASSIFICATION OF BLOOD PRESSURE FOR ADULTS AGED 18 YEARS AND OLDER*		
CATEGORY	**SYSTOLIC PRESSURE (mmHg)**	**DIASTOLIC PRESSURE (mmHg)**
Normal	< 130	< 85
High normal	130-139	85-89
Hypertension		
Stage 1 (mild)	140-159	90-99
Stage 2 (moderate)	160-179	100-109
Stage 3 (severe)	180-209	110-119
Stage 4 (very severe)	210	120

*Not taking antihypertensive medication and not acutely ill. When systolic and diastolic pressures fall into different categories, the higher category should be selected.

Reprinted with permission from the Joint National Committee on Detection, Evaluation, and Treatment of High Blood Pressure: The Fifth Report of the Joint National Committee on Detection, Evaluation, and Treatment of High Blood Pressure (JNC V). *Arch. Intern. Med.* 153: 154-83, 1993.

aldosteronism), and coarctation of the aorta. Persons who are elderly have a higher frequency of renal parenchymal disease and renovascular hypertension. Medications, including oral contraceptives, may elevate BP.

Effects on the Exercise Response

A single session of dynamic exercise usually evokes a normal rise in systolic BP from baseline levels in unmedicated persons with hypertension, although the response may be exaggerated or diminished in certain individuals. However, because of an elevated baseline level, the absolute level of systolic BP attained during dynamic exercise is usually higher in persons with hypertension. In addition, their diastolic BP may not change, or may even slightly rise, during dynamic exercise, probably as a result of an impaired vasodilatory response.

Recent studies have documented a 10 to 20 mmHg reduction in systolic BP during the initial 1 to 3 hours following 30 to 45 minutes of moderate-intensity dynamic exercise in persons with hypertension. This response, which may persist for up to 9 hours, appears to be mediated by a transient decrease in stroke volume rather than peripheral vasodilation.

Untreated hypertension may be accompanied by some limitation in exercise tolerance. The use of certain antihypertensive drugs may further impair exercise performance. However, exercise tolerance may be enhanced by control of hypertension with lifestyle modification and, if warranted, well-tolerated antihypertensive medications.

Effects of Exercise Training

Existing evidence indicates that endurance exercise training reduces the magnitude of rise in BP that can be expected over time in persons at increased risk for developing hypertension. Longitudinal studies further show that endurance training may elicit an average reduction of about 10 mmHg in both systolic and diastolic BP in persons with stage 1 or 2 hypertension. Both the Joint National Committee and ACSM (1993) advocate regular aerobic exercise as a preventive strategy to reduce the incidence of high BP, and indicate that exercise training can be effectively used as definitive or adjunctive therapy for hypertension.

The mechanisms by which exercise training lowers BP are unclear. Possibilities include

- decrease in plasma norepinephrine levels,
- increase in circulating vasodilator substances,
- amelioration of hyperinsulinemia, and
- alteration in renal function.

Physically active persons with hypertension and those with higher levels of cardiorespiratory fitness have been shown to have markedly lower mortality rates than sedentary and less fit persons.

The cardiovascular responses to a single session of resistance exercise differ from those for endurance exercise in several fundamental ways. In particular, heavy-resistance exercise elicits a pressor response that involves only moderate increases in heart rate and cardiac output, relative to those seen with dynamic exercise, but a greater elevation in systolic and diastolic BP. With the exception of circuit weight training, chronic strength or resistive training has not consistently been shown to lower resting BP.

Management and Medications

According to the Joint National Committee, the goal of treating persons with hypertension is to prevent morbidity and mortality associated with high BP and to control BP by the least intrusive means possible. To accomplish this, BP should be lowered and maintained below 140/90 mmHg while other modifiable cardiovascular risk factors are controlled concurrently.

For hypertension control or overall cardiovascular risk reduction, or both, it is recommended that people make the following lifestyle modifications:

- Lose weight if overweight.
- Limit alcohol intake to < 1 ounce per day of ethanol (24 ounces of beer, 8 ounces of wine, or 2 ounces of 100-proof whiskey).
- Exercise (aerobic) regularly.
- Reduce sodium intake to less than 2.3 grams per day.
- Maintain adequate dietary potassium, calcium, and magnesium intake.
- Stop smoking and reduce dietary fat, saturated fat, and cholesterol intake.

The decision to initiate drug therapy requires consideration of several factors:

- Severity of BP elevation
- Presence or absence of target-organ disease
- Presence or absence of other medical conditions and cardiovascular disease risk factors

Beta blockers and, to a lesser degree, the calcium antagonists diltiazem and verapamil reduce the heart rate response to submaximal and maximal exercise. In contrast, dihydropyridine-derivative calcium antagonists and direct vasodilators may increase the heart rate response to submaximal exercise.

With the exception of beta blockers, most antihypertensive agents do not substantially alter the systolic BP response to a single session of dynamic exercise. However, they do lower the resting BP and therefore the absolute level attained. Beta blockers have been shown to attenuate the magnitude of rise in systolic BP from the baseline level as well as to reduce the resting BP. Unfortunately, the usefulness of beta blockers, especially nonselective agents, is often considerably limited by a concomitant impairment of exercise tolerance in persons without myocardial ischemia, and by a possible blunting of exercise training-induced lowering of BP and triglycerides as well as by increases in high-density lipoprotein cholesterol.

Antihypertensive agents that reduce total peripheral resistance by vasodilation may predispose to postexercise hypotension. This potential adverse effect can usually be prevented by avoidance of abrupt cessation of exercise and use of a longer cool-down period. Diuretics may result in serum potassium derangements and thereby accentuate the risk for exercise-induced dysrhythmias.

Recommendations for Exercise Testing

Standard exercise testing methods and protocols may be used for persons with hypertension. Individuals with an additional coronary risk factor, and those who are male and > 40 years or female and > 50 years, should perform an exercise test with ECG monitoring before starting a vigorous exercise program. Irrespective of the intensity of exercise training, persons with symptoms of cardiovascular disease or with known cardiovascular disease should perform an exercise test with ECG monitoring before commencing an exercise program. When exercise testing is performed for the purpose of exercise prescription, the individual should be taking his or her usual antihypertensive medications. A resting systolic BP > 200 mmHg or diastolic BP > 115 mmHg is considered a relative contraindication to exercise testing. Attainment of a systolic BP > 260 mmHg or diastolic BP > 115 mmHg is an indication for exercise test termination.

Recommendations for Exercise Programming

It is recommended that people with more marked elevations in BP (> 180/110) add endurance training to their treatment regimen only after initiating drug therapy. The mode (large muscle, aerobic activities), frequency (three to seven days per week), duration (20-60 minutes), and intensity of exercise (50-85% of maximal oxygen consumption) recommended for persons with hypertension are similar to those for healthy adults. Interestingly, exercise training at somewhat lower intensities (40-70% of maximal oxygen consumption) appears to lower BP as much as, if not more than, exercise at higher intensities. The latter is especially important in certain specific populations of persons with hypertension, such as those who are elderly or who have chronic diseases in addition to hypertension.

Strength or resistive training is not recommended as the only form of exercise training for persons with hypertension because, with the exception of circuit weight training, it has not consistently been shown to lower BP. Thus, resistive exercise training is recommended when done as one component of a well-rounded exercise program, but not when done independently. Resistive training using low resistances and high repetitions should be prescribed.

Suggested Readings

American College of Sports Medicine. 1993. Position stand. Physical activity, physical fitness, and hypertension. *Med. Sci. Sports Exerc.* 25: i-x.

American College of Sports Medicine. 1995. *ACSM's guidelines for exercise testing and prescription*, ed. W.L. Kenney, R.H. Humphrey, C.X. Bryant, D.A. Mahler, V. Froehlicher, N.H. Miller, and T. D. York. 5th ed. Baltimore: Williams & Wilkins.

Blair, S.N., H.W. Kohl, C.E. Barlow, and L.W. Gibbons. 1991. Physical fitness and all-cause mortality in hypertensive men. *Ann. Med.* 23: 307-12.

Fletcher, G.F., V.F. Froelicher, L.H. Hartley, W.L. Haskell, and M.L. Pollock. 1990. Exercise standards. A statement for health professionals from the American Heart Association. *Circulation* 82: 2286-322.

Gordon, N.F., C.B. Scott, W.J. Wilkinson, J.J. Duncan, and S.N. Blair. 1990. Exercise and mild essential hypertension: Recommendations for adults. *Sports Med.* 10: 390-404.

Hagberg, J.M. 1990. Exercise, fitness, and hypertension. In *Exercise, Fitness, and Health*, ed. C. Bouchard, R.J. Shephard, T. Stephens, J.R. Sutton, and B.D. McPherson, 455-466. Champaign, IL: Human Kinetics.

Joint National Committee on Detection, Evaluation, and Treatment of High Blood Pressure. 1993. The fifth report of the Joint National Committee on Detection, Evaluation, and Treatment of High Blood Pressure (JNC V). *Arch. Intern. Med.* 153: 154-83.

Kaplan, N.M., R.B. Deveraux, and H.S. Miller, Jr. 1994. Task force 4: Systemic hypertension. *Med. Sci. Sports Exerc.* 26: S268-S270.

Paffenbarger, R.S., Jr., R.T. Hyde, A.L. Wing. and C.-C. Hsieh. 1986. Physical activity, all-cause mortality, and longevity of college alumni. *N. Engl. J. Med.* 314: 605-13.

HYPERTENSION: EXERCISE TESTING

METHODS	MEASURES	ENDPOINTS*	COMMENTS
Aerobic power **Cycle** (17 watts/min) ramp protocol (25-50 watts/3 min stage) **Treadmill** (1-2 METs/3 min stage)	• 12-lead ECG, heart rate • Blood pressure • RPE • Respired gas analysis	• Serious dysrhythmias • > 2 mm ST-segment depression or elevation • Ischemic threshold • T-wave inversion with significant ST change • SBP > 260 mmHg or DBP > 115 mmHg • Headache or other significant symptoms • $\dot{V}O_2$ max/ventilatory threshold	• Medications should be taken at usual time relative to the exercise bout.
Strength **Free weights, machines**	• 1 repetition maximum or maximal voluntary contraction		• Observe for exaggerated pressor response (SBP > 260 mmHg or DBP > 115 mmHg).

*Measurements of particular significance; do not *always* indicate test termination.

MEDICATIONS

• See table on testing in chapter 3.
• Beta blockers: Cause low chronotropic response of about 30 contractions/min.

HYPERTENSION: EXERCISE PROGRAMMING

MODES	GOALS	INTENSITY/ FREQUENCY/DURATION	TIME TO GOAL
Aerobic • Large muscle activities	• Increase $\dot{V}O_2$ max and ventilatory threshold. • Increase peak work and endurance. • Increase caloric expenditure. • Control blood pressure.	• 50-85% peak HR. • RPE of 11-13. • 3-7 days/week. • 30-60 minutes/session. • 700-2000 kcal/week.	• 4-6 months
Strength • Circuit training	• Increase strength.	• High repetitions, low resistance.	

MEDICATIONS	SPECIAL CONSIDERATIONS
• Beta blockers: Attenuate HR by about 30 contractions per minute. • Alpha$_1$ blockers, alpha$_2$ blockers, calcium channel blockers, and vasodilators: May cause postexertional hypotension.	• See table on programming in chapter 3. • Do not exercise if resting systolic BP > 200 mmHg or diastolic BP > 115 mmHg. • Exercise when pressor response is best controlled by medications. • Exercise at 40-70% $\dot{V}O_2$ max appears to lower resting blood pressure as much as, if not more than, exercise at higher intensities. • 700 kcal/week should be the initial goal; 2000 kcal/week should be the long-term goal.

CHAPTER 11

Peripheral Arterial Disease

Andrew W. Gardner, PhD

Baltimore VA Medical Center

Overview of the Pathophysiology

Peripheral arterial disease (PAD) results from stenoses and occlusions of the arteries of the lower extremities, causing a reduction in blood flow beyond the obstructions. The severity of PAD may be classified into the following categories according to recent guidelines:

- Grade 0 = asymptomatic
- Grade 1 = intermittent claudication
- Grade 2 = ischemic rest pain
- Grade 3 = minor or major tissue loss from the foot

Effects on the Exercise Response

The primary effect of PAD on acute exercise is the development of claudication pain in the leg musculature during exercise because of insufficient blood flow. Ankle systolic blood pressure is measured to noninvasively assess the peripheral circulation and is expressed relative to the brachial systolic pressure, termed the ankle/brachial systolic pressure index (ABI). Ankle systolic pressure and ABI are obtained while the client is supine at rest and following exercise.

- The time and/or distance to onset and to maximal claudication pain during walking are used as criteria for assessing the functional severity of disease.
- Ankle systolic pressure and ABI are reduced following exercise because blood flow is shunted into the proximal leg musculature at the expense of the periphery and distal areas of the leg.

Effects of Exercise Training

The clinical status of intermittent claudication in clients with PAD is improved through physical conditioning. Proposed mechanisms for an increase in exercise tolerance include the following adaptations:

- An increase in leg blood flow
- A more favorable redistribution of blood flow
- Improved hemorheological properties of blood (e.g., reduced viscosity)
- Greater reliance upon aerobic metabolism because of a higher concentration of oxidative enzymes
- Less reliance upon anaerobic metabolism
- An improvement in the efficiency of walking

Management and Medications

Common medications for intermittent claudication include

- pentoxifylline (Trental),
- dipyridamole (Persantine),

- warfarin (Coumadin), and
- aspirin.

Either clients should not take these medications until the exercise test procedures have been completed, or the time of day at which the medications were taken should be recorded and kept consistent upon repeated tests. In terms of exercise programming, little information is available on the interaction between exercise training and medication therapy for the treatment of intermittent claudication.

Recommendations for Exercise Testing

The primary objectives of a treadmill test for clients with PAD are to

- obtain reliable measures of claudication pain times,
- obtain reliable measures of ankle pressure following exercise, and
- assess whether coronary artery disease is present.

The procedures for treadmill testing clients with PAD are as follows:

- Ankle and brachial systolic blood pressures are measured and ABI is calculated after the client has been in a supine position for 15 minutes.
- Blood pressure is measured in both arms and in the posterior tibial and dorsalis pedis arteries of both legs (via Doppler). The artery yielding the higher systolic pressure in each leg is used for the measurement of ankle systolic pressure, and the higher pressure between the two arms is used to calculate ABI.
- An exercise test with gradual increments in grade is then performed. Small increments in grade allow claudication times of clients to be stratified according to disease severity. A highly reliable protocol uses a constant speed of 2 mph and an increase in grade of 2% every two minutes beginning at 0% grade.
- A validated pain scale ranging from 0 to 4 (0 = no pain, 1 = onset of pain, 2 = moderate pain, 3 = intense pain, and 4 = maximal pain) is used to assist clients in identifying progression of claudication pain during the test to maximal pain (a score of 4). The time elapsed from the start of

exercise to each pain score is recorded. Holding on to the handrails is discouraged, except for brief moments to maintain balance, because it alters metabolic demands, resulting in changes in physiological responses that cause variability in claudication times. Heart rate and brachial blood pressure are recorded during the last minute of each two-minute exercise stage.

- The client recovers in a supine position for 15 minutes. The time elapsed from the start of recovery to the relief of claudication pain (a pain score of 0) is recorded. Ankle and brachial blood pressures are recorded throughout the recovery period.

Recommendations for Exercise Programming

Exercise programs for clients with PAD should be designed with a goal of improving claudication pain symptoms and reducing cardiovascular risk factors. Most persons should do interval walking or stair climbing three times a week, at an intensity that causes pain of a score of 3 on a 4-point scale. The onset of claudication should occur in approximately five minutes; full recovery is allowed between intervals. This type of program may start with 20 minutes of exercise per session at 40% of heart rate reserve, and gradually progress to 40 minutes at 70% of heart rate reserve, over a period of about six months. Non-weight-bearing tasks (e.g., bicycling) may be used for warming up and cooling down. There are circumstances in which it is inappropriate for clients with PAD to exercise:

- Exercise training should not be performed until medical clearance, based on a physical exam, blood screening, and graded exercise test (GXT) results, has been completed.
- Exercise should not be performed when there are concomitant co-morbidities that may limit exercise tolerance.

Special Considerations

The most common potential complications for exercise testing are cardiovascular and orthopedic problems. These include

- angina (with ST depression on ECG),
- dyspnea,

- fatigue,
- dizziness, and
- leg pain not of vascular origin (e.g., neuropathy, arthritis, and orthopedic-related pain).

Special considerations for exercise programming are the following:

- Increases in intensity and duration should be made every three to four weeks during the program.
- Treadmill tests should be performed every two months for adjustment of the exercise prescription.

Several additional considerations should be noted:

- Psychologic status: The psychologic status of clients should be evaluated before enrollment into an exercise program. Use questionnaires to assess cognitive function, dementia, depression, and perceived quality of life and health status. For better adherence during the program, clients should be informed of the potential long-term benefits of exercise.
- Progression: Gradually increase exercise duration before increasing intensity.
- Personnel: A physician and an exercise physiologist should be involved for exercise testing, and exercise physiologists or nurses (or both) for exercise training.
- Safety: Changes in co-morbidities need to be carefully monitored.
- Supervision/monitoring: Clients with coronary disease should be monitored by ECG.
- Appropriate follow-up: A home maintenance exercise program should be recommended with periodic treadmill tests to determine long-term compliance.
- Environmental factors: Because cold weather causes peripheral vasoconstriction, clients with PAD need to spend more time warming up before exercising on cold days.

Suggested Readings

Ad hoc Committee on Reporting Standards. 1986. Suggested standards for reports dealing with lower extremity ischemia. *J. Vasc. Surg.* 4: 80-94.

American College of Sports Medicine. 1995. *ACSM's guidelines for exercise testing and prescription,* ed. W.L. Kenney, R.H. Humphrey, C.X. Bryant, D.A. Mahler, V. Froehlicher, N.H. Miller, and T.D. York. 5th ed. Baltimore: Williams & Wilkins.

Gardner, A.W., J.S. Skinner, B.W. Cantwell, and L.K. Smith. 1991. Progressive vs single-stage treadmill tests for evaluation of claudication. *Med. Sci. Sports Exerc.* 23: 402-08.

Gardner, A.W., J.S. Skinner, and L.K. Smith. 1991. Effects of handrail support on claudication and hemodynamic responses to single-stage and progressive treadmill protocols in peripheral vascular occlusive disease. *Am. J. Cardiol.* 68: 99-105.

Skinner, J.S., and D.E. Strandness, Jr. 1967. Exercise and intermittent claudication: I. Effect of repetition and intensity of exercise. *Circulation* 36: 23-29.

Yao, S.T., T.N. Needham, C. Gourmoos, and W.T. Irvine. 1972. A comparative study of strain-gauge plethysmography and Doppler ultrasound in the assessment of occlusive arterial disease of the lower extremities. *Surgery* 71: 4-9.

PERIPHERAL ARTERIAL DISEASE: EXERCISE TESTING

METHODS	MEASURES	ENDPOINTS*	COMMENTS
Aerobic power **Treadmill (preferred)** (1-2 METs/stage) **Cycle** (17 watts/min) ramp protocol (25-50 watts/3 min stage)	• 12-lead ECG • Blood pressure • 4-point claudication scale	• Serious dysrhythmias • > 2 mm ST-segment depression or elevation • Ischemic threshold • T-wave inversion with significant ST change • SBP > 260 mmHg or DBP > 115 mmHg	• When screening for CAD, use the treadmill protocol. • Record time of pain onset and maximal pain.
Endurance **Constant work rate**	• Time to maximal pain	• Maximal pain	• Record time of pain onset and maximal pain.
Neuromuscular **Gait analysis**	• Speed • Step rate • Step length		• May change with disease progression.
Functional capacity **6-minute walk (majority of patients)** **Time to maximal pain (severe disease)**	• Distance	• Time • Maximal pain	• Record time of pain onset and maximal pain.

*Measurements of particular significance; do not *always* indicate test termination.

MEDICATIONS	SPECIAL CONSIDERATIONS
• Pentoxyphylline, dipyridamole, aspirin, and warfarin: May improve time to claudication. • Beta blockers: May decrease time to claudication.	• Hish risk for CAD. • High prevalence of smoking/COPD. • Diabetic neuropathy can mimic claudication. • Skin ulcers common in persons with pain at rest (grade 2).

PERIPHERAL ARTERIAL DISEASE: EXERCISE PROGRAMMING

MODES	GOALS	INTENSITY/ FREQUENCY/DURATION	TIME TO GOAL
Aerobic • Large muscle activities	• Improve pain response; perform longer in time trials. • Decrease CAD risk factors.	• 40-70% $\dot{V}O_2$ peak HR reserve, or grade achieved on GXT. • Intermittent walk to 3 out of 4 on claudication scale (monitor HR). • 3 days/week. • 20-40 minutes/session.	• 4-6 months
Neuromuscular • Walking	• Improve gait.		
Functional • Walking	• Increase daily living activities, work potential, quality of life.		

MEDICATIONS	SPECIAL CONSIDERATIONS
• Pentoxyphylline, dipyridamole, aspirin, and warfarin: May improve time to claudication. • Beta blockers: May decrease time to claudication.	• Improvement may unmask angina pectoris. • Aggressive lifestyle and lipid management necessary.

CHAPTER 12

Aneurysms and Marfan Syndrome

Reed E. Pyeritz, MD, PhD

Medical College of Pennsylvania
and Hahnemann University

Overview of the Pathophysiology

Many diseases may cause enlargement (dilation) or tearing (dissection) of arteries. Marfan syndrome is an example of this type of disease. Regardless of cause, enlargement is usually painless and progressive, so substantial dilation (commonly called an aneurysm) can be present before the diagnosis is suspected. Aneurysms are often discovered when their size causes a complication. Unfortunately, dissection or rupture can be one of those complications, both of which often cause death, even if treated promptly. As a general rule, the larger the diameter of the aneurysm, the greater the risk of dissection or rupture. Aneurysms are much more common in later life, but can appear in early childhood if the underlying structure of the arterial wall is defective.

The most common site for aneurysms is in the brain, where sac-like bulges in the wall of a cerebral artery (berry aneurysm) occur in perhaps 2% to 5% of the population. Most berry aneurysms cause no symptoms or illness during the person's entire life. When a berry aneurysm enlarges, however, it takes up space within the skull; this can squeeze on that area of the brain and cause neurologic problems. A rupture (cerebral hemorrhage) can cause severe disability or death, or it may cause mild, reversible damage and be treatable by medicines, surgery, or

both. Unfortunately, except for some associations with polycystic kidney disease and coarctation of the aorta, there is generally no way of knowing who has a berry aneurysm until it ruptures.

The aorta is the next most common artery site of aneurysms. The enlargement usually occurs in a well-defined location, although some regions of this long artery are more susceptible than others. The aortic root (just where the vessel leaves the heart) is one such region. The abdominal aorta (in the region of the branches to the kidneys) is the most common site, affecting about 3% of older adults and particularly men over the age of 60. Other regions of the aorta can enlarge at different ages depending on the disease process.

- High blood pressure greatly increases the chances that a berry aneurysm will rupture.

- Aneurysm enlargement is usually without symptoms.

Causes of Aortic Enlargement and Dissection

The principal diseases that cause aortic aneurysms can be grouped into (1) structural defects present at birth (congenital), (2) diseases or events that damage the vessel wall, and (3) combinations of these groups. Genetic disease plays an important role in early-onset enlargement, although the problem sometimes does not appear until later in life. High blood pressure and cigarette smoking are the most common coincidental medical problems in older adults with abdominal aortic aneurysms. Other causes of aneurysms include inflammation (aortitis), infection (syphilis), and injury to the aorta (especially deceleration injuries as in automobile accidents). The main congenital cause is Marfan syndrome, which is usually discovered because persons with this disease are often tall and lanky, have deformity of the chest such as scoliosis (curvature of the spine) and pectus excavatum (inward-shaped chest), overly flexible joints, and dislocation of the eye lens, or, alternatively, because a close relative is affected. Marfan syndrome is caused by a genetic defect in the microfibrils forming the elastic fibers of large arteries as well as in similar microfibrils that give strength and structure to some connective tissues.

- Marfan syndrome causes the aortic root to dilate immediately above the aortic valve.
- As dilatation progresses, the aortic valve begins to leak (aortic regurgitation), and the risk of dissection increases.

Effects on the Exercise Response

Early in the course of Marfan syndrome, or when aneurysmal disease is minimal, there is usually no effect on the exercise response. In persons with existing aneurysms, there is likely to be little change in the exercise response other than a delay and blunting in pulse pressure.

Effects of Exercise Training

To the extent that exercise increases blood pressure, exercise increases the tension on the wall of an aneurysm, so exercise increases the risk of dissection or rupture for an already weakened aneurysm. Also, the progression of enlargement, or worsening, of the aneurysm is likely to be increased by exercise. These complications may be attributable to an increase in heart rate as well as blood pressure, since rapid heart rates cause more pulsations acting on the weakened wall in a given period of time. Thus, exercise training is relatively contraindicated in persons with aneurysmal disease.

Management and Medications

Does all this mean that people with aneurysms should not exercise? In the ideal situation, a risk profile should be generated for each individual. This approach has at least three limitations. First,

there has been little scientific work, in humans or animals, on the actual risk of a given degree of dilatation. Second, many people with aneurysms are asymptomatic (or even undiagnosed) and may *want* to exercise. Third, exercise offers benefits that people with aneurysms should not be denied, if the risks are not too high.

For people diagnosed with an aneurysm, the key step in medical management is to follow the progress of the enlarged area. This might involve echocardiography, abdominal ultrasound, magnetic resonance imaging, or (less and less commonly) angiography. The next most important step is lowering blood pressure to the low-normal range. A beta-adrenergic blocking drug, like atenolol or propranolol, is ideally suited to blood pressure management because it will also reduce the strength of arterial pulses. Even people with a low-normal baseline blood pressure should be treated with a beta blocker if there is not a contraindication to this medicine. Finally, when the vessel wall reaches about double the diameter it would ordinarily be, strong consideration is given to surgical repair. Some people, such as those with a strong family history of dissection, should have surgery even sooner.

- Stress tests can help adjust medications so that pulse rate does not rise above 100 contractions per minute (adults).
- The larger the aneurysm, the less active a person should be, in both lifestyle and the exercise laboratory.

Recommendations for Exercise Testing

In general, people with known aneurysms of any type *should not undergo maximal exercise testing.* Submaximal stress tests can be used to optimize therapeutic control of heart rate and blood pressure. In particular, it is important to avoid raising the heart rate-blood pressure product (heart rate multiplied by systolic blood pressure), which is a measure of stress on the arteries. There are no good exercise data on the likelihood that an increase in rate-pressure product will cause an aneurysm to rupture, but it is thought that the larger the aneurysm, the greater the likelihood of exercise to cause a rupture. Maximal strength testing should similarly be avoided since resistance exercise can markedly increase blood pressure.

Recommendations for Exercise Programming

The recommended modes of exercise are limited. In general, contact sports and competition should be avoided. Sports that have low cardiovascular demand, such as bowling, are recommended by the American College of Cardiology (1994) for clients with no evidence of aneurysmal disease. The larger the diameter of the aneurysm relative to the normal diameter of the vessel, the more exercise should be restricted. In any case, any aerobic isotonic activity should be performed at a moderate to low intensity. For individuals taking beta-adrenergic blocking drugs, the heart rate is not a good guide of intensity unless the peak heart rate has been ascertained by way of a graded exercise test. If peak heart rate is unknown, perceived exertion scales should be used. Resistance exercise should also be performed at moderate to low intensity. In persons with Marfan syndrome, flexibility training (e.g., some yoga positions) should not be done by persons with joint involvement, since this may risk joint dislocation. Some yoga activities may be useful, however, for blood pressure control.

Special Considerations

One management difficulty with aneurysmal disease is in advising persons who want to exercise. In particular, what about people who want to engage in sports? Indeed, some people with Marfan syndrome may be particularly suited to sport because of their stature and flexibility. Unfortunately, the very sports for which these individuals are predisposed to have talent involve body contact and extreme elevation of the rate-pressure product. Most notable in this regard is basketball. Furthermore, high doses of beta-blocking medications are likely to decrease aerobic performance needed for an intense fast-break style of play. The psychological characteristics that lead to athletic success may present problems with adherence to recommendations of limiting this activity, and may warrant the involvement of an expert in sport medical psychology.

Suggested Readings

Cheitlin, M.D., P.S. Douglas, and W.M. Parmley. 1994. Task force 2: Acquired valvular heart disease. In 26th Bethesda Conference: Recommendations for determining eligibility for competition in athletes with cardiovascular abnormalities. *J. Am. Coll. Cardiol.* 24 (4): 874-80.

Graham, T.P., Jr., J.T. Bricker, F.W. James, and W.B. Strong. 1994. Task force 1: Congenital heart disease. In 26th Bethesda Conference: Recommendations for determining eligibility for competition in athletes with cardiovascular abnormalities. *J. Am. Coll. Cardiol.* 24 (4): 867-73.

Pyeritz, R.E., and U. Francke. 1993. Conference report: The second international symposium on the Marfan's syndrome. *Am. J. Med. Genet.* 47: 127-35.

Pyeritz, R.E., and V.A. McKusick. 1979. The marfan syndrome: Diagnosis and management. *New Engl. J. Med.* 300 (14): 772-77.

ANEURYSMS AND MARFAN SYNDROME: EXERCISE TESTING

METHODS	MEASURES	ENDPOINTS*	COMMENTS
Aerobic power **Not recommended**			• Raises HR and BP too high.
Endurance **6-minute walk**	• Distance	• Time	• Assesses low-level exercise endurance.
Strength **Not recommended**			• Raises HR and BP too high.
Flexibility **Goniometry** **Sit-and-reach**			• Assesses range of motion (see Special Considerations below).
Functional capacity **Balance**			• Assesses the need for occupational/physical therapy.

*Measurements of particular significance; do not *always* indicate test termination.

MEDICATIONS	SPECIAL CONSIDERATIONS
• Beta blockers: Limit chronotropic response.	• Elevated HR and BP (double product) potentially harmful (risk of dissection). • HR should never go above 100 beats/min. • In Marfan syndrome, joint contractures, hypermobility, scoliosis, hyperlordosis, kyphosis, and protrusio acetabuli are possible.

ANEURYSMS AND MARFAN SYNDROME: EXERCISE PROGRAMMING

MODES	GOALS	INTENSITY/ FREQUENCY/DURATION	TIME TO GOAL
Aerobic • Large muscle activities (e.g., walking, swimming)	• Increase peak work and endurance.	• Do not exceed HR of 100 contractions/minute. • 3-4 days/week. • 30 minutes/session. • Emphasize duration over intensity.	• 4-6 months
Strength • Isokinetic/isotonic—large muscle groups	• Increase stability of hypermobile joints and spine.	• Do not exceed 30-40 pounds. • 2-3 days/week. • 15-30 minutes/session. • Emphasize consistency over intensity.	• 4-6 months
Flexibility • Stretching	• Maintain/increase range of motion.		
Functional • Activity-specific exercise	• Maintain daily living activities.		

SPECIAL CONSIDERATIONS

• See table on testing.
• Some persons with Marfan syndrome may be prone to *joint laxity*. Flexibility training should be limited in these individuals.

CHAPTER 13

Pulmonary Disease

Christopher B. Cooper, MD, FACSM
UCLA School of Medicine

Overview of the Pathophysiology

Chronic pulmonary disease imposes multiple pathophysiological problems, not only through obvious ventilatory and gas exchange impairments, but also through complex interactions with the cardiovascular and muscular systems. To appreciate the nature of these impairments it is instructive to divide the pathophysiology into a number of categories.

Ventilatory Impairments

• *Increased airway resistance* as seen in obstructive pulmonary diseases such as chronic bronchitis and asthma. Airflow obstruction is compromised mainly during expiration since the airways tend to become smaller as lung volume decreases. While smoking-related chronic bronchitis is slowly progressive, asthma can be intermittent and of varying severity. In the special case of exercise-induced bronchoconstriction, pulmonary function can be normal between attacks.

• *Reduced compliance* as seen in restrictive pulmonary diseases—for example, reduced lung compliance as seen in pulmonary fibrosis or reduced chest wall compliance as seen in kyphoscoliosis.

• *Increased work of breathing*, which occurs in both obstructive and restrictive diseases.

• *Ventilatory muscle weakness* due to either hyperinflation or neuromuscular weakness. Hyperinflation occurs with expiratory airflow obstruction placing the inspiratory muscles at a mechanical disadvantage. Neuromuscular weakness of the respiratory muscles also causes a restrictive ventilatory defect as seen in poliomyelitis or muscular dystrophy.

• *Ventilatory inefficiency* due to increased dead space and an inappropriately high ratio between physiological dead space and tidal volume (VD/VT).

• *Ventilatory muscle fatigue* resulting from increased work of breathing, ventilatory muscle weakness, ventilatory inefficiency, or a combination of these factors.

• *Ventilatory failure* with inadequate alveolar ventilation, hypoxemia, and hypercarbia. This condition arises in the later stages of many chronic pulmonary diseases.

Abnormalities of Gas Exchange

• *Destruction of the alveolar-capillary membrane* as seen in emphysema and pulmonary fibrosis. Due to diffusion impairment, both conditions can result in hypoxemia during exercise or even at rest in advanced disease.

• *Ventilation-perfusion inequality* as seen particularly in chronic obstructive pulmonary disease (COPD) and recurrent pulmonary emboli. These conditions can also result in hypoxemia, which usually worsens during exercise.

Cardiovascular Impairments

• *Cardiovascular deconditioning*, which is an inevitable consequence of reduced physical activity in chronic pulmonary disease. Individuals may experience an accumulation of lactic acid at low work rates.

• *Reduced pulmonary vascular conductance* as seen in chronic hypoxemia and pulmonary vascular disease such as thromboembolism and emphysema. As a result of increased pulmonary vascular resistance, the right ventricle is unable to respond adequately to the demand for increased cardiac output during exercise.

Muscular Impairments

- *Peripheral muscle deconditioning*, which is an inevitable consequence of reduced physical activity in chronic pulmonary disease.

- *Muscle wasting and weakness* due to inactivity and malnutrition.

Symptomatic Limitations

- *Breathlessness (dyspnea)* is a frightening symptom with a complex etiology. Dyspnea results from a summation of neurological inputs from pulmonary receptors, chemoreceptors, and mechanoreceptors in the chest wall and limbs. Some individuals have dyspnea that is disproportional to their ventilatory limitations.

Psychological Disturbances

- *Chronic anxiety* afflicts many individuals with chronic pulmonary disease because of the frightening nature of their symptoms.

- *Depression* follows from limited ability to pursue normal daily activities with resulting social isolation, feelings of helplessness, and despair.

Effects on the Exercise Response

Some, but not all, people with chronic pulmonary disease have true ventilatory limitation whereby the ventilatory requirement at maximum exercise equals the ventilatory capacity that can be measured over 12 or 15 seconds (maximal voluntary ventilation) or calculated from spirometry. Individuals with obstructive disease have impeded expiration requiring a longer time for adequate lung emptying. In these persons, increased breathing frequency during exercise tends to lead to hyperinflation and smaller tidal volumes, circumstances that worsen breathing efficiency by increasing VD/VT. Individuals with restrictive diseases characteristically have limited inspiratory capacity (i.e., tidal volume constraint) but usually have unimpeded or even accelerated expiration. These persons characteristically exhibit rapid respiratory rates (e.g., > 50 per minute) at maximum exercise.

In the absence of true ventilatory limitation, exercise can be limited by cardiovascular factors such as deconditioning, impaired left ventricular function due to hypoxemia, or reduced pulmonary blood flow secondary to chronic hypoxemia. Peripheral muscle deconditioning can lead to lactic acid accumulation at low work rates, increased CO_2 output from bicarbonate buffering, and consequently an increased ventilatory requirement (which compounds the situation).

Impairment of gas exchange occurs in emphysema because of destruction of the alveolar-capillary membrane and in pulmonary fibrosis because of loss of functioning lung units. Both conditions might cause hypoxemia during exercise, particularly when increases in pulmonary blood flow increase shunting through areas of incomplete gas exchange. Chronic hypoxemia also causes erythrocytosis, and the resulting increase in blood viscosity can further compromise the circulation during exercise. In smokers, increases in carboxyhemoglobin, which does not carry oxygen, will impair blood oxygen transport. Finally, in some individuals, symptoms (predominantly dyspnea) and psychological factors might limit exercise capacity independently.

Effects of Exercise Training

Regular participation in physical activity can manifest beneficial changes in persons with chronic pulmonary disease. These changes include

- cardiovascular reconditioning,
- desensitization to dyspnea,
- improved ventilatory efficiency,
- increased muscle strength,
- improved flexibility,
- improved body composition,
- better balance, and
- enhanced body image.

The accomplishment of these changes requires careful attention to medications to obtain optimal respiratory mechanics, and may require use of oxygen therapy to maintain adequate oxygenation during exercise.

Management and Medications

Since individuals with chronic pulmonary disease have some degree of physical deconditioning, exercise training is a crucial aspect of clinical management and rehabilitation. The specific goals of management are the following:

- *Optimization of respiratory system mechanics* by careful attention to bronchodilator therapy, inhaler dosage, and technique
- *Correction of hypoxemia* whether it occurs at rest, during exercise, or during sleep
- *Desensitization to dyspnea, fear, and other potentially limiting symptoms*
- *Breathing retraining* to improve ventilatory efficiency
- *Energy conservation* by improved coordination, balance, and mechanical efficiency during activities of daily living
- *Exercise training* to correct physical deconditioning, reduce lactic acidosis, and reduce ventilatory requirement during exercise

The first five goals listed are directed toward enabling an individual to perform exercise at higher intensity, thus increasing the potential for obtaining a reconditioning effect from exercise training.

Individuals with chronic pulmonary disease are often taking several medications that could have implications for exercise testing and training. Furthermore, chronic pulmonary disease often coexists with cardiovascular diseases such as coronary artery disease, hypertension, and peripheral arterial disease. The potential effects of medications for these conditions are described in chapters 3, 4, 5, 10, and 11.

- *Sympathomimetic agonists* (e.g., albuterol, metaproterenol, and salmeterol). These drugs are selective beta$_2$-adrenoceptor agonists intended to produce bronchodilation. However, they also reduce peripheral vascular resistance and tend to cause tachycardia, palpitations, and tremulousness. Nonselective sympathomimetic drugs (e.g., epinephrine and isoprenaline) should not be used because of unwanted effects on the cardiovascular system.
- *Methylxanthines* (e.g., theophylline and aminophylline). These drugs have potent bronchodilator action but also cause tachycardia, cardiac dysrhythmias, and central nervous system stimulation with increased respiratory drive and the risk of seizures.
- *Thiazide diuretics* (e.g., hydrochlorothiazide) and *loop diuretics* (e.g., furosemide). These drugs are prescribed to control fluid retention in cor pulmonale. Intravascular volume depletion might cause hypotension during exercise. Hypokalemia might predispose to cardiac dysrhythmias and muscle weakness.

- *Glucocorticoids* (e.g., prednisone). Many individuals with chronic pulmonary disease end up on long-term glucocorticoid therapy. These drugs are prescribed for COPD and idiopathic pulmonary fibrosis with the hope of reducing inflammation and improving pulmonary function. Important side effects that influence exercise include skin atrophy and fragility, osteoporosis, muscle atrophy, and myopathy (including the ventilatory muscles).
- *Antidepressants* (e.g., tricyclics). Many psychotropic drugs cause resting and exercise tachycardia.

Recommendations for Exercise Testing

Exercise testing is extremely valuable in persons with chronic pulmonary disease to distinguish between several possible causes of limited exercise capacity as described in the section on the pathophysiology. It is also essential to identify coexistent exercise-induced hypoxemia, hypertension, cardiac dysrhythmias, or myocardial ischemia.

Maximal exercise testing is safe with appropriate monitoring and gives the best definition of the limitations, including psychological problems and symptoms. The cycle ergometer offers the best means of controlling external work rate, measuring gas exchange, and blood sampling. A typical protocol might include 3 minutes of unloaded pedaling followed by a ramp increase in work rate of 5, 10, 15 or 20 watts per minute, depending on the degree of impairment. The aim should be to obtain between 8 and 10 minutes of exercise data. A constant work rate protocol on a cycle ergometer can be used repetitively to allow accurate comparison of physiological responses and to show improvements after therapeutic interventions including exercise training.

Treadmill exercise testing is helpful for the oxygen-dependent person and can be repeated with different oxygen systems and flows to determine the best means of correcting hypoxemia.

Recommendations for Exercise Programming

Exercise is to be encouraged in persons with chronic pulmonary disease. The exercise prescription should be individualized and flexible to account for fluctuations in clinical status. Any significant change in the medical condition of the person requires reassessment of the goals and risks of the exercise program. Exercise rehabilitation should involve several different professionals. Respiratory therapists evaluate, teach, and ensure effective use of bronchodilator medications and oxygen therapy. Physical therapists and exercise professionals evaluate exercise endurance, muscle strength, flexibility, and body composition. They determine and adjust the exercise prescription and demonstrate and supervise techniques for improving flexibility, balance, and muscle strength. Occupational therapists evaluate activities of daily living and quality of life. They teach energy conservation and improved body mechanics aimed at reducing the oxygen requirement for specific activities. All therapists teach improved breathing efficiency using methods such as pursed lips and diaphragm breathing, which slow the respiratory rate.

The recommended mode of exercise training can be walking, cycling, swimming, or conditioning exercises based on energy centering and balance, such as tai chi. The mode of exercise selected should be one that is enjoyable and one that directly improves ability to perform usual daily activities. In addition to the accepted specificity of training effect in terms of muscle performance, there is some evidence that desensitization to dyspnea is task-specific.

Oxygen should be administered during exercise to individuals who have had a fall in arterial oxygen tension to less than 55 mmHg or in oxyhemoglobin desaturation to less than 88%. Prevention of exercise-induced hypoxemia is likely not only to improve exercise capacity but also to enhance the effects of exercise training. The goal of oxygen therapy during exercise is to maintain an oxyhemoglobin saturation over 90%.

Modifications to the duration and frequency of exercise might be necessary. Commonly the person with chronic respiratory disease is unable to sustain 20 or 30 minutes of exercise, and interval exercise consisting of 5- or 10-minute sessions might be necessary until adaptations have occurred that allow reduction of the rest intervals and gradual increases in the work intervals.

An intensive six-week exercise program with group interaction is helpful to begin the process of physical reconditioning. However, the importance of maintaining a higher level of physical activity cannot be overemphasized. The individual with chronic pulmonary disease is at particular risk of relapsing into a state of inactivity and physical deconditioning. Membership in a health and fitness facility is worth considering.

Suggested Readings

Casaburi, R., A. Patessio, F. Ioli, S. Zanaboni, C.F. Donner, and K. Wasserman. 1991. Reductions in exercise lactic acidosis and ventilation as a result of exercise training in patients with obstructive lung disease. *Am. Rev. Respir. Dis.* 143: 9-18.

Cochrane, L.M., and C.J. Clark. 1990. Benefits and problems of a physical training program for asthmatic patients. *Thorax* 45: 345-51.

Cooper, C.B. 1993. Long term oxygen therapy. In *Principles and practice of pulmonary rehabilitation*, ed. R. Casaburi and T.L. Petty, 183-203. Philadelphia: Saunders.

Cooper, C.B. 1995. Determining the role of exercise in patients with chronic pulmonary disease. *Med. Sci. Sports Exerc.* 27: 147-57.

Criner, G.J., and B.R. Celli. 1988. Effect of unsupported arm exercise on ventilatory muscle recruitment in patients with severe chronic airflow obstruction. *Am. Rev. Respir. Dis.* 138: 856-61.

Davidson, A.C., R. Leach, R.J.D. George, and D.M. Geddes. 1988. Supplemental oxygen and exercise ability in chronic obstructive airways disease. *Thorax* 43: 965-71.

Mahler, D.A. 1992. The measurement of dyspnea during exercise in patients with lung disease. *Chest* 101 (suppl. 5): 2425-75.

Ries, A.L. 1990. Position paper of the American Association of Cardiovascular and Pulmonary Rehabilitation. Scientific basis of pulmonary rehabilitation. *J. Cardiopulmonary Rehabil.* 10: 418-41.

PULMONARY DISEASE: EXERCISE TESTING

METHODS	MEASURES	ENDPOINTS*	COMMENTS
Aerobic power **Cycle (preferred)** (10, 15, or 20 watts/min) **Ramp protocol** (25-50 watts/3 min stage) **Treadmill** (1-2 METs/stage)	• 12-lead ECG	• Serious dysrhythmias • > 2 mm ST-segment depression or elevation • Ischemic threshold • T-wave inversion with significant ST change	• Patients with COPD often have coexistent CAD.
	• Blood pressure	• SBP > 260 mmHg or DBP > 115 mmHg	
	• RPE, dyspnea scales		
	• Pulse oximetry/ arterial P_aO_2		
	• Respired gas analysis • Blood lactate	• Maximum ventilations • $\dot{V}O_2$ peak • Lactate/ventilatory threshold	• Breathing pattern analysis may also be helpful. • Lactic acidosis may contribute to exercise limitation in some patients.
Endurance **6-minute walk** **Isokinetic/isotonic**	• Distance • Same measures as with aerobic power testing • Maximum number of repetitions	• Time	• Useful for measurement of improvement throughout conditioning program.
Strength **Isokinetic/isotonic**	• Peak torque • Maximum number of repetitions • 1 repetition maximum		• Angular range must be constant when making pre- and/or post-training comparisons of peak torque.
Flexibility **Sit-and-reach**	• Hip, hamstring, and lower back flexibility		
Neuromuscular **Gait analysis** **Balance**			• Body mechanics, coordination, and work efficiency are often impaired.
Functional capacity **Sit-to-stand** **Stair climbing** **Lifting**			

*Measurements of particular significance; do not *always* indicate test termination.

MEDICATIONS	SPECIAL CONSIDERATIONS
All of the following medications, despite potential side effects, may improve exercise capacity through bronchodilation, relief of congestive heart failure, and psychotropic effects. • Methylxanthines: May cause tachycardia, cardiac dysrhythmias, and increased dyspnea. • Sympathomimetic bronchodilators: May cause tachycardia. • Loop and thiazide diuretics: May cause hypokalemia leading to dysrhythmias and muscle weakness. • Antidepressants: May cause tachycardia at rest and during exercise.	• High risk for CAD. Worsening hypoxia during exertion may induce angina and/or dysrhythmias. • Monitoring of 12-lead ECG, blood pressure, and oxygen saturation is essential. • Spirometry, especially maximal voluntary ventilation, is helpful in defining ventilatory limitations. • Exercise testing in mid- to late morning or afternoon is desirable. Pulmonary patients often have worse symptoms in the early morning. • Medications should be taken as usual to obtain best exercise performance, especially when using test results for exercise prescription purposes. • Patients may become more dyspneic when lifting objects. Specific evaluation and training may be necessary.

PULMONARY DISEASE: EXERCISE PROGRAMMING

MODES	GOALS	INTENSITY/ FREQUENCY/DURATION	TIME TO GOAL
Aerobic/Endurance • Large muscle activities (e.g., walking, cycling, swimming)	• Increase $\dot{V}O_2$ peak work, and endurance. • Increase lactate threshold and ventilatory threshold. • Become less sensitive to dyspnea. • Develop more efficient breathing patterns. • Facilitate improvement in daily living activities.	• RPE 11-13 (comfortable, pace to ensure compliance). • Monitor dyspnea. • 1-2 sessions 3-7 days/week. • 30 minutes/session (shorter intermittent sessions may be necessary initially). • Emphasize progression of duration over intensity.	• 2-3 months
Strength • Free weights • Isotonic/isokinetic machines	• Increase maximal number of repetitions. • Increase isokinetic torque/ work. • Increase lean body mass.	• Low resistance, high repetitions. • 2-3 days/week.	• 2-3 months
Flexibility • Stretching • Tai chi	• Increase range of motion.	• 3 sessions/week.	
Neuromuscular • Walking, balance exercises • Breathing exercises	• Improve gait, balance. • Improve breathing efficiency.	• Daily.	

(continued)

PULMONARY DISEASE: EXERCISE PROGRAMMING (continued)

MODES	GOALS	INTENSITY/ FREQUENCY/DURATION	TIME TO GOAL
Functional • Activity-specific exercises	• Increase/maintain daily living activities. • Return to work. • Improve quality of life. • Recreation/fun.	• Daily.	

MEDICATIONS	SPECIAL CONSIDERATIONS
• Corticosteroids: May contribute to psychological disturbances. • See table on testing.	• RPE and dyspnea are the preferred methods of monitoring intensity. Many patients are unable to achieve a "training" heart rate, but still show physiological improvement. • Coronary artery disease, peripheral artery disease, and musculoskeletal problems (e.g., arthritis, osteoporosis) are common in patients with COPD. • Muscular myopathy (including respiratory muscles) may be present due to corticosteroids and disuse atrophy. • Patients usually respond to exercise best in mid- to late morning. • Avoid extremes in temperature and humidity. • Supplemental O_2 flow rate should be adjusted to maintain $S_aO_2 > 90\%$. • Anxiety, depression, and/or fear are common due to dyspnea and physical disability.

CHAPTER 14

Cystic Fibrosis

Patricia A. Nixon, PhD, FACSM
University of Pittsburgh
School of Medicine

Overview of the Pathophysiology

Cystic fibrosis (CF) is the most common inherited life-shortening disease in white populations, occurring in 1 in 2500 live white births. The genetic defect causes abnormal epithelial transport of chloride ions, excessive sodium ion reabsorption, and subsequent extracellular dehydration that results in abnormally salty sweat and thick mucus that clogs ducts, tubes, and tubules. The two organs most adversely affected by the mucus blockage are the pancreas and the lungs. In the pancreas, mucus prevents digestive enzymes from reaching the small intestine to digest fats and proteins, leading to malnutrition and poor growth. In the lungs, the thick mucus blocks the airways and leads to infection, inflammation, and eventually, fibrosis and irreversible loss of pulmonary function. The pulmonary involvement accounts for over 90% of the mortality.

Effects on the Exercise Response

Many healthier persons with CF have normal aerobic fitness and normal cardiorespiratory responses to a single session of exercise. However, as the disease progresses and pulmonary function deteriorates, exercise tolerance diminishes. During exercise, individuals must use greater minute ventilation to compensate for airway obstruction and increased dead space. Consequently, the ratio of peak minute ventilation to maximal voluntary ventilation (peak $\dot{V}_E$/MVV) often exceeds the normal range of 60% to 70%, limiting mechanical ventilatory reserve. Most persons with mild-to-moderate lung disease are able to maintain adequate gas exchange, although those with more severe lung disease may exhibit oxyhemoglobin desaturation and carbon dioxide retention during exercise. The likelihood that oxyhemoglobin desaturation will fall below 91% during exercise increases in persons with a forced expiratory volume for one second (FEV_1) that is less than 50% of the predicted value. Peak heart rate may reach age-predicted maximal levels in healthier persons. However, ventilatory factors may prevent the cardiovascular system from being maximally stressed in persons with worse lung disease, resulting in peak heart rates that are below age-predicted maximal values. In addition, exercise capacity may be limited by peripheral factors associated with deconditioning and malnutrition. Furthermore, in people with very severe lung disease, $\dot{V}_E$/MVV and heart rate at peak exercise may be well below normal, suggesting that other factors such as chest pain, sensations of dyspnea, excessive coughing, or other peripheral factors may limit exercise. During submaximal exercise, oxygen consumption, minute ventilation, and heart rate may be disproportionately high, possibly as a result of physical deconditioning, increased work of breathing, hypoxemia, or any combination of these factors.

Effects of Exercise Training

To date there has been no report of a well-controlled, randomized study, with sufficient statistical power, to establish the effects of long-term aerobic exercise intervention in persons with CF. Existing research suggests that individuals with CF *may* derive the following benefits from aerobic exercise training:

- Increase in physical work capacity and peak oxygen consumption

- Increase in ventilatory muscle endurance
- Improvement in cardiopulmonary *efficiency* for a given submaximal work rate
- Greater mucus clearance
- Temporary increase or delayed deterioration in some indices of pulmonary function (although most studies show no benefit)

Higher levels of aerobic fitness have been associated with better quality of well-being and with eight-year survival. However, it is not known whether quality of well-being and survival probability can be improved via exercise training. Individuals *may* also benefit from upper-body weight training through an increase in muscle strength as well as a decrease in air trapping in the lungs. Interventions aimed at improving nutritional status *may* also improve exercise capacity.

Management and Medications

Standard treatment for individuals with CF now includes

- oral pancreatic enzyme supplements to enhance digestion of dietary fats and proteins and improve nutritional status,
- chest physical therapy to facilitate mucus clearance from the airways,
- bronchodilator therapy to open airways, and
- antibiotic therapy to fight pulmonary infection.

With the exception of supplemental oxygen, the effects of the following medications on exercise tolerance and responses to exercise have not been studied specifically in persons with CF. Consequently, these effects are speculative:

- *Pancreatic enzyme* supplements may indirectly improve exercise capacity by improving nutrition and growth.
- *Inhaled bronchodilator* (albuterol, ipratropium) therapy may improve exercise tolerance and gas exchange and may reduce exercise-induced bronchospasm, but can also cause tachycardia and cough.
- *Oral bronchodilator* (theophylline) therapy can cause tachycardia, ventricular dysrhythmia, and tachypnea.
- *Anti-inflammatory agents* may improve exercise tolerance by reducing airway inflammation and bronchial hyperreactivity.

- *Sodium cromolyn and Nedocromil* (inhaled) in chronic and acute administration may improve exercise tolerance by diminishing or preventing bronchoconstriction, particularly exercise-induced bronchoconstriction.
- *Corticosteroids* (inhaled) used on a long-term basis may improve exercise tolerance by reducing bronchial hyperreactivity, but may cause effects similar to those of oral corticosteroids if systemically absorbed.
- *Corticosteroids* (oral) used on a long-term basis may improve exercise tolerance by reducing bronchial hyperreactivity, but can cause weight gain, retard growth, and result in below-normal exercise capacity for age; prolonged use of oral steroids may result in skeletal muscle (including ventilatory muscle) weakness and myopathy that may reduce exercise capacity; prolonged use may also result in elevated blood pressure at rest and during exercise.
- *Mucolytic* therapy reduces viscosity of mucus.
- *Recombinant human DNase* effects on exercise tolerance are not known.
- *Insulin* may improve exercise tolerance in individuals with diabetes.
- *Supplemental oxygen* improves oxyhemoglobin saturation at rest and during exercise; improves cardiopulmonary efficiency (i.e., lower heart rate and minute ventilation) during submaximal and maximal exercise; and does not appear to increase peak oxygen consumption or physical work capacity.

Optimal exercise test results *may* be obtained if persons undergo testing after chest physiotherapy and bronchodilator therapy. It should be noted, however, that some have a negative or adverse response to bronchodilator therapy and consequently should not include it as part of their treatment.

Recommendations for Exercise Testing

The primary objectives for exercise testing persons with CF are to

- assess disease severity,
- assess physical work capacity and aerobic fitness,
- observe cardiorespiratory and metabolic responses to exercise,

- observe oxyhemoglobin saturation during exercise,
- provide a basis for prescribing exercise within safe limits, and
- assess changes in fitness and cardiorespiratory responses to exercise that occur with disease progression or medical intervention (e.g., pharmacologic, exercise).

Physical work capacity and aerobic fitness are ideally evaluated by a progressive maximal exercise test. Peak heart rate cannot be estimated from age-predicted equations and therefore must be obtained from a maximal exercise test. Pediatric clients should be tested with use of a standard pediatric protocol that has established normative data for comparison (e.g., Godfrey protocol). Exercise testing equipment may need to be modified to accommodate children and smaller individuals.

Oxyhemoglobin saturation should be monitored particularly in clients with an FEV_1 less than 50% of the predicted value. If the purpose of the exercise test is to provide a basis for prescribing exercise, persons who exhibit oxyhemoglobin desaturation at rest or during exercise should be tested while breathing supplemental oxygen. To terminate the test because of marked oxyhemoglobin desaturation (for instance, < 80%) may be overly cautious, since no irreversible or harmful effects of short-term hypoxemia have been reported in this population. Submaximal steady state exercise testing or self-paced walk tests (e.g., six minute) may be useful for examining cardiorespiratory responses to exercise or changes in response to intervention, particularly in severely ill persons for whom a maximal exercise test may be unduly stressful and provide limited information. Exercise may induce excessive coughing in some individuals, causing them to terminate exercise. However, the majority of persons, despite their obstructive lung disease, report leg fatigue as the reason for terminating exercise, particularly on the cycle ergometer.

Recommendations for Exercise Programming

The primary aim of exercise training is to improve aerobic fitness. The majority of individuals with CF should be able to engage in continuous aerobic exercise for 20 to 30 minutes at moderate intensity (heart rates = 60-80% of peak heart rate). Persons with severe lung disease may need to intersperse rest periods with exercise and may also require supplemental oxygen during training. Training may be better tolerated and optimal benefits gained if training is performed after chest physiotherapy and bronchodilator therapy (in persons who have a positive response to bronchodilator therapy). Standard exercise equipment may need to be adapted to fit children and smaller individuals. However, clients should be encouraged to adopt lifestyle changes that include aerobic activities such as walking, jogging, bike riding, and swimming. Exercise intensity may need to be altered during an exacerbation of pulmonary infection commonly experienced by individuals with CF. At such times, clients are most likely to attain their target heart rates at a less intense work rate.

Special Considerations

Exercise training in a supervised and monitored setting is not necessary for the majority of persons with CF. However, it may be prudent initially to monitor oxyhemoglobin saturation in hypoxemic persons to determine the desired amount of oxygen supplementation. Some persons with CF may also have asthma or exercise-induced asthma, and may require bronchodilator therapy prior to physical activities that might provoke bronchoconstriction. Despite losing excessive salt through sweating, people with CF appear to be able to maintain adequate thermoregulation during shorter periods of exercise in the heat. Longer periods of exercise in the heat may warrant increased fluid and dietary salt intake.

Some persons with more severe lung disease may experience bone or joint pain in the legs, particularly in the knees. The pain may be attributed to hypertrophic pulmonary osteoarthropathy, seen as an elevated periosteum upon x-ray examination.

With increasing age, it is estimated that nearly 50% of persons with CF develop impaired glucose tolerance and that 6% to 10% develop overt diabetes. The risk of diabetes increases with each decade of life and may be exacerbated by oral corticosteroid treatment. Exercise testing and training for these individuals should follow the recommendations outlined in chapter 16.

Finally, some persons with severe or end-stage lung disease may have evidence of cor pulmonale (right ventricular hypertrophy) and even right ventricular failure. For these individuals, submaximal exercise testing may be indicated, and exercise training should be of low intensity and aimed at improving functional capacity with respect to activities of daily living.

Suggested Readings

Cerny, F.J., T.P. Pullano, and G.J. Cropp. 1982. Cardiorespiratory adaptations to exercise in cystic fibrosis. *Am. Rev. Respir. Dis.* 126 (2): 217-20.

Godfrey, S. 1974. *Exercise testing in children.* Philadelphia: Saunders.

Nixon, P.A. 1996. Role of exercise in the diagnosis and management of pulmonary disease in children and youth. *Med. Sci. Sports Exerc.* 28 (4): 414-20.

Nixon, P.A., D.M. Orenstein, S.E. Curtis, and E.A. Ross. 1990. Oxygen supplementation during exercise in cystic fibrosis. *Am. Rev. Respir. Dis.* 142 (4): 807-11.

Nixon, P.A., D.M. Orenstein, S.F. Kelsey, and C.F. Doershuk. 1992. The prognostic value of exercise testing in patients with cystic fibrosis. *N. Engl. J. Med.* 327: 1785-88.

Orenstein, D.M., K.G. Henke, D.L. Costill, C.F. Doershuk, P.J. Lemon, and R.C. Stern. 1983. Exercise and heat stress in cystic fibrosis patients. *Pediatr. Res.* 17: 267-69.

Orenstein, D.M., and P.A. Nixon. 1989. Patients with cystic fibrosis. In *Exercise in modern medicine,* ed. B.A. Franklin, S. Gordon, and C.G. Timmis, 204-14. Baltimore: Williams & Wilkins.

Orenstein D.M., and B.E. Noyes. 1993. Cystic fibrosis. In *Principles and practice of pulmonary rehabilitation,* ed. R. Casaburi and T.L. Petty, 439-58. Philadelphia: Saunders.

Wood R.E., T.F. Boat, and C.F. Doershuk. 1976. State of the art: Cystic fibrosis. *Am. Rev. Respir. Dis.* 113: 833-78.

CYSTIC FIBROSIS: EXERCISE TESTING

METHODS	MEASURES	ENDPOINTS*	COMMENTS
Aerobic power **Cycle** 10, 15, or 20 watts/min or 0.15, 0.35 watts/kg/min **Treadmill** (1-2 METs/3 min stage) (Suggest modified Balke or Bruce protocol)	• 12-lead ECG, heart rate	• Serious dysrhythmias • > 2 mm ST-segment depression or elevation • Ischemic threshold • T-wave inversion with significant ST change	• Peak HR may be below age-predicted level. • ECG usually normal, but may show cor pulmonale in end-stage cystic fibrosis.
	• Blood pressure	• Hypertensive response	• Corticosteroids may increase BP.
	• Oximetry (S_aO_2)		• An increased risk of decreased S_aO_2 and/or CO_2 retention exists if FEV_1 is < 50% of predicted value.
	• Respired gas analysis	• $\dot{V}O_2$ peak • Peak $\dot{V}_E$ • End-tidal CO_2	
	• Spirometry (forced vital capacity (FVC), FEV_1, maximal midexpiratory flow rate (MMEFR), MVV)		

METHODS	MEASURES	ENDPOINTS*	COMMENTS
Anaerobic power **Wingate protocol**	• Peak and mean power output • Percent of fatigue	• 30 seconds	• May reflect nutritional status.
Endurance **6-minute walk**	• Distance walked • HR, S_aO_2	• 6 minutes	• Most useful in persons with very limited exercise tolerance.

*Measurements of particular significance; do not *always* indicate test termination.

MEDICATIONS	SPECIAL CONSIDERATIONS
• Beta$_2$ agonists and ipratropium bromide: Have a bronchodilator effect in most persons, but may cause tachycardia. • Corticosteroids (inhaled or oral): Reduce airway inflammation and bronchospasm. Oral steroids may cause myopathy, diabetes, and hypertension. • Sodium cromolyn: Diminishes or prevents exercise-induced bronchospasm. • Theophylline: Has a bronchodilator effect, but may cause tachycardia, ventricular ectopy, and tachypnea. • Supplemental oxygen: May prevent desaturation, attenuate HR and V_E, and cause relative hypoventilation. • Intravenous aminoglycosides: May cause auditory and vestibular ototoxicity resulting in deafness, dizziness, and/or unsteady gait.	• May need to adapt equipment to small persons. • Use supplemental O_2 in persons with hypoxemia if exercise tests are being used for exercise programming. • Premedication with bronchodilator therapy may provide optimal results in persons who respond positive to bronchodilator therapy.

CYSTIC FIBROSIS: EXERCISE PROGRAMMING

MODES	GOALS	INTENSITY/FREQUENCY/DURATION	TIME TO GOAL
Aerobic • Large muscle activities (e.g., walking, biking, rowing, swimming, jogging—whatever the participant enjoys most)	• Increase peak $\dot{V}O_2$, peak work capacity, and endurance. • Decrease $\dot{V}_E$, HR, and RPE and increase S_aO_2 at a given work rate. • Increase respiratory muscle endurance. • Facilitate mucus clearance.	• 60-80% peak $\dot{V}O_2$ or 55-90% HR reserve. • 3-4 days/week; sicker clients may need 2 daily sessions. • Start with 10 minutes, build in 1 minute increments up to 20-30 minutes. • Emphasize duration rather than intensity. • RPE, dyspnea scales sometimes useful.	• 4-6 months
Strength • Large muscle exercises	• Increase muscular strength and endurance. • Possibly diminish steroid-induced muscle weakness and myopathy. • Possibly decrease air-trapping with upper-body strength training.	• Start with 3 sets of 10 repetitions, light resistance. • Optimal programming not established.	• 6-12 weeks
Functional • Activity-specific exercise	• Increase/maintain functional capacity and daily living activities.	• Optimal programming not established.	

MEDICATIONS	SPECIAL CONSIDERATIONS
• Brochodilators: Premedication may enhance training effect in persons who respond to bronchodilators. • Steroids: Myopathy may not reverse with training and may cause diabetes/hypertension complications for exercise. May also cause muscle weakness and myopathy. • Supplemental oxygen: May enhance training effect by increasing oxygenation and attenuating HR and $\dot{V}_E$, but can also cause CO_2 retention.	• May need to adapt equipment to smaller persons and children. • Persons with reactive airways may require premedication with an inhaled beta agonist or sodium cromolyn. • Use supplemental O_2 in persons with resting or exertional hypoxemia ($S_aO_2 < 91\%$). • Some persons complain of bone and joint (primarily knee) pain due to hypertrophic pulmonary osteoarthropathy. • Chest physical therapy may increase mucus clearance in conjunction with exercise. • Decrease exercise intensity during exacerbations of pulmonary infection. • Increase fluid and salt intake for prolonged exercise or when in a warm environment.

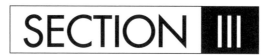

SECTION III

Metabolic Diseases

Section Editor:

Patricia L. Painter, PhD, FACSM

University of California at San Francisco

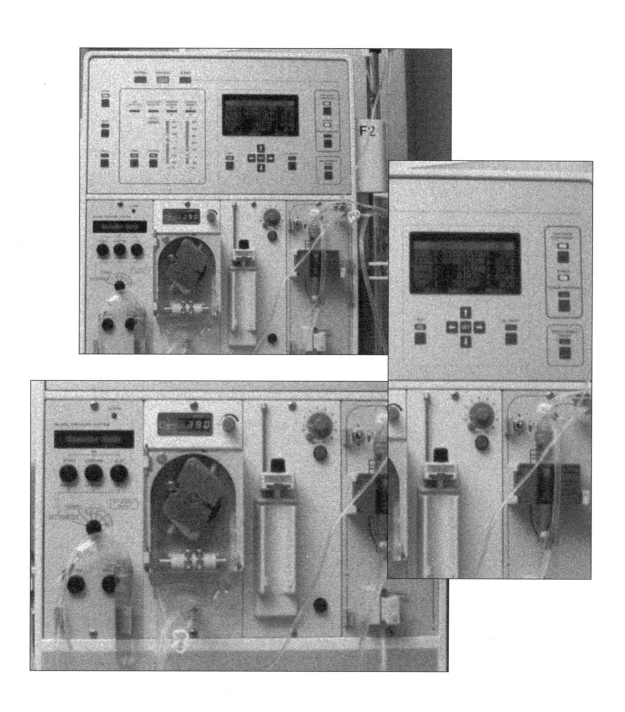

CHAPTER 15

Renal Failure

Patricia L. Painter, PhD, FACSM

University of California at San Francisco

Overview of the Pathophysiology

End-stage renal disease (ESRD) is the loss of kidney function to the point of severe reduction of clearance of necessary waste products from the blood. End-stage renal disease results in severe metabolic abnormalities that affect nearly all physiologic systems. The following are common consequences of renal failure:

- Metabolic acidosis
- Hypertension
- Left ventricular hypertrophy
- Anemia
- Secondary hyperparathyroidism
- Peripheral neuropathy
- Muscle weakness
- Autonomic dysfunction
- Elevated triglycerides and reduced high-density lipoprotein cholesterol

Thirty percent of dialysis patients are diabetic. Most dialysis patients are inactive and possess low functional capacities.

Effects on the Exercise Response

Exercise intolerance is well documented in individuals on dialysis, with the average peak $\dot{V}O_2$ being about 20 ml·kg^{-1}·min^{-1}. Exercise responses are characterized by a blunted heart rate response and excessive blood pressure increases. The primary reason for termination of exercise is leg fatigue. The limitations to exercise in these individuals could be any one of a number of factors, including

- reduced peak cardiac output due to a blunted heart rate response,
- reduced oxygen-carrying capacity due to anemia, and
- subnormal capacity to extract oxygen related to weakness and structural and functional changes in muscle.

Effects of Exercise Training

The level of exercise tolerance that can be achieved in these individuals is unclear, and it is probable that some individuals on dialysis will not improve their peak $\dot{V}O_2$ levels with training. Aerobic exercise training usually improves peak $\dot{V}O_2$ by about 20% to 25%. This increase in peak $\dot{V}O_2$ is the result of increased oxygen extraction in the muscle, because stroke volume or cardiac output does not change after training. Low oxygen delivery to the skeletal muscle is improved by erythropoeitin (EPO) therapy that increases hemoglobin as well as peak $\dot{V}O_2$ and quality of life. Because peak $\dot{V}O_2$ in these persons correlates with muscle strength more closely than with hemoglobin, it is thought that skeletal muscle dysfunction is a major limiting factor for exercise capacity.

It has been reported that exercise training improves blood pressure control, lipid profiles, and psychological profiles in some patients. The peak exercise capacity of many people on dialysis is such that the energy requirements of common activities of daily living are challenging to them. Thus, increasing functional capacity should be a major objective of exercise therapy for people with renal failure. Since limitations may be related to muscle weakness, it is reasonable to try both resistance and aerobic training programs to improve functional capacity.

Management and Medications

Some form of renal replacement therapy is required for maintenance of life. The main form of maintenance therapy is hemodialysis. Other treatment options include peritoneal dialysis and renal transplantation. Medical management issues include assuring adequate dialysis therapy, which is monitored through urea kinetics and other blood testing; adequate blood pressure control, which often requires a variety of antihypertensive agents; control of the anemia using recombinant human erythropoeitin (EPO); control of secondary hyperparathyroidism through use of phosphate-binding agents; and adequate access for dialysis, that is, either blood access (for hemodialysis via arteriovenous fistula) or peritoneal catheter (for peritoneal dialysis). Patients may develop any of the following problems:

- Congestive heart failure before the initiation of dialysis (due to fluid overload) or in the case of inadequate dialysis or fluid intake indiscretion

- Accelerated atherosclerosis

- Pericardial effusion resulting from inadequate dialysis and uremia

- Abnormal electrocardiogram due to electrolyte abnormalities or structural changes

- Dysrhythmias due to abnormal electrolytes

- Cardiomegaly resulting from fluid and/or pressure overload, coronary artery disease, pericardial disease, uremic toxins, or other conditions

- Renal osteodystrophy resulting from secondary hyperparathyroidism

- Persistent anemia due to iron deficiency, nonresponse to EPO, or both

- Peritonitis due to catheter infection (in patients treated with peritoneal dialysis)

Many patients are hypertensive and are treated with antihypertensive agents. During hemodialysis there is a complex interaction of antihypertensive medications and dialysis itself that can lead to either inadequate drug levels or severe hypertension. For this reason, antihypertensive medications are often not taken on dialysis days. Nearly all dialysis patients take recombinant EPO for anemia, although hematocrits are only partially corrected (usually up to 35%). Phosphate binders are prescribed for virtually all dialysis patients to prevent hyperparathy-

roidism and renal osteodystrophy. Insulin is administered to diabetic patients requiring it, with those on peritoneal dialysis receiving medication in their dialysis fluid. Other medications may be required for coexisting medical concerns.

Recommendations for Exercise Testing

The utility of exercise testing for diagnostic purposes is questioned in this patient group since they are limited primarily by muscle fatigue. Thus, for screening before beginning an exercise training program, maximal diagnostic exercise testing may not be beneficial, and in most cases requiring such testing may present an unnecessary barrier to beginning a program of exercise training. Since these individuals experience continuing and intensive medical care, such testing probably does not provide any additional information.

Recommendations for Exercise Programming

There is no guarantee that all individuals on dialysis will respond to exercise training with an increase in peak $\dot{V}O_2$ or an increase in functional capacity. The optimal program of exercise training has not been identified for this patient group. Additionally, the interactions between morbidity, the adequacy of dialysis and other unknown factors, and the response to exercise training have not been completely defined. The chronicity of the disease and the multiple medical problems present in these individuals often become the focus of the health care professionals who are caring for them. Information or referral for exercise training in the past has typically not been part of the routine patient care plan. Although it is difficult to integrate an exercise program into an already complex and intensive medical schedule, exercise training does provide the only possible chance to increase functional capacity in these individuals. Increased awareness of the potential exercise benefits for the dialysis patient on the part of the nephrology community is needed.

Suggested Readings

Diesel, W., T.D. Noakes, C. Swanepoel, and M. Lambert. 1990. Isokinetic muscle strength predicts maximum exercise tolerance in renal patients on chronic hemodialysis. *Am J. Kidney Dis.* 16: 109-14.

Goldberg, A.P., E.M. Geltman, J.M. Hagberg, J.R. Gavin, J.A. Delmez, R.M. Carney, A. Naumowicz, M. Holdfield, and H.R. Harter. 1983. Therapeutic benefits of exercise training for hemodialysis patients. *Kidney Int.* 516: S303-S309.

Moore, G.E., K.R. Brinker, and J. Stray-Gundersen. 1993. Determinants of $\dot{V}O_2$ peak in patients with end-stage renal disease: On and off dialysis. *Med. Sci. Sports Exerc.* 25: 18-23.

Painter, P.L. 1988. Exercise in end stage renal disease. *Exerc. Sport Sci. Rev.* 16: 305-39.

Painter, P.L., D.L. Messer-Rehak, P. Hanson, S.W. Zimmerman, and N.R. Glass. 1986. Exercise capacity in hemodialysis, COPD and renal transplant patients. *Nephron.* 42: 47-51.

Painter, P.L., and G.E. Moore. 1994. The impact of rHuErythropoetin on exercise capacity in hemodialysis patients. *Advances in Renal Replacement Therapy* 1 (1): 55-65.

Painter, P.L., J.N. Nelson-Worel, M.M. Hill, D.R. Thornberry, A.R. Harrington, and A.B. Weinstein. 1986. The effects of exercise training during dialysis. *Nephron.* 43: 87-92.

Robertson, H.T., N.R. Haley, M. Guthrie, D. Cardenas, J.W. Eschbach, and J.W. Adamson. 1990. Recombinant erythropoietin improves exercise capacity in anemic hemodialysis patients. *Am. J. Kidney Dis.* 15: 325-32.

RENAL FAILURE: EXERCISE TESTING

METHODS	MEASURES	ENDPOINTS*	COMMENTS
Aerobic power **Treadmill** (1-2 METs/stage) **Cycle** (5-25 watts/min) ramp protocol	• 12-lead ECG, heart rate	• Serious dysrhythmias • > 2 mm ST-segment depression or elevation • Ischemic threshold • T-wave inversion with significant ST change	
	• Blood pressure	• SBP > 260 mmHg or DBP > 115 mmHg	
	• RPE	• Onset of muscle fatigue	• Most patients terminate test because of skeletal muscle fatigue.
Strength **Isotonic/isokinetic**	• 10-12 repetition maximum, peak torque		• 1 repetition maximum not recommended.
Flexibility **Goniometry** **Sit-and-reach**			
Neuromuscular **Gait analysis** **Balance**			• Indicated for peripheral neuropathy, prosthetic devices, and/or severe muscle wasting.
Functional capacity **Timed sit-to-stand** **Gait speed** **Functional lifting tests**			• Used for assessment of capacity for daily living activities.

*Measurements of particular significance; do not *always* indicate test termination.

MEDICATIONS	SPECIAL CONSIDERATIONS
• Antihypertensive agents: Administer as needed. Depends on dialysis schedule and compliance to fluid restrictions. • Erythropoietin: Use for anemia. Hematocrit should be maintained between 30% and 35%.	• Hemodialysis patients should be tested on a non-dialysis day. • Patients treated with continuous ambulatory peritoneal dialysis should be tested without fluid in the abdomen. • Do not measure blood pressure in the arm with the arteriovenous fistula. • Spontaneous tendon rupture may be possible in patients with long-standing renal bone disease (usually have been on dialysis > 5 years). • 30% of dialysis patients are diabetic; see testing table in chapter 16. • Fatigue is a common concern.

RENAL FAILURE: EXERCISE PROGRAMMING

MODES	GOALS	INTENSITY/ FREQUENCY/DURATION	TIME TO GOAL
Aerobic • Large muscle activities	• Increase aerobic capacity. • Increase time to exhaustion. • Increase work capacity. • Improve blood pressure.	• 50-90% peak HR. • 50-85% peak $\dot{V}O_2$. • Monitor RPE, discomfort. • 4-7 days/week. • 20-60 minutes/session.	• 4-6 months
Strength • Free weights, weight machines, isokinetic machines	• Increase maximal number of repetitions.	• Avoid high weights. • Concentrate on low weight/ high repetition program.	• 4-6 months
Flexibility • Stretching/yoga	• Maintain/increase range of motion. • Improve gait, balance, and coordination.		
Functional • Activity-specific exercise	• Increase daily living activities. • Increase vocational potential. • Increase physical self-confidence.		

MEDICATIONS	SPECIAL CONSIDERATIONS
• Antihypertensive agents: Administer as needed. Depends on dialysis schedule and compliance to fluid restrictions. • Erythropoietin: Use for anemia. Hematocrit should be maintained between 30% and 35%.	• Individuals receiving hemodialysis may not tolerate exercise after dialysis treatment. • Patients treated with continuous ambulatory peritoneal dialysis may be more comfortable exercising without fluid in the abdomen. • Be aware of the arteriovenous fistula and IV access lines. • Spontaneous tendon rupture may occur in patients with long-standing renal bone disease (usually have been on dialysis > 5 years). • 30% of dialysis patients are diabetic; see programming table in chapter 16. • Fatigue is a common concern. • Gradual progression is essential. • Patients frequently experience medical setbacks; program may have to be adjusted accordingly. • Exercise during hemodialysis treatment is recommended and should be encouraged when possible (in conjunction with the dialysis unit staff).

CHAPTER 16

Diabetes

Ann L. Albright, PhD
UCSF/California Department of
Health Services

Overview of the Pathophysiology

Diabetes is a chronic metabolic disease characterized by an absolute or relative deficiency of insulin resulting in hyperglycemia. Individuals with diabetes are at risk for developing microvascular complications including retinopathy and nephropathy, macrovascular disease, and various neuropathies (both autonomic and peripheral). Silent ischemia is common in persons with diabetes, particularly if the disease is long-standing (refer to chapter 5 for management of this problem). Several forms of diabetes exist, and they may be divided into the following major classifications.

Diabetes Mellitus; Type I (Insulin-Dependent or Juvenile Onset)

In diabetes mellitus type I there is an absolute deficiency of insulin due to a marked reduction in insulin-secreting beta cells of the pancreas. Consequently, insulin *must* be supplied by injection or an insulin pump. Because of the absolute deficiency of insulin, those with type I diabetes are prone to developing ketoacidosis when marked hyperglycemia occurs. The cause of type I diabetes is thought to involve an autoimmune response directed at the beta cells that ultimately leads to their destruction in genetically susceptible individuals. The factors that trigger the autoimmune response have not been specifically identified, but may include viruses or toxins. The precise nature of the genetic influence in the pathogenesis of type I diabetes is

also unclear, but the histocompatibility (human lymphocyte antigen) types DR3 and DR4 are associated with increased risk for type I diabetes. This form of diabetes usually occurs before the age of 30, but can occur at any age. Of the 16 million people with diabetes mellitus, approximately 10% to 15% have type I diabetes.

Type II (Non-Insulin-Dependent or Adult Onset)

Individuals with type II diabetes are considered to have a relative insulin deficiency since they may have elevated, reduced, or normal insulin levels but still present with hyperglycemia. The pathophysiology of type II diabetes remains unclear and is probably multifactorial. In this form of diabetes, peripheral tissue insulin resistance and defective insulin secretion are common features. With insulin resistance, glucose does not readily enter the insulin-sensitive tissues (primarily muscle and adipose tissue), and blood glucose rises. The increase in blood glucose causes the beta cells of the pancreas to secrete more insulin in an attempt to maintain a normal blood glucose concentration. Unfortunately, this additional endogenous insulin is usually ineffective in lowering blood glucose and may further contribute to insulin resistance. In some people, the beta cells may become exhausted over time and insulin secretion decreases. The mechanisms underlying insulin resistance remain unclear, but probably involve defects in the binding of insulin to its receptor and in postreceptor events such as glucose transport. Obesity significantly contributes to insulin resistance, and the majority (80%) of people with type II diabetes are obese at onset. Several varieties of abnormalities in insulin secretion have been identified, but virtually all people with type II diabetes have lost the acute (first) phase insulin release. Insulin therapy may or may not be required, depending upon the degree of functional insulin and/or insulin sensitivity/responsiveness remaining. Those with type II diabetes do not develop ketoacidosis except under conditions of unusual stress (e.g., trauma). Type II diabetes is clearly genetically influenced, since it occurs in identical twins with almost total concordance. The onset is insidious, with few or no classic symptoms, and many people go undiagnosed until organ damage has occurred. This form of diabetes usually occurs after the age of 40, although a small number of people under age 30 have a form of type II diabetes called maturity-onset diabetes of youth. Type II diabetes affects approximately 85% to 90% of the 16 million people with diabetes mellitus.

Gestational Diabetes

Gestational diabetes occurs during pregnancy because of the contrainsulin effects of pregnancy. Gestational diabetes is usually diagnosed by an oral glucose tolerance test (OGTT) done during the second and possibly the third trimester. Risk factors for the development of gestational diabetes include family history of gestational diabetes, previous delivery of a large birth-weight baby, and obesity. The term gestational diabetes does not apply to those who have diabetes prior to pregnancy or to those with type II diabetes who may have been undiagnosed until pregnancy. The classic characteristic of gestational diabetes is that it resolves postpartum. This characteristic separates it from previously undiagnosed type II diabetes that remains following the pregnancy. Approximately 50% of the women who develop gestational diabetes develop type II diabetes later in life.

Secondary Diabetes

Other diseases, injuries, or medications may result in a diabetic condition that is referred to as secondary diabetes. Secondary diabetes may or may not require insulin treatment depending upon the pathophysiology of the condition and the degree of functional insulin. These conditions include

- pancreatic disease such as chronic pancreatitis and pancreatectomy,
- hormonal conditions such as Cushing's syndrome and acromegaly,
- drugs such as prednisone and chlorothiazides,
- insulin receptor abnormalities such as acanthosis nigricans and lipodystrophy, and
- genetic syndromes such as Laurence-Moon-Bardet-Biedl syndrome and myotonic dystrophy.

Impaired Glucose Tolerance

Impaired glucose tolerance (IGT) applies to those in whom fasting plasma glucose is lower than that required for diagnosis of diabetes, but in whom the two-hour oral glucose tolerance test (OGTT) value lies between the normal and diabetic values (140 and 200 mg ·dl^{-1}). Those with IGT are at increased risk for developing diabetes, but progression to diabetes is not a certainty.

Effects on the Exercise Response

Under normal conditions there is a precise coordination of hormonal and metabolic events that results in maintenance of glucose homeostasis. Insulin concentrations in people with diabetes do not respond to exercise in the normal manner, and the balance between peripheral glucose utilization and hepatic glucose production may be disturbed. The effect of diabetes on a single session of exercise is dependent upon several factors, including

- use and type of medication to lower blood glucose (insulin or oral hypoglycemic agents);
- timing of medication administration;
- blood glucose level prior to exercise;
- timing, amount, and type of previous food intake;
- presence and severity of diabetic complications;
- use of other medication secondary to diabetic complications; and
- intensity, duration, and type of exercise.

Effects of Exercise Training

Exercise is considered by many to be one of the cornerstones of diabetes care. An exercise training program has the potential to provide several benefits for the person with diabetes. These benefits may include the following:

- **Possible improvement in blood glucose control**: Exercise should be a part of diabetes therapy (in addition to diet and medication) to improve blood glucose control for those with type II diabetes, but exercise is not considered a component of treatment in type I diabetes to lower blood glucose. Those with type I diabetes are encouraged to exercise to gain other benefits, but blood glucose must be in reasonable control (< 250 mg·dl^{-1}, no ketones) if the individual is to exercise safely.

- **Improved insulin sensitivity/lower medication requirement**: Exercise training results in improved insulin sensitivity, and for many with diabetes this translates into a reduction in dose of insulin or oral hypoglycemic agents (OHAs).

- **Reduction in body fat**: Weight loss increases insulin sensitivity and may allow those with diabetes to reduce the amount of insulin or oral hypoglycemic agents needed. Exercise coupled with moderate caloric intake is considered the most effective way to lose weight.

- **Cardiovascular benefits**: Regular exercise decreases the risk of cardiovascular disease. It is likely that this is true to some extent for persons with diabetes.

- **Stress reduction**: Stress can disrupt diabetes control by increasing counterregulatory hormones, ketones, free fatty acids, and urine output, making stress reduction an important part of diabetes care.

- **Prevention of type II diabetes**: Epidemiological studies have indicated that exercise may play a role in preventing type II diabetes. Those with IGT, gestational diabetes, or a family history of type II diabetes may especially benefit from a regular aerobic exercise program.

Nearly everyone with diabetes can derive some benefit from an exercise program, although not all benefits will necessarily be realized by each person with diabetes. Careful monitoring of blood glucose and attention to balancing food intake and medication administration are necessary in order for the person to participate safely in an exercise program.

Management and Medications

The management of diabetes depends upon the form of diabetes, blood glucose goals, and the presence and severity of diabetic complications. The goal of diabetes management is to normalize blood glucose to the extent that it is safe to do so. This is accomplished by insulin, OHAs, or both if necessary, by an individual nutrition care plan, and by participation in regular aerobic exercise as appropriate.

Medications used in diabetes management not only include glucose-lowering agents, but also may include antihypertensives, lipid-lowering agents, and pain medications. Please refer to the material in this volume on hypertension (chapter 10) and hyperlipidemia (chapter 17) for information on these medications.

Table 16.1 TYPES OF INSULIN			
INSULIN TYPE	**ONSET (hours)**	**PEAK (hours)**	**EFFECTIVE DURATION (hours)**
Animal			
Regular	0.5-2.0	3-4	4-6
NPH	4-6	8-14	16-20
Lente	4-6	8-14	16-20
Ultralente	8-14	minimal	24-36
Human			
Regular	0.5-1.0	2-3	3-6
NPH	2-4	4-10	10-16
Lente	3-4	4-12	12-18
Ultralente	6-10	?	18-20

A new insulin is being developed called lys-pro that will have a more rapid onset and shorter duration than regular insulin.

Table 16.2 ORAL HYPOGLYCEMIC AGENTS

NAME	USUAL DAILY DOSAGE (mg)	DURATION (hours)
First Generation Sulfonylureas		
Acetohexamide	250-1500	12-18
Chlorpropamide	100-750	60+
Tolazamide	100-1000	18-24
Tolbutamide	500-3000	6-10
Second Generation Sulfonylureas		
Glipizide	2.5-40	16-24
Glyburide	1.25-20	12-24
Biguanides*		
Metformin	500-1500	12-24

*This agent does not increase insulin secretion, but increases the cells' sensitivity to insulin, lowers plasma cholesterol concentration, and suppresses appetite.

- *Insulin* allows glucose to enter the cells of insulin-sensitive tissue. There are several different types of insulin available pharmaceutically that vary in onset, peak, duration, and source (see table 16.1).

- *Oral hypoglycemic agents (sulfonylureas)* are medications that help the pancreas secrete more insulin, reduce liver glycogenolysis, and increase insulin sensitivity (see table 16.2).

The most significant effect of both insulin and OHAs on exercise testing and exercise training is their ability to cause hypoglycemia. Attention to timing of medication, food intake, and blood glucose level before and after exercise is necessary. If exercise is of long duration (> 60 minutes), blood glucose should be tested during exercise.

Recommendations for Exercise Testing

Recommendations for exercise testing depend upon age, duration of diabetes, and presence of diabetic complications. Exercise testing using protocols for populations at risk for coronary artery disease is recommended in people who

- have type I diabetes and are over 30 years old,

- have had type I diabetes longer than 15 years,

- have type II diabetes and are over 35 years old,

- have either type I or type II diabetes and one or more of the other coronary artery disease risk factors,

- have suspected or known coronary artery disease, and/or

- have any microvascular or neurological diabetic complications.

People with diabetes who do not meet any of these criteria may be tested with use of protocols for the general, healthy population. The primary objectives of exercise testing in those with diabetes are to

- identify the presence and extent of coronary artery disease, and

- determine appropriate intensity range for aerobic exercise training.

Recommendations for Exercise Programming

The exercise prescription for people with diabetes must be individualized according to medication schedule, presence and severity of diabetic complications, and goals and expected benefits of the exercise program. Food intake with exercise must also be considered. In general, one hour of exercise requires an additional 15 grams of carbohydrate either before or after exercise. If exercise is vigorous and of longer duration, an additional 15 to 30 grams of carbohydrate every hour may be required. Exercise is contraindicated if

- there is active retinal hemorrhage or there has been recent therapy for retinopathy (e.g., laser treatment),
- illness or infection is present,
- blood glucose is > 250 to 300 mg·dl⁻¹ and ketones are present (blood glucose should be lowered before initiation of exercise), or
- blood glucose is 80 to 100 mg·dl⁻¹, since the risk of hypoglycemia is great (in this situation carbohydrate should be eaten and blood glucose allowed to increase before initiation of exercise).

Exercise precautions include

- keeping source of rapidly acting carbohydrate available during exercise;
- consuming adequate fluids before, during, and after exercise;
- practicing good foot care and wearing proper shoes and cotton socks; and
- carrying medical identification.

Suggested Readings

American Diabetes Association. 1994. Nutrition recommendation and principles for people with diabetes mellitus. *J. Am. Dietetic Assoc.* 94: 504-06.

American Diabetes Association Council on Exercise. 1990. Position statement: Diabetes mellitus and exercise. *Diabetes Care* 13: 804-05.

American Diabetes Association Council on Exercise. 1994. *The fitness book for people with diabetes,* ed. W.G. Hornsby. Richmond, Virginia: American Diabetes Association.

Grahm, C., and P. Lasko-McCarthey. 1988. Exercise options for persons with diabetic complications. *Diabetes Educator* 16: 212-20.

Horton, E.S. 1988. Role and management of exercise in diabetes mellitus. *Diabetes Care* 11: 201-11.

Ruderman, N.B., and S.H. Scheneider. 1992. Diabetes, exercise and atherosclerosis. *Diabetes Care* 15: 1787-93.

Sherman, W.M., and A.L. Albright. 1992. Exercise and type II diabetes. *Exerc. and Sports Science Exchange* 4 (37): 1-5.

Vitug, A., S.H. Schneider, and N.B. Ruderman. 1988. Exercise and type I diabetes mellitus. *Exerc. Sport Sci. Rev.* 16: 285-304.

DIABETES: EXERCISE TESTING

METHODS	MEASURES	ENDPOINTS*	COMMENTS
Aerobic power **Treadmill** (1-2 METs/stage) **Cycle** (17 watts/min) ramp protocol (25-50 watts/3 min stage)	• 12-lead ECG, heart rate • Blood pressure • RPE	• Serious dysrhythmias • > 2 mm ST-segment depression or elevation • Ischemic threshold • T-wave inversion with significant ST change • SBP > 260 mmHg or DBP DBP > 115 mmHg • Onset of peripheral pain	
Strength **Isotonic/isokinetic**	• Maximal number of repetitions, peak torque		• Excessive blood pressure increases may be problematic if macrovascular complications exist.
Flexibility **Goniometry** **Sit-and-reach**			
Neuromuscular **Gait analysis** **Balance** **Nerve conduction**			• Indicated for peripheral neuropathy and/or prosthetic devices.

*Measurements of particular significance; do not *always* indicate test termination.

MEDICATIONS	SPECIAL CONSIDERATIONS
• Insulin/hypoglycemic agents: May result in hypoglycemia. • Antihypertensives: See appendix A. • Lipid-lowering agents: See appendix A.	• Test should be postponed if blood glucose concentration is > 250 mg/dl and ketones are present. • If blood glucose is < 80-100 mg/dl, then carbohydrate should be administered. • Autonomic neuropathy is common; may be associated with silent ischemia, postural hypotension, and/or blunted HR response to exercise. • Peripheral neuropathy is common; may cause numbness, tingling in extremities, Charcot's joint, reduced balance. • Microvascular complications may be affected by excessively high blood pressure. • Peripheral vascular disease may result in intermittent claudication and/or infections or ulcers in the lower extremities with poor wound healing. • Insulin and meal schedule should be considered when testing. • Hypoglycemia can still occur several hours after exercise. • If angina and/or silent ischemia is present, see chapter 5.

DIABETES: EXERCISE PROGRAMMING

MODES	GOALS	INTENSITY/ FREQUENCY/DURATION	TIME TO GOAL
Aerobic • Large muscle activities	• Increase aerobic capacity. • Increase time to exhaustion. • Increase work capacity. • Improve blood pressure response to exercise. • Reduce cardiovascular risk factors.	• 50-90% peak HR*. • 50-85% peak $\dot{V}O_2$*. • Monitor RPE. • 4-7 days/week. • 20-60 minutes/session.	• 4-6 months
Strength/anaerobic • Free weights, weight machines, isokinetic machines • Interval training	• Increase maximal number of repetitions. • Improve performance for patients interested in competition.		• 4-6 months
Flexibility • Stretching/yoga	• Maintain/increase range of motion. • Improve gait, balance, and coordination.		• 4-6 months
Functional • Activity-specific exercise • Weight management	• Increase daily living activities. • Increase vocational potential. • Increase physical self-confidence.		

*If complications are present and/or diabetes is of long duration, lower-intensity activity may be necessary.

MEDICATIONS	SPECIAL CONSIDERATIONS
• See table on testing.	• A snack may be needed and/or insulin dosage change may be needed 30-60 minutes before exercise. • Monitor blood glucose before and after exercise. • Exercising late in the evening increases risk of nocturnal hypoglycemia. • If angina and/or silent ischemia is present, see chapter 5.

CHAPTER 17

Hyperlipidemia

J. Larry Durstine, PhD, FACSM
University of South Carolina

Geoffrey E. Moore, MD, FACSM
University of Pittsburgh

Overview of the Pathophysiology

Lipids are not soluble in an aqueous solution such as plasma and must combine with various proteins (apolipoproteins) to form micelle structures called lipoproteins. Lipoproteins are spherical in shape with apolipoproteins surrounding a lipid core that contains triglyceride, phospholipid, and free and esterified cholesterol. Lipoproteins are separated by ultracentrifugation into different gravitational density ranges. There are four principal lipoprotein classes:

- **Chylomicrons** are derived from intestinal absorption of exogenous (dietary) triglyceride.

- **Very low density lipoprotein (VLDL or pre-*b*-lipoprotein)** is synthesized in the liver and is the primary transport mechanism for endogenous triglyceride.

- **Low-density lipoprotein (LDL or *b*-lipoprotein)** represents the final stage in the catabolism of VLDL and is the principal carrier of cholesterol. Intermediate-density lipoprotein (IDL) and lipoprotein(a) are subfractions of LDL.

- **High-density lipoprotein (HDL or *a*-lipoprotein)** is involved in the reverse transport of cholesterol and is typically studied as two separate subfractions: HDL_2 and the more dense HDL_3.

Triglyceride and cholesterol move between the intestine, liver, and extrahepatic tissue by a complex transport system with plasma lipoproteins as the prominent element. This system is facilitated by several important enzymes: lipoprotein lipase (LPL), hepatic lipase, lecithin:cholesterol acyltransferase (LCAT), and cholesteryl ester transfer protein (CETP). These enzymes and lipoproteins interact to create several metabolic pathways. Chylomicrons, VLDL, IDL, and LDL are involved in the pathways that move lipids from the intestine or liver to peripheral tissues. High-density lipoprotein, however, is involved in the reverse transport of cholesterol. Alterations in these pathways can change lipoprotein composition and modify coronary artery disease (CAD) risk.

A variety of environmental, genetic, and pathologic factors can alter cholesterol and triglyceride transport. Some factors are gender, age, body fat distribution, dietary composition, cigarette smoking, some medications, genetic inheritance, and routine participation in physical activity. When these factors combine to yield elevated blood lipid and lipoprotein concentrations, the condition is referred to as *dyslipidemia* and has several forms:

- *Hyperlipidemia* indicates elevated blood triglyceride and cholesterol.

- *Hypertriglyceridemia* denotes only elevated triglyceride concentration.

- *Hypercholesterolemia* implies only elevated blood cholesterol concentration.

- *Hyperlipoproteinemia* or *dyslipoproteinemia* denotes elevated lipoprotein concentrations. Hyperlipoproteinemia either is associated with genetic abnormalities, or may be secondarily related to an underlying disease such as diabetes mellitus, renal insufficiency, hypothyroidism, biliary obstruction, dysproteinemia, or nephrotic kidney disease.

When one considers risk of CAD and peripheral arterial disease, the principal concerns are hypertriglyceridemia (elevated VLDL triglyceride), hypercholesterolemia (increased LDL cholesterol [LDL-C]), and mixed hyperlipidemia (increased LDL-C and VLDL triglyceride).

Effects on the Exercise Response

Generally, dyslipidemia does not alter the exercise response to a single session of exercise unless the dyslipidemia is long-standing and has led to CAD or secondary illness. When this occurs, the secondary disease process alters the exercise response in accordance with that problem (e.g., angina and claudication). In such cases, attention must be given to the exercise response in view of these other conditions. Possible exceptions to this rule include individuals with genetic disorders. Individuals who have extraordinarily high lipid concentrations may have inadequate oxygen supply to vital tissues such as heart or brain and be at great risk for stroke, myocardial infarction, or both. Medical management to gain control of the dyslipidemia before the client begins an exercise program would be prudent, and in these cases exercise should be supervised. In addition, since dyslipidemic clients may have prescribed medications for other conditions, the type and dose of these medications should be noted before the person undergoes exercise testing or training.

Effects of Exercise Training

Regular participation in physical activity can manifest beneficial changes in persons with normal lipid and lipoprotein concentrations as well as most persons with dyslipidemia. These changes include the following:

- Triglyceride concentrations are generally lower.
- High-density lipoprotein cholesterol concentrations are typically higher (but not always).
- Enzyme activity (LPL, LCAT, and CETP) in the metabolism of lipoproteins is increased.

These exercise training changes will enhance reverse cholesterol transport, and can be augmented further by a low-fat diet, weight loss, and reduction in adiposity. Thus, exercise training can directly (e.g., by increased LPL activity) or indirectly (e.g., by reductions in body weight and body fat) improve blood lipid and lipoprotein profiles.

Congenital deficiencies in lipid transport can cause abnormal blood lipid and lipoprotein profiles, and these clients may have a substantially different response to routine physical activity from that seen in healthy individuals. For example, exercise training does not amplify LPL activity in clients with LPL deficiency, nor does HDL concentration increase in individuals with low HDL (hypoalphalipoprotein syndrome). The mechanisms responsible for changes in dyslipidemic conditions as a consequence of exercise training are unclear and in many cases are likely to be different from those reported for healthy subjects.

Management and Medications

Diet, weight loss, and drug therapy are the mainstay of treatment for dyslipidemia while exercise training is used as adjunctive therapy. Low-fat, low-calorie diets that lead to weight loss aid in lowering blood lipids and lipoproteins when used in conjunction with an exercise program.

- Low-fat and high-carbohydrate diets lower HDL cholesterol (HDL-C) and increase triglyceride concentrations.
- Exercise diminishes these effects of diet on HDL-C and triglyceride concentrations.
- Low-calorie diets that cause weight loss decrease total cholesterol and LDL-C and increase HDL-C.
- The effects of low-calorie diets are complex (e.g., low-calorie diets decrease HDL-C in obese women, but increase HDL-C in distance runners).

Lipid-lowering medications act by a variety of mechanisms, but generally have few hemodynamic or electrocardiographic effects. A combination of lipid-lowering drugs is frequently used. This practice can cause substantial reductions in dyslipidemia with reductions in cost and side effects while compliance is enhanced. A major risk of combination therapy is muscle toxicity and damage (rhabdomyolysis) with use of fibric acid derivatives and hepatic hydroxymethylglutaryl coenzyme A (HMG CoA) reductase inhibitors. Recent data suggest that exercise potentiates the propensity to develop drug-induced muscle damage.

- **Nicotinic acid** (niacin) suppresses VLDL synthesis by the liver. Niacin can cause vasodilatory flushing and lower blood pressure.

- **Bile acid-binding resins** (e.g., cholestyramine and colestipol) absorb bile acids in the small intestine, decreasing bile acid resorption, and thus lower LDL-C.

- **Fibric acid derivatives** (e.g., gemfibrozil and clofibrate) increase LPL activity and result in an increased catabolism of VLDL and IDL. Clofibrate may provoke dysrhythmias and/or angina in individuals with prior myocardial infarction.

- **Hepatic hydroxymethylglutaryl coenzyme A reductase inhibitors** (e.g., lovastatin) inhibit the synthesis of cholesterol that results in a compensatory increase in LDL receptors. The combined effect is to decrease LDL-C. The HMG CoA reductase inhibitors can cause damage to skeletal muscle (rhabdomyolysis), particularly when used in combination with fibric acid derivatives.

- **Probucol** may increase lipid clearance by the macrophage pathway. This medication may cause QT-interval prolongation.

Some medications used to treat other medical problems also affect plasma lipid and lipoprotein; these include beta antagonists (beta blockers), thiazide diuretics, oral hypoglycemic agents, insulin, estrogen, and progesterone.

- **Beta blockers** increase triglyceride concentrations and reduce HDL-C concentrations, with the exception of those with intrinsic sympathomimetic activity.

- **Thiazide diuretics** increase total plasma cholesterol, VLDL cholesterol, LDL-C, and triglyceride without an effect on HDL-C concentration.

- **Oral hypoglycemic agents or insulin therapy** may reduce triglyceride and increase HDL-C in diabetic individuals in whom blood glucose is not well controlled. These benefits are secondary to the improvement in blood glucose.

- **Levothyroxine** increases hepatic LDL receptor activity and thereby lowers LDL-C in clients who are hypothyroid. This medication may produce elevations of heart rate and blood pressure as well as cardiac dysrhythmias, and can lead to angina in patients with CAD.

- **Sex steroids** in combinations (as in oral contraceptives) tend to increase cholesterol depending on the estrogen:progesterone ratio.

- **Estrogens** tend to raise HDL-C and VLDL tri-

glyceride concentrations especially in postmenopausal women.

- **Progesterone** decreases triglyceride as well as HDL-C concentrations.

To date, few studies have examined the interaction of these medications with exercise training. Some preliminary results suggest that exercise training may attenuate the increased triglyceride concentration and reduced HDL-C concentrations associated with the use of beta blockers. Thus, it is possible that exercise may counteract the adverse effect of some medications.

Recommendations for Exercise Testing

If the dyslipidemia condition is congenital, but the client does not have any signs or symptoms of some other primary condition (e.g., CAD or renal insufficiency), exercise testing can follow normal protocols used for populations at risk for CAD. However, if signs or symptoms of other primary diseases are present, exercise testing should follow recommendations for that particular disorder.

The primary objectives of exercise testing of these clients are to

- uncover hidden CAD,

- determine functional capacity, and

- determine appropriate intensity range for *aerobic* exercise training.

Recommendations for Exercise Programming

The exercise prescription for the client with dyslipidemia should be adjuvant to therapy that restricts energy intake and dietary fat consumption as well as the appropriate therapy of lipid-lowering medications. Presently available information suggests that there may be different energy expenditure thresholds for different lipids and lipoproteins. For example, triglyceride concentrations are lower in hypertriglyceridemic men after two weeks of *aerobic* exercise (45 minutes per day) on consecutive days, whereas total plasma cholesterol concentration usually remains unchanged even after one year of exercise training. On the other hand, HDL-C concentrations are frequently increased by exercise regimens requiring 1000 to 1200 kilocalories of energy expenditure per week (minimal training period of 12 weeks). Inactive subjects may also have a lower threshold than physically active persons for change in HDL-C concentration. In any case, inactive persons may expect a favorable change in blood lipids within several months.

The primary goal for exercise training is to *expend* calories by *aerobic* exercise training, with exercise that is

- performed at moderate intensities (40-70% of maximal functional capacity),

- performed often (preferably five days a week), and

- performed once a day—although exercising twice a day may be necessary to increase total energy expenditure and may be useful in persons with time constraints or severe exercise intolerance from chronic disease or morbid obesity.

Suggested Readings

Durstine, J.L. 1995. Exercise and optimization of the lipid profile. In *Current therapy in sports medicine,* ed. J.S. Torg and R.J. Shephard, 668-76. 3rd ed. St. Louis: Mosby.

Durstine, J.L., and W.L. Haskell. 1994. Effects of exercise-training on plasma lipids and lipoproteins. *Exerc. Sport Sci. Rev.* 22: 477-521.

Haskell, W.L., and J.L. Durstine. 1992. Impact of exercise training on lipoprotein metabolism. In *Diabetes mellitus and exercise,* ed. J. Devlin, E.S. Horton, and M. Vranic, 205-16. London: Smith-Gordon.

Kokkinos, P.F., and B.F. Hurley. 1990. Strength training and lipoprotein-lipid profiles: A critical analysis and recommendations for further study. *Sports Med.* 9 (5): 266-72.

Shepherd, J. 1992. Lipoprotein metabolism: An overview. *Ann. Acad. Med.* 21 (1): 106-13.

Superko, H.R. 1991. Exercise training, serum lipids, and lipoprotein particles: Is there a change threshold? *Med. Sci. Sports Exerc.* 23 (6): 677-85.

Superko, H.R. 1993. Advances in lipoprotein metabolism: Applications in the cardiac rehabilitation setting. In *Clinical cardiac rehabilitation: A cardiologist's guide,* ed. F.J. Pashkow and W.A. Dafoe, 196-226. Baltimore: Williams & Wilkins.

Superko, H.R, and W.L. Haskell. 1987. The role of exercise training in the therapy of hyperlipoproteinemia. *Cardiology Clinics* 5 (2): 285-310.

Tall, A.R. 1990. Plasma high density lipoproteins: Metabolism and relationship to atherogenesis. *J. Clin. Invest.* 86: 379-84.

Tikkanen, M.J. 1990. Plasma lipoproteins and atherosclerosis. *J. Diabetes Complications* 4 (2): 35-38.

HYPERLIPIDEMIA: EXERCISE TESTING

METHODS	MEASURES	ENDPOINTS*	COMMENTS
Aerobic power **Cycle** (17 watts/min) ramp protocol (25-50 watts/3 min stage) **Treadmill** (1-2 METs/3 min stage)	• 12-lead ECG, heart rate • Blood pressure	• Peak $\dot{V}O_2$/work rate • Serious dysrhythmias • > 2 mm ST-segment depression or elevation • Ischemic threshold • T-wave inversion with significant ST change • Exaggerated or hypotensive response	• See chapters on hypertension and diabetes (chapters 10 and 16, tables on exercise testing).
Endurance **6-minute walk**	• Distance	• 6 minutes	• Useful for duration of training.

*Measurements of particular significance; do not *always* indicate test termination.

MEDICATIONS	SPECIAL CONSIDERATIONS
• HMG CoA reductase inhibitors and fibric acid: May cause muscle damage. • See chapters on hypertension and diabetes (tables on testing).	• High risk of cardiac and arterial insufficiency. • Xanthomas may cause biomechanical problems. • Very high triglyceride/cholesterol may cause intravascular sludging and ischemia. • See chapters on hypertension and diabetes (tables on testing).

HYPERLIPIDEMIA: EXERCISE PROGRAMMING

MODES	GOALS	INTENSITY/ FREQUENCY/DURATION	TIME TO GOAL
Aerobic • Large muscle activities	• Increase work capacity. • Increase endurance. • Decrease cholesterol and triglyceride concentrations. • Increase caloric expenditure. • Decrease adiposity.	• 40-70% of peak work rate or RPE of 11-16. • Monitor HR or RPE. • 1-2 sessions 5-7 days/week. • 40 minutes. • Emphasize increasing duration rather than intensity.	• 4 months (fitness) • 9-12 months (lipids)

MEDICATIONS	SPECIAL CONSIDERATIONS
• See appendix A. • See table on testing.	• Obesity may limit training choices. • See table on testing in this chapter and table on programming for people with obesity (chapter 18).

Obesity

Janet P. Wallace, PhD, FACSM

Indiana University

Overview of the Pathophysiology

Obesity is excess body fat frequently resulting in a significant impairment of health. The prevalence of obese and overweight adults varies depending on the measurement technique. According to height/weight tables, 14% of all United States men and 24% of all United States women are obese. An additional 31% of men and 24% of women are overweight. With use of the most conservative criteria, which would be met by 5% of men and 8% of women, the total number of obese adults in this country is between 5 and 10 million.

Although the causes of obesity include hypothalamic, endocrine, and genetic disorders, diet and physical inactivity are the primary causes of the more common form of obesity found in this country. The accumulation of excess fat is not just a simple balance of caloric intake and caloric expenditure. Caloric intake and expenditure may be likened to opposing forces balanced on a fulcrum of physiological and metabolic functions that control fat storage and fat release. The balance can be altered by the lifestyle factors of diet and physical inactivity, but once the fulcrum of the balance is displaced, the caloric balance between intake and expenditure is no longer even. Excess dietary fat and sugar and physical inactivity, in combination, are the lifestyle factors that contribute to the instability of caloric balance. This altered physiological fulcrum in obesity includes

- increased fasting insulin,
- increased insulin response to glucose,
- decreased insulin sensitivity,
- decreased growth hormone,
- decreased growth hormone response to insulin stimulation,
- increased adrenocortical hormones,
- increased cholesterol synthesis and excretion, and
- decreased hormone-sensitive lipase.

Altered insulin function may be a primary mechanism in the etiology and maintenance of obesity.

Obesity has been defined many ways. The most common systems for defining obesity have been height/weight tables, body mass index (BMI), and body fat percentage.

- Height/weight tables: People are considered obese when they weigh more than twenty percent of their desirable weight as listed in the tables.

- Body mass index: Although different BMI standards have been published for increased risk of disease for men [>27.8 kg/m^2] and women [27.3 kg/m^2], a combined categorization has been derived from the epidemiologic literature:

  - Acceptable range (low risk)—20.0-25.0 kg/m^2

  - Mildly overweight (increased risk)—25.1-27.0 kg/m^2

  - Moderately overweight/obese—27.1-30.0 kg/m^2

  - Markedly overweight/obese—30.1-40.0 kg/m^2

  - Morbidly obese—> 40.0 kg/m^2

    (BMI = body weight [kg]/height [m]^2)

- Percentage body fat:

	Men	Women
Minimal fat	5%	8%
Below average	5% to 15%	14% to 23%
Above average	16% to 25%	24% to 32%
At risk	> 25%	> 32%

Classification systems of obesity have also been based on phenotype, fat cell morphology, and health status.

- **Phenotype**
  - Type I — Excess body mass or percentage fat
  - Type II — Excess subcutaneous truncal-abdominal fat (android)
  - Type III — Excess abdominal visceral fat
  - Type IV — Excess gluteal-femoral fat (gynoid)

- **Cell Morphology**
  - Hyperplastic obesity
  - Hypertrophic obesity

- **Health Status**
  - Mild obesity
  - Morbid obesity

Obesity increases not only the risk of disease, but also the severity of disease. Body fat distribution may contribute more to disease than total body fat. Upper body fat distribution has been associated with increased risk of coronary artery disease, hypertension, hyperlipidemia, and diabetes, as well as hormone and menstrual dysfunction. For example, truncal adipocytes have a higher metabolic activity than other sites. This increased activity has been associated with glucose intolerance, hypertension via increased sodium retention, sympathetic nervous system activation, increased intracellular calcium, and hypertrophy of smooth muscle vessels. Abdominal adipocytes are associated with increased very low density lipoprotein, triglyceride, and adipose lipoprotein lipase activity. Thus, excess fat in specific deposits may contribute to the diseases associated with obesity.

Body fat distribution can be estimated by the measurement of waist-to-hip ratio. The waist-to-hip ratio is not well standardized. The most common and most often recommended technique may be the ratio of the minimal waist to the largest gluteal. Standards for this method of calculating waist-to-hip ratio are as follows:

- Lower body fat distribution for men < 0.776 and women < 0.776

- Upper body fat distribution for men > 0.913 and women > 0.861

Effects on the Exercise Response

The effects of obesity on exercise testing are not always straightforward. The obvious effect of obesity on exercise testing is low physical work capacity because of excess body weight. However, because obesity is associated with other diseases, any of the confounding influences of these diseases may be involved in exercise testing. For example, obese adults have a higher risk of coronary artery disease and may exhibit myocardial ischemia during exercise testing. A hypertensive response to graded exercise may be exhibited despite the absence of hypertension at rest. Consideration of glucose intolerance is essential for the obese diabetic patient.

Effects of Exercise Training

Exercise training is very effective in reducing body weight in moderate obesity, but may not be as effective in morbid obesity. When body weight is reduced through regular dynamic exercise, body fat is reduced while lean body weight is either maintained or increased. Populations that have low lean body weight are the most likely to gain lean body weight with exercise training. This excludes the obese, because in these people lean weight has been increased to support the excess fat. On the other hand, resistance training can increase the lean body weight of almost any population.

Physical activity affects body fat distribution by promoting regional fat loss in the abdominal sites. Fat loss through exercise is more efficient for individuals with upper body fat distribution. The resultant reduction of regional fat in the abdominal sites significantly decreases the risk of the diseases associated with upper body fat distribution. The influence of physical activity on food intake is unclear in human studies. Non-obese people may increase food intake with exercise, whereas obese people may not.

Physical activity may be one of the most important factors in the maintenance of weight loss. This maintenance may occur directly through increase in energy expenditure, or the positive behavior change of exercise could act indirectly by influencing the participant to decrease caloric intake.

The effects of exercise training on metabolism are not well established. Metabolic rate does decline with weight reduction via caloric restriction. However, in the starvation state, the maintenance of metabolic rate through exercise may not always counteract the reduction mediated by food restriction. In any case, exercise training has profound effects on glucose metabolism in both the moderately and the morbidly obese; these include

- decreased fasting glucose,
- decreased fasting insulin,
- increased glucose tolerance, and
- decreased insulin resistance.

These changes have been found, in some instances, without changes in body weight or body fat. Others have reported that the more dramatic changes in glucose metabolism occurred in those who exhibited the greatest reduction in deep abdominal fat.

Management and Medications

Reduction of fat weight with the preservation of lean body weight is the primary objective of obesity management. The individual who is most likely to be *successful in weight loss*

- is slightly or moderately obese,
- has upper body fat distribution,
- has no history of weight cycling,
- has a sincere desire to lose weight, and
- became overweight as an adult.

Behavior change focuses on dietary and activity habits toward weight reduction, whereas more invasive interventions have been used in morbid obesity (BMI > 40).

Dietary Objectives
- Reduction in total calories
- Reduction in fat intake

Physical Activity Objectives
- Increase in daily activity
- Physical conditioning

Other Medical Techniques
- Starvation diets

- Gastroplasties
- Jejunoileal bypass
- Jaw wiring
- Intragastric balloons
- Fat excision
- Anti-obesity medications

Medications

There are prescriptions and over-the-counter medications for weight control that act by suppressing appetite. Such FDA-approved medications include sympathomimetic drugs (medications that stimulate the sympathetic nervous system) such as amphetamines, other synthetic amines, isoindoles, and caffeine. Serotonin uptake inhibitors have been tried as appetite suppressants but do not have FDA approval for that purpose. The contribution that these pharmacologic appetite suppressants will make to weight loss in obese persons is not well understood; it is thought that these agents have little clinical value. Thyroid hormone has been used in the past, but since drug-induced hypothyroidism can cause dangerous cardiovascular side effects as well as osteoporosis, thyroid hormone *should not* be used as a weight control medication.

Recommendations for Exercise Testing

Evaluation of the client who is obese includes more than just exercise testing. Additional assessments include medical and weight histories, nutrition and eating habits, and body composition. Body composition assessment includes a measure of the extent of obesity, distribution of body fat, and a reasonable target weight. An additional assessment for potential for injury would also be prudent.

Obesity is not considered one of the major risk factors for safety in exercise testing, nor is exercise testing always necessary for obese adults who want to start an exercise program. However, exercise testing plays an important role in the optimal management of exercise treatment for persons who are obese. The primary objective of exercise testing with individuals who are obese is exercise prescription. Disease diagnosis is a secondary, yet essential, objective. A determination of physical work capacity is important for selecting the intensity of exercise.

Recommendations for Exercise Programming

Although the primary objective of exercise in the treatment of obesity is to expend more calories, the optimal approach to increased energy expenditure is debatable. The exercise prescription must optimize the energy expenditure yet minimize potential for injury. On the other hand, exercise should be enjoyable and practical and should fit into the lifestyle of the individual. The energy expenditure of the actual exercise as well as that of the recovery period, often referred to as *excess postexercise oxygen consumption (EPOC)*, should be considered in the total energy expenditure of a single exercise session. The debate is whether two short sessions a day will produce a higher total energy expenditure (exercise plus EPOC) than one longer session of the same intensity. The use of two shorter sessions has been recommended because the elevated energy expenditure of recovery may be sustained for a longer period of time than after a single session even though it is longer. On the other hand, the single longer exercise session may have an advantage for substrate utilization and also be easier to incorporate into some individuals' lifestyles. For this reason, recommendations for both types of prescriptions are listed.

- Mode
  - Non-weight-bearing exercise
  - Walking
  - Increase in daily living activities
  - Resistance training
- Frequency
  - Daily or at least five sessions per week
- Duration
  - Forty to sixty minutes per day *or*
  - Twenty to thirty minutes twice daily
- Intensity
  - Fifty to seventy percent of maximal oxygen consumption

Exercise programs that include high-resistance activities (i.e., free weights, resistance machines) can lead to maintenance or to gain in fat-free body weight. However, aerobic activity has more potential to decrease fat weight (maintain or increase fat-free weight) than does resistance training because the former can be sustained for a longer time, allowing more energy to be expended.

Special Considerations

Injury prevention is the most important consideration in exercise for adults who are obese; physical injury may be one of the primary reasons for discontinuation of exercise. Excess body weight may exacerbate existing joint conditions. Another concern is thermoregulation. The following considerations and guidelines are relevant for programming with people who are obese:

- Considerations for prevention of overuse injury
  - Injury history
  - Adequate flexibility, warm-up, and cooldown
  - Gradual progression of intensity and duration
  - Low-impact or non-weight-bearing exercises
- Thermoregulation considerations
  - Exercising in neutral environment
  - Exercising during cool times of the day
  - Drinking plenty of water
  - Wearing loose-fitting clothes

Other considerations may be dependent on associated diseases that result from obesity.

Suggested Readings

Atkinson, R.L., and J. Walberg-Rankin. 1994. Physical activity, fitness, and severe obesity. In *Physical activity, fitness and health,* ed. C. Bouchard, R.J. Shephard, and T. Stephens, 696-711. Champaign, IL: Human Kinetics.

Buskirk, E.R. 1993. Obesity. In *Exercise testing and exercise prescription for special cases: Theoretical basis and clinical application,* ed. J.S. Skinner, 185-210. Philadelphia: Lea & Febiger.

Hill, J.O., H.J. Drougas, and J.C. Peters. 1994. Physical activity, fitness, and moderate obesity. In *Physical activity, fitness and health,* ed. C. Bouchard, R.J. Shephard, and T. Stephens, 684-95. Champaign, IL: Human Kinetics.

Verrill, D., E. Shoup, L. Boyce, B. Fox, A. Moore, and T. Forkner. 1994. Recommended guidelines for body composition assessment in cardiac rehabilitation: A position paper by the North Carolina Cardiopulmonary Rehabilitation Association. *J. Cardiopulmonary Rehabil.* 14: 104-121.

Wallace, J.P., P.G. Bogle, K.T. Murray, and W.C. Miller. 1994. Variation in the anthropometric dimensions for estimating upper and lower body obesity. *Am. J. of Human Biol.* 6: 699-709.

OBESITY: EXERCISE TESTING

METHODS	MEASURES	ENDPOINTS*	COMMENTS
Aerobic power **Treadmill** (1-2 METs/stage) **Cycle** (17 watts/min) ramp protocol (25-50 watts/3 min stage)	• 12-lead ECG, heart rate • Blood pressure • RPE	• Serious dysrhythmias • > 2 mm ST-segment depression or elevation • Ischemic threshold • T-wave inversion with significant ST change • SBP > 260 mmHg or DBP > 115 mmHg • Volitional fatigue	• Patients are at higher-than-normal risk for CAD/hypertension.
Flexibility **Goniometry**	• Range of motion		• Used to determine joints that need stretching exercise.
Neuromuscular **Gait analysis** **Balance analysis** **Balance**			• Useful in identifying individuals with poor balance who may require more supervision during exercise and to assess improvement in balance after training and/or weight reduction.

*Measurements of particular significance; do not *always* indicate test termination.

MEDICATIONS	SPECIAL CONSIDERATIONS
• For patients with hypertension, refer to chapter 10. • For patients with diabetes, refer to chapter 16. • For patients with hyperlipidemia, refer to chapter 17.	• Increased risk of orthopedic injury. • Increased risk of cardiovascular disease. • Increased risk of heat intolerance.

OBESITY: EXERCISE PROGRAMMING

MODES	GOALS	INTENSITY/ FREQUENCY/DURATION	TIME TO GOAL
Aerobic • Large muscle activities (walking, rowing, cycling, water aerobics, etc.)	• Reduce weight. • Increase functional performance. • Reduce risk of CAD.	• 50-70% peak $\dot{V}O_2$. • Monitor RPE and HR. • 5 days/week. • 40-60 minutes/session (or 2 sessions/day of 20-30 min). • Emphasize increasing duration rather than intensity.	• 9-12 months
Flexibility • Stretching	• Increase range of motion.	• Daily or at least 5 sessions/ week.	
Functional • Activity-specific exercise	• Increase ease of performing daily living activities. • Increase vocational potential. • Increase physical self-confidence.		

MEDICATIONS	SPECIAL CONSIDERATIONS
• For patients with hypertension, refer to chapter 10. • For patients with diabetes, refer to chapter 16. • For patients with hyperlipidemia, refer to chapter 17.	• Use low-impact modes of activity. • Increased risk of hyperthermia. • Equipment modification may be necessary, e.g., wide seats on cycle ergometers and rowers. • Strength training may serve as a valuable adjunct to aerobic training when trying to maintain or gain lean body weight. Begin with guidelines listed in table on programming in chapter 3. For further strength gain, heavier resistance with fewer repetitions may be employed as the client adapts to the program.

CHAPTER 19

Frailty

Connie Bayles, PhD, FACSM
Mercy Hospital, Pittsburgh, PA

Overview of the Pathophysiology

Physical decline associated with aging can be attributed to a number of complex interactions including normal aging, disease, and disuse. Frail health can be found across the entire age spectrum, but adults who are elderly are especially prone to becoming *frail* (weak, vulnerable, slight). The frail older adult is generally identified as having one or more of the following: extreme old age, some type of disability, and the presence of multiple chronic diseases or geriatric syndromes. Adults who are older and frail are more dependent, recover slowly from illness, undergo more falls and injuries, have more acute illnesses, and are more often institutionalized or hospitalized. All these factors can result in increased mortality. Approximately 10% to 20% of adults older than 65 are considered frail; 46% of adults over 85 also are considered frail. According to the National Center for Health Statistics (1992), the fastest-growing segment of our population comprises people over 85 years of age. Many older adults who are considered frail tend to have the most serious health problems and disabilities and/or are functionally impaired. Functional impairment for the individual who is elderly means a restriction in or lack of ability to perform the activities of daily life required for independent living.

The elderly person is often confronted with disease that results in disuse and may accelerate the development of frailty. The body is in constant change throughout life, with changes occurring in the cardiovascular, respiratory, nervous, musculoskeletal, renal, and metabolic systems as part of the normal aging process (see table 19.1). Along with normal aging, the presence of multiple chronic diseases also contributes to increased physical decline (table 19.2). The presence of these diseases does not in itself define frailty, but may place an individual at greater risk of becoming frail.

Effects on the Exercise Response

Persons who are elderly and frail are faced with a variety of medical problems that can put them at risk for a medical emergency during exercise testing. As a result, the following should be kept in mind with respect to exercise testing in persons who are frail.

- Medical history and present medications should be reviewed before the person undergoes testing.

- Exercise tests should be individualized, starting at low work rates, and in many cases should incorporate longer warm-up periods.

- Since older frail persons usually will take a longer time to reach steady state, the exercise test should focus on longer work stages with increases in grade rather than speed.

- Caution should be taken that the exercise stages are not too long, since older frail persons are more quickly fatigued. Notwithstanding, if the test is needed for diagnostic purposes, a more aggressive protocol may be used.

- In addition, older frail persons are susceptible to dehydration and insulin insensitivity, and care should be taken to identify physiologic features associated with these conditions.

Effects of Exercise Training

Physical activity appears to be of critical importance for delaying the metabolic disorders associated with

	Table 19.1 PHYSIOLOGIC CHANGES ASSOCIATED WITH AGING	
SYSTEM	**FUNCTION**	**CHANGE**
Cardiovascular	Resting Heart Rate	No change
	Maximal Heart Rate	Decrease
	Resting Cardiac Output	Decrease
	Maximal Cardiac Output	Decrease
	Resting Stroke Volume	Decrease
	Maximal Stroke Volume	Decrease
	Resting Blood Pressure	Increase
	Exercise Blood Pressure	Increase
	Maximal Oxygen Consumption	Decrease
Respiratory	Residual Volume	Increase
	Vital Capacity	Decrease
	Total Lung Capacity	No Change
	Respiratory Frequency	Increase
Nervous	Reaction Time	Decrease
	Nerve Conduction Time	Increase
	Sensory Deficits	Increase
Musculoskeletal	Muscular Strength	Decrease
	Muscle Mass	Decrease
	Flexibility	Decrease
	Balance	Decrease
	Bone Density	Decrease
Renal	Kidney Function	Decrease
	Acid-Base Control	Decrease
	Glucose Tolerance	Decrease
	Drug Clearance	Decrease
	Cellular Water	Decrease
Metabolic	Basal Metabolic Rate	Decrease
	Lean Body Mass	Decrease
	Body Fat	Increase

aging. In older populations, physical activity can produce increased muscle strength, muscular endurance, and maximal aerobic power. Flexibility, coordination, and balance are also improved, resulting in a decreased risk for falling while enhancing mobility. Also, exercise has been shown to increase socialization and self-esteem. These benefits have important implications for the frail elderly in maintaining or promoting independence in daily living activities.

Management and Medications

The person who is elderly and frail is usually taking more medications than are people in any other segment of the population. Since renal excretion of chemicals is reduced in the elderly, drugs will remain in the body for longer periods of time. This increases the importance of recognizing conditions such as polypharmacy and self-medication. Exercise

Table 19.2 COMMON MEDICAL DISORDERS THAT CONTRIBUTE TO FRAILTY IN INDIVIDUALS THAT ARE ELDERLY

SYSTEM	MEDICAL DISORDER
Cardiovascular	Hypertension, Hypotension, Coronary Artery Disease, Valvular Heart Disease, Failure, Dysrhythmias, Peripheral Arterial Disease
Pulmonary	Asthma, Chronic Pulmonary Disease, Pneumonia
Musculoskeletal	Arthritis, Degenerative Disk Disease, Polymyalgia Rheumatica, Osteoporosis, Degenerative Joint Disease
Metabolic/Endocrine	Diabetes, Hypercholesterolemia
Gastrointestinal	Dental, Malnutrition, Incontinence, Diarrhea
Genitourinary	Urinary Tract Infection, Cancer
Hematologic/Immunologic	Anemia, Leukemia, Cancer
Neurologic	Dementia, Alzheimer Disease, Cerebrovascular Disease, Parkinson Disease, Disorders
Eye and Ear	Cataracts, Glaucoma, Hearing Disorders
Psychiatric	Anxiety Disorders, Hypochondria, Depression, Alcohol Abuse

professionals working with this group must be able to identify individuals who do not follow medication instructions. Before one develops an exercise program for an elderly person, a comprehensive list of the client's medications is necessary.

Many medications have side effects. Side effects and the type of medicines associated with these side effects are

- *dizziness* (sedatives, hypnotics, anticonvulsants, tricyclic antidepressants, antipsychotics),

- *confusion/depression* (sedatives, hypnotics, anticonvulsants, antipsychotics, antidepressants, diuretics, antihypertensives),

- *fatigue and weakness* (beta blockers, diuretics, tricyclic antidepressants, antipsychotics, barbiturates, benzodiazepines, antihistamines, antihypertensives),

- *postural hypotension* (tricyclic antidepressants, antipsychotic antihypertensives, diuretics, nitrates, narcotic analgesics, vasodilators, and levodopa),

- *involuntary muscle movements* (antipsychotics, levodopa, tricyclic antidepressants, adrenergics),

- *urinary incontinence* (benzodiazepines, barbiturates, phenothiazines, chlorpromazines, anticholinergics, diuretics), and

- *increases in heart rate* (antiglaucoma agents/miotics, bronchodilators/antiasthmatic agents).

Recommendations for Exercise Testing

Cardiorespiratory, strength, neuromuscular, flexibility, and functional performance tests enable the exercise leader to assess the current functional levels of participants and are important for recommending an appropriate exercise program. The client who has cardiac problems and exhibits coronary heart disease risk factors should be assessed by a graded exercise test. Various testing modalities, including treadmill and bicycle tests, can be used depending upon the client's medical status. For clients who are free from any coronary heart disease and who have physician clearance, a simple 6- or 12-minute or 20-foot walk test is recommended. Heart rate, blood pressure, ratings of perceived exertion, and distance walked are monitored and recorded to ensure a proper exercise prescription.

Maintaining or improving muscle strength can improve functional ability in persons who are elderly. A hand-held dynamometer is often used to assess muscle strength because it is easy to use and is a reliable means of obtaining an objective measurement of strength. Baseline measures of strength enable the exercise leader to chart progress and provide feedback information to participants as they progress in an exercise program.

In the development of a physical activity program for individuals who are frail and elderly, neuromuscular and functional performance tests are sometimes important for use in evaluating progress. Information obtained from gait, balance, and coordination tests enables the exercise leader to plan appropriate intervention programs as well as to target those individuals who are at risk for falling. Flexibility training can increase joint flexibility and mobility. The goniometer is an important tool for measuring flexibility, and information gained from such tests can be employed as feedback information that participants can use to note improvements.

Recommendations for Exercise Programming

The exercise prescription for persons who are elderly and frail should reflect medical and social needs. Past exercise experience and the setting of goals are major contributors to the success of a program. Since in many instances persons who are elderly have lost the right to choose, the choice of activity by the participant is very important. Compliance to exercise programming is enhanced when the exercise leader and the client work together.

Prescribing the mode of exercise for persons who are elderly must be done with care. The primary goal for this population is to increase functional capacity and independence. The medical history of the participant and past exercise experience are important indicators of the type of exercise to be recommended. Although walking is the easiest and least expensive form of exercise, this activity may not be best for everyone. Bicycling, swimming, and chair activities are most appropriate for people with degenerative joint disease, hip replacements, and knee replacements. Low-level strength training programs in the frail elderly can incorporate ankle and wrist weights as an essential component. Flexibility, eye-hand coordination, reflex training, and fall prevention activities are also important.

Special Considerations

Exercise programming for frail and elderly persons must be individualized and progressive. Since exercise intensity is not necessarily as important as participation, care should be taken in regulating exercise intensity so that compliance to the program is not compromised. This population is faced with physiologic, psychologic, and social problems each day that may interfere with their normal activities of daily living and impact on their participation in regular physical activity.

Emergency procedures should be outlined and posted in the exercise room and reviewed by all participants. Medical occurrence reports and equipment safety checks should be current and filed in a locked cabinet with the participant's charts. Records of attendance and of medical problems that occur during exercise must be maintained. Body weight as well as resting and exercise heart rate and blood pressure measurements should be monitored and recorded. Progression of the exercise prescription should be discussed by the exercise leader and the client. Motivational techniques are recommended to enhance compliance and create an atmosphere of fun. Variations in the exercise program are helpful; these could include music, modified team sports (low competition), and special events such as Olympics. It is important to focus on compliance to an exercise program and not as necessary to rigidly regulate the mode, intensity, and duration of the exercise. Nonetheless, the overall exercise setting should promote physical activity participation and optimize functional capacity of persons who are frail and elderly.

If exercise programming is not possible in a group environment, a very low-level home exercise program can be recommended. Simple flexibility exercises and walking, preferably with assistance, may be used to meet the person's needs. A more progressive program may be implemented if in-home assistance is available.

Suggested Readings

Abrass, I.B. 1990. The biology and physiology of aging. *West. J. Med.* 153: 641-45.

American College of Sports Medicine. 1993. *ACSM'S resource manual for guidelines for exercise testing and prescription,* ed. J.L. Durstine, A.C. King, P.L. Painter, J.L. Roitman, L.D. Zwiren, and W.L. Kenney. 2nd ed. Philadelphia: Lea & Febiger.

American College of Sports Medicine. 1995. *ACSM's guidelines for exercise testing and prescription,* ed. W.L. Kenney, R.H. Humphrey, C.X. Bryant, D.A. Mahler, V. Froehlicher, N.H. Miller, and T. D. York. 5th ed. Baltimore: Williams & Wilkins.

Chapron D.J., and R.W. Besdine. 1987. Drugs as an obstacle to rehabilitation of the elderly: A primer for therapists. *Topics in Geriatr. Rehab.* 2 (3): 63-81.

Fried, L.P. 1994. Frailty. In *Principles of geriatric medicine and gerontology,* ed. W.R. Hazzard, E.L. Bierman, J.P. Blass, W.H. Ettinger, and J.B. Halter, 1149-55. New York: McGraw-Hill.

Lord, S., R. Clark, and I. Webster. 1991. Physiological factors associated with falls in an elderly population. *J. Am. Geriatr. Soc.* 39 (12): 1194-1200.

Schwartz, R.S., and D.M. Buchner. 1994. Exercise in the elderly: Physiologic and functional effects. In *Principles of geriatric medicine and gerontology,* ed. W.R. Hazzard, E.L. Bierman, J.P. Blass, W.H. Ettinger, and J.B. Halter, 95-105. New York: McGraw-Hill.

Silverstone, B. 1994. Public policies on aging: Reconsidering old-age eligibility. *Gerontologist* 34 (6): 724-25.

Tinetti, M.E. 1986. Performance-oriented assessment of mobility problems in elderly patients. *J. Am. Geriatr. Soc.* 34: 119-26.

Tinetti, M.E., and S.F. Ginter. 1988. Identifying mobility dysfunctions in elderly patients: Standard neuromuscular examination or direct assessment? *JAMA* 259: 1190-93.

United States Department of Health and Human Services. National Center for Health Statistics. 1992. *Highlights from health data on older Americans.* Washington, D.C.: U.S. Government Printing Office.

Vitti, K.A., C.M. Bayles, W.J. Carender, J.M. Prendergast, and F.J. D'Amico. 1993. A low-level strength training exercise program for frail elderly adults living in an extended attention facility. *Aging, Clinical and Experimental Research* 5 (5): 363-69.

FRAILTY: EXERCISE TESTING

METHODS	MEASURES	ENDPOINTS*	COMMENTS
Aerobic power **Treadmill** Low-level ramp protocol (such as Naughton-Balke-Ware) **Cycle** (17 watts/min) ramp protocol (25-50 watts/3 min stage) **6- or 12-minute walk** **20-foot walk**	• 12-lead ECG, heart rate • Blood pressure • RPE • METs • Distance • Speed • Number of steps	• Serious dysrhythmias • > 2 mm ST-segment depression or elevation • Ischemic threshold • T-wave inversion with significant ST change • SBP > 260 mmHg or DBP > 115 mmHg • Volitional fatigue • Unsteadiness	• 6- or 12-minute walk good for measuring progress in exercise programs. • Walk tests are good for measuring gait and balance disorders and progress in exercise programs.
Strength **Hand-held dynamometer**	• 3 repetition maximum		• Used to determine intensity of strength training and progress in strength training programs. • Sometimes contraindicated in people with osteoporosis.
Fall risk **Chair stand** **One-legged stance** **8-step tandem gait** **360° turn**	• Mobility/balance	• Volitional fatigue • Unsteadiness	
Flexibility **Sit-and-reach**	• Distance		

*Measurements of particular significance; do not *always* indicate test termination.

MEDICATIONS	SPECIAL CONSIDERATIONS
• May be taking one or more of the following: Diuretics, antihypertensives, anti-anginal agents, antiarrhythmic agents, psychotropic medications, insulin, and anticoagulants. See appendix A for effects.	• Observe client for balance difficulties to prevent falls. • Clients may be prone to fractures due to osteoporosis. • Increased risk of cardiovascular and cerebrovascular diseases. • Low tolerance for hot and cold environments; reduced effectiveness of sweating, susceptible to heat cramps, exhaustion, stroke, and dehydration. • Make sure that regular medication schedule is followed. • Assess the participant for any cognitive deficits. • Adapt the test if the participant is using an assistive device.

FRAILTY: EXERCISE PROGRAMMING

MODES	GOALS	INTENSITY/ FREQUENCY/DURATION	TIME TO GOAL
Aerobic • Large muscle activities (e.g., walking, cycling, rowing, swimming; chair exercise may be indicated for some clients)	• Increase aerobic capacity.	• Monitor RPE (intensity should not be main focus). • 3-5 days/week. • 5-60 minutes/session.	• Average about 3 months
Strength • Low-level, progressive resistance exercise (free weights, weight machines, isokinetic machines) • Ball squeeze	• Increase overall muscular strength. • Decrease risk of falling. • Increase hand strength.	• Start program without weight. Add weight slowly. • 3 days/week. • Approximately 20 minutes/ session.	• Average about 3 months
Flexibility • Stretching/yoga/ tai chi	• Increase range of motion.		
Neuromuscular • 1-foot stand • Stair climbing • Practice falling techniques • Balloon activities • Tandem gait • Chair stand exercise	• Increase neuromuscular coordination, gait, balance, flexibility, and lower-body strength. • Prevent falls. • Increase hand-eye coordination, reaction time.		

MEDICATIONS	SPECIAL CONSIDERATIONS
• See table on testing.	• Target HR should not be main focus. • Avoid ballistic exercises. • Avoid neck circumduction. • Avoid isometric and static resistance exercises. • See table on testing.

Immunological/ Hematological Disorders

Section Editors:

Geoffrey E. Moore, MD, FACSM
University of Pittsburgh

J. Larry Durstine, PhD, FACSM
University of South Carolina

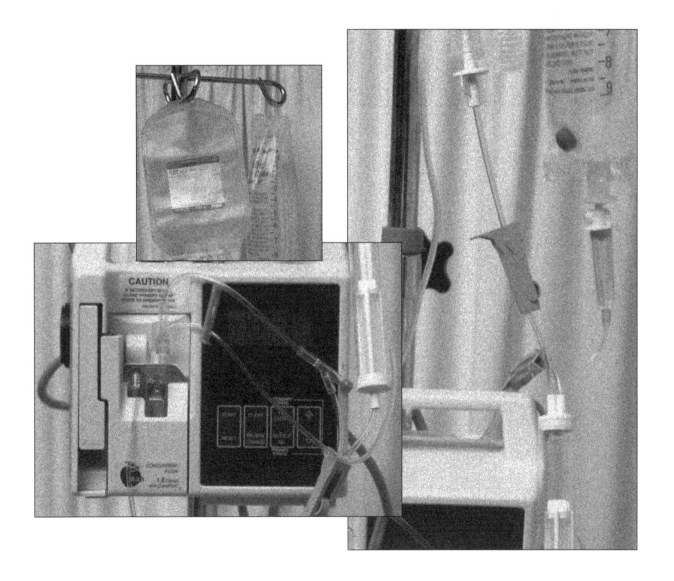

CHAPTER 20

Cancer

George Selby, MD
University of Oklahoma Health Science Center

Overview of the Pathophysiology

Cancer is not a single disease; it is a collection of hundreds of diseases that share the common feature of inappropriate cellular proliferation and the potential for these cells to spread to distant anatomical sites. Symptoms of cancer can be either local, such as the cough of the person with lung cancer, or systemic, as in the drenching night sweats of Hodgkin's lymphoma. The treatment of cancer involves surgery, radiation, and chemotherapy either singly or in combination. All three modes are attempts to make the person cancer-free (remission), although sometimes remission is not possible. There are recurrences when a few cancer cells escape being eradicated and subsequently grow back over time. Cancer is cured when the remission is thought to be permanent. Patients in remission have the most to gain from rehabilitation and exercise training, but some patients who are undergoing treatment may receive benefit as well.

Effects on the Exercise Response

In general, formal exercise testing is appropriate for persons whose cancer is in remission. Persons undergoing intensive chemotherapy or radiation therapy may benefit from routine physical therapy, occupational therapy, and ambulation, as well as strength and flexibility exercises. These people are usually easily fatigued by their cancer therapy and easily worn out. Thus, formal laboratory testing is probably not necessary, but bedside assessment for routine daily exercises may help maintain function and speed recovery after therapy is complete.

Formal exercise testing should be individualized, since each malignancy and mode of therapy carries its own group of complications (see the section on management and medications). Exercise testing is useful to quantitatively assess the effects of these complications and to help monitor progress during training and rehabilitation.

Effects of Exercise Training

Exercise training for persons with cancer is somewhat dependent on individual circumstances. For survivors of cancer (in remission or after cure), exercise training should have the objective of returning them to their former level of physical and psychological function. For persons who are undergoing therapy for cancer, exercise training should have the objective of maintaining endurance, strength, and level of function. Cancer therapy exhausts physical and emotional reserves, so a good use of exercise training is an attempt to maintain these resources. Also, exercise training may have profound psychologic benefits for persons in cancer therapy, particularly with regard to depression. It is not known whether exercise training helps individuals to withstand the rigors of therapy.

Persons with (and survivors of) cancer may have disease- or treatment-specific obstacles to exercise training. The side effects of anti-cancer therapy are often permanent; amputations cause permanent disability; radiation and chemotherapy can cause permanent scar formation in joints and lung and heart tissues; drug-induced cardiomyopathies (see section on management and medications) usually cause a permanent limitation on cardiovascular function. However, many cancer survivors can reap rewards from exercise training, because many of the benefits occur in skeletal muscle and in psychological status. There is a paucity of information on the role of exercise training in persons with cancer, but given that most patients are affected by limited strength and endurance, it seems logical that exercise should be directed at improving these parameters.

The effects of exercise in persons with cancer have been best studied in women with breast cancer. Exercise training in women who have had breast removal results in

- improved shoulder range of motion,
- enhanced self-image and sense of control, and
- increased muscle mass in women receiving postoperative chemotherapy.

Children who have been cured of leukemia may have persistent mild cardiovascular compromise as a result of therapy. This does not usually impair function at moderate exercise levels but, by logical extension, *may* prevent outstanding athletic performance at a later age. Nonetheless, aerobic capacity and submaximal performance should significantly improve after routine exercise training programs. Adult cancer survivors are less well studied; however, their response to exercise training should be similar to that of children, although they are more likely to have co-morbid conditions such as coronary artery disease, high blood pressure, diabetes, or high blood lipids. These conditions may influence exercise management more than the history of cancer does.

Management and Medications

The most common problems encountered with each treatment category are as follows:

- Surgery can cause pain, loss of flexibility, amputation, and motor and sensory nerve damage.
- Radiation can cause loss of flexibility in irradiated joints and cardiac or lung scarring, or both.
- Chemotherapy uses several drugs that have characteristic side effects:
  - *Vinca alkaloids*—Vincristine, Velban. *Effects*—peripheral nerve damage.
  - *Daunorubicin*—Cerubidine. *Effects*—cardiomyopathy.
  - *Doxorubicin*—Adriamycin. *Effects*—cardiomyopathy.
  - *Mitoxantrone*—Novantrone. *Effects*—cardiomyopathy.

- *Bleomycin*—Blenoxane. *Effects*—pulmonary fibrosis.
- *Corticosteroids*—Decadron, prednisone. *Effects*—myopathy.
- Many others. *Effects*—anemia.

Some side effects of anti-cancer treatment are acute: for example, radiation can cause acute inflammatory response in lung tissue and impair oxygen transfer. However, many of the effects are quite delayed in onset, occurring months to years after therapy. For example, radiation can also cause lung scarring many months after therapy, and daunorubicin-induced cardiomyopathy typically occurs months after treatment. Virtually all anti-cancer drugs cause anemia, and of course, persons who are treated with combinations of surgery, radiation, and chemotherapy can develop any or all of the problems noted.

Recommendations for Exercise Testing

Exercise testing can usually be performed with use of standard protocols but may need modification to suit the individual. Many cancer survivors will be extremely deconditioned or emaciated, or both, and will require very low level protocols. Persons who have received chest irradiation or chemotherapy that is toxic to the heart or lungs must be monitored for cardiopulmonary decompensation via frequent vital signs and arterial oximetry. The primary objectives of exercise testing are to

- assess aerobic capacity, submaximal endurance, strength, and functional performance, and
- reveal other co-morbidity such as coronary artery disease.

Recommendations for Exercise Programming

Recommendations for exercise programming are dependent on whether the person is undergoing treatment for cancer or is a survivor who is in remission or has been cured. For survivors, the goal is to return to a healthy, active lifestyle. There may be disease- or treatment-specific obstacles to the mode of exercise (needs of amputees, requirement for portable oxygen, and so on). The optimal frequency and duration are not known, but these probably depend somewhat on any aftereffects (such as cardiomyopathy). Unless the effects of therapy leave severe degradation in metabolic function, adaptations should occur as in normal individuals. For persons in therapy the goals should be to improve strength, endurance, and psychological status and possibly to maintain physical reserves. The optimal frequency, duration, and time course of adaptation are not known. Adaptation may be very blunted, or not apparent (especially if exercise training merely slows down physical wasting). Avoid exhaustion in persons undergoing therapy.

Suggested Readings

Gaskin, T.A., A. LoBuglio, P. Kelly, M. Doss, and N. Pizitz. 1989. STRETCH: A rehabilitative program for patients with breast cancer. *South. Med. J.* 82: 467-69.

Mathys, D., H. Verhaaren, Y. Benoit, G. Laureys, A. DeNaeyer, and M. Craen. 1993. Gender differences in aerobic capacity in adolescents after cure from malignant disease in childhood. *Acta Paediatr.* 82: 459-62.

Sharkey, A.M., A.B. Casey, C.T. Heise, and G. Barber. 1993. Cardiac rehabilitation after cancer therapy in children and young adults. *Am. J. Cardiol.* 71: 1488-90.

St. Pierre, B., C.E. Kaspar, and A.M. Lindsey. 1992. Fatigue mechanisms in patients with cancer: Effects of tumor necrosis factor and exercise on skeletal muscle. *Oncology Nurs. Forum* 19: 419-25.

Winningham, M.L., M.G. MacVicar, M. Bondoc, J.I. Anderson, and J.P. Minton. 1989. Effect of aerobic exercise on body composition in patients with breast cancer on adjuvant chemotherapy. *Oncology Nurs. Forum* 16: 683-89.

CANCER: EXERCISE TESTING

METHODS	MEASURES	ENDPOINTS*	COMMENTS
Aerobic power **6-minute walk**	• Distance covered	• 6 minutes	• Endurance often limited.
Strength **Isotonic/isokinetic**	• 1 repetition maximum, maximal voluntary contraction		• Atrophy and frailty common.
Flexibility **Goniometry**			• Assess upper-extremity range of motion after mastectomy. • Atrophy can limit range of motion.
Functional capacity **Gait analysis**			• Assess for neuropathy after vincristine or radiation.

*Measurements of particular significance; do not *always* indicate test termination. (*continued*)

CANCER: EXERCISE TESTING *(continued)*

MEDICATIONS	SPECIAL CONSIDERATIONS
• Radiation: May cause cardiomyopathy and/or accelerated atherosclerosis. • Bleomycin: May cause pulmonary fibrosis. • Vincristine: May cause neuropathy in extremities. • Daunorubicin: May cause cardiomyopathy.	• Amputee may need special prosthetics or may have residual bone disease. • If the patient has CAD complications, see chapters 3, 4, and 5.

CANCER: EXERCISE PROGRAMMING

MODES	GOALS	INTENSITY/ FREQUENCY/DURATION	TIME TO GOAL
Aerobic • Large muscle activities	• Increase $\dot{V}O_2$, peak work, and endurance.	• Unknown (see Special Considerations).	• Unknown
Strength • Circuit training	• Increase muscular strength and endurance.	• Unknown (see Special Considerations).	• Unknown
Flexibility • Stretching/yoga • Upper extremity range-of-motion exercises	• Increase range of motion.	• Passive range-of-motion exercises 1-2 sessions/day.	• 6-12 weeks
Neuromuscular • Walking • Balance exercises	• Improve gait, balance, and overall coordination.	• Unknown (see Special Considerations).	• Unknown
Functional • Activity-specific exercises	• Increase daily living activities. • Return to work. • Improve quality of life.	• Unknown (see Special Considerations).	• Unknown

MEDICATIONS	SPECIAL CONSIDERATIONS
• See table on testing.	• See table on testing. • Intensity, frequency, and duration recommendations are difficult to make. Very little research information is available. The guidelines presented in chapters 3, 4, and 5 can be used with caution and may need adjustment according to treatment and state of disease.

CHAPTER 21

Anemia

George Selby, MD

University of Oklahoma Health Science Center

Overview of the Pathophysiology

Red blood cells carry oxygen from the lungs to the skeletal muscles to fuel the furnaces of physical activity. Anemia is a shortage of red blood cells, so anemic blood cannot carry as much oxygen as normal blood. Anemia is the common manifestation of several disorders that affect red blood cell formation or life span:

- **Nutritional deficiencies**—iron (the most common), vitamin B-12, folic acid

- **Decreased production**—chronic kidney failure, chronic inflammation, some hormonal disorders

- **Shortened red cell life span**—hemolytic anemias, sickle cell disease, thalassemias

The primary symptoms of anemia are easy fatigability with exercise, shortness of breath, and decreased work capacity, so aerobic exercise tests are virtually always abnormal. These symptoms are related primarily to the low oxygen-carrying capacity of anemic blood, but severe iron deficiency may also reduce the activity of iron-containing muscle enzymes and impair the intrinsic ability of skeletal muscle.

Effects on the Exercise Response

At rest, the anemic person compensates for low oxygen- and carbon dioxide–carrying capacity by increasing cardiac output and breathing rate. Also, there is often a "rightward shift" of the oxyhemoglobin dissociation curve, as well as an increased percentage of oxygen extraction by the tissues. During exercise, heart rate and ventilation increase more rapidly than in nonanemic persons because the reduction in oxygen-carrying capacity is overcome by increasing blood flow. Unfortunately, some of the physiologic reserve is used by the compensatory mechanisms during rest, so there is less potential for an increase in performance. As a result, peak aerobic performance is always reduced in persons with anemia.

Anemia has some specific risks related to exercise. In middle-aged people with iron-deficiency, B-12-deficiency, and folate-deficiency anemias, vigorous exercise may unmask occult coronary artery disease and cause angina (chest discomfort). For this reason, exercise testing should be carefully monitored until such individuals have been adequately treated for their specific deficiency. The use of iron to treat all types of anemias is discouraged because it may mask serious underlying disorders such as gastrointestinal bleeding or may accelerate the damaging effects of undiagnosed hemochromatosis. Similarly, the universal use of folic acid to treat macrocytic anemias of unknown cause results in the partial correction of the anemia of B-12 deficiency (pernicious anemia) but does nothing to arrest development of the severe neurological damage that accompanies pernicious anemia.

While individuals with sickle cell anemia and thalassemia will be severely limited by their low hemoglobin, it is reported that they can exercise to exhaustion without precipitating any complications (such as sickle pain crisis). On the other hand, persons with sickle cell trait (heterogeneous hemoglobin S) are not limited, because their hemoglobin levels are normal. In fact, the percentage of African-American professional athletes with sickle cell trait is about the same as in the general population. However, this does not mean that sickle cell trait is not dangerous. Over the last several years, there have been numerous reports of sudden death in young men with sickle cell trait. These incidents seem to have occurred after sudden increases in activity, a rapid increase in altitude, or prolonged very high intensity exercise. Dehydration may have been part of these tragic deaths.

Effects of Exercise Training

The adaptations to exercise training in anemia varies to some extent, depending on the kind of anemia. When deficiency anemias have been adequately treated with iron, B-12, or folate replenishment, the individual should be able to respond to exercise training as if there had never been any anemia. The person with sickle cell anemia, however, will always have an abnormal response to exercise. On the other hand, data gathered from animals suggest that aerobic exercise training in anemic individuals can improve exercise endurance to levels superior to those of nonanemic sedentary normals. Thus, persons with refractory anemia will always have their peak aerobic performance limited by the anemia, but submaximal performance is largely a parameter of skeletal muscle function, which can be markedly improved by endurance training.

Management and Medications

The causes for anemia include blood loss, nutritional deficiencies, decreased red cell production, and shortened red cell life span. In women, the most common cause of anemia is loss of blood during the menstrual cycle. Management of blood loss through gastrointestinal bleeding consists of finding and stopping the source of bleeding. In persons with nutritional deficiencies the treatment is to identify, prevent, and/or supplement the deficiency (whether with iron, folate, or B-12). When red cell production is decreased, as in renal failure for example, the hormone erythropoietin may be used to stimulate red blood cell production. In persons in whom red cell life span is shortened (as in sickle cell anemia for example), transfusions are at risk for an iron overload (hemochromatosis), which can ultimately lead to severe consequences for many organs. For this reason most persons with congenital anemia are allowed to be chronically anemic. Treatments for the different types of anemia include the following:

- Iron: Replace deficiency (iron-poor diet), increase intake (often to match menstrual losses).

- Folic acid: Supplement folic acid-deficient diet.
- Vitamin B-12: Supplement B-12-deficient diets; pernicious anemia.
- Erythropoietin: Stimulate bone marrow to make red blood cells.

Recommendations for Exercise Testing

The exaggerated heart rate response to exercise and limited peak performance in persons with anemia suggest that aerobic exercise tests will be likely to end sooner than predicted by age and gender. Thus, one should consider choosing a low-level exercise protocol. Although there are no data to confirm the theory, persons with sickle cell anemia might be at risk for inducing a sickle cell crisis during intense anaerobic exercise. It seems prudent to be cautious about testing a person with sickle cell anemia or trait. These people should not be allowed to become dehydrated.

Recommendations for Exercise Programming

The main goal of the exercise program is to improve endurance. Any form of large muscle exercise is acceptable, although intensity of exercise should be moderate. In persons with sickle cell anemia, high-intensity exercise leading to dehydration may cause a sickle cell crisis. Persons with either sickle cell anemia or trait must maintain liberal fluid intake in order to avoid dehydration. The optimal frequency and duration of training sessions are not known. Adaptability is not known, but the time course of improvement in performance is presumably normal after anemia is corrected.

Special Considerations

Avoid high-intensity exercise and dehydration in persons with sickle cell disease or trait.

Suggested Readings

Gozal, D., P. Thiriet, E. Mbala, D. Wouassi, H. Galas, A. Geyssant, and J. Lacour. 1992. Effect of different modalities of exercise and recovery on exercise performance in subjects with sickle cell trait. *Med. Sci. Sports Exerc.* 24: 1325-31.

Gregg, S.G., W.T. Willis, and G.A. Brooks. 1989. Interactive effects of anemia and muscle oxidative capacity on exercise endurance. *J. Appl. Physiol.* 67: 765-70.

Jones, S., R. Binder, and E. Donowho. 1970. Sudden death in sickle cell trait. *N. Engl. J. Med.* 282: 323-25.

McConnell, M., S. Daniels, J. Lobel, F. James, and S. Kaplan. 1989. Hemodynamic responses to exercise in patients with sickle cell anemia. *Pediatr. Cardiol.* 10: 141-44.

Sproule, B., J.H. Mitchell, and W. Miller. 1960. Cardiopulmonary physiological responses to heavy exercise in patients with anemia. *J. Clin. Invest.* 39: 378-88.

ANEMIA: EXERCISE TESTING

METHODS	MEASURES	ENDPOINTS	COMMENTS
Endurance **6-minute walk**	• Distance covered	• 6 minutes	• Useful throughout training program.

SPECIAL CONSIDERATIONS

• Occult peripheral artery disease may be unmasked with increased claudication.
• Other tests (e.g., aerobic power) may be used. See table on testing in chapter 3.

ANEMIA: EXERCISE PROGRAMMING

MODES	GOALS	INTENSITY/ FREQUENCY/DURATION	TIME TO GOAL
Aerobic • Large muscle activities	• Increase $\dot{V}O_2$ max, peak work, and endurance.	• 40-70% peak HR. • RPE 11-13. • 3-7 days/week. • 30-60 minutes/session. • Emphasize increased duration over intensity.	• 4-6 months

SPECIAL CONSIDERATIONS

• Do not exercise if resting BP > 180/110 mmHg.
• Exercise when pressor response is controlled by medications, see chapter 10 on hypertension.

CHAPTER 22

Bleeding Disorders

George Selby, MD

University of Oklahoma Health Science Center

Overview of the Pathophysiology

The ability of the body to control bleeding after trauma requires the intricate coordination of coagulation and platelet aggregation. When a vessel is torn or cut, the open ends spasm, and this reduces blood flow and allows blood cells called platelets to aggregate at the site of bleeding. Substances released from the damaged vessel wall, as well as the activated platelets, initiate a series of interactions involving the coagulation proteins present in blood. The combination of platelet plugging and coagulation produces a durable clot at the site of injury. Subnormal coagulation or platelet plugging produces inappropriate or uncontrolled bleeding or both, so that bleeding disorders come in two main forms: those due to platelet abnormalities and those due to coagulation protein abnormalities.

The most common platelet disorder that causes bleeding is called thrombocytopenia. This is a condition with insufficient number of platelets. The hemorrhages seen in thrombocytopenia are called petechiae, which are pinpoint-sized red spots, too small to feel, that are commonly confused with a rash. Normal platelet counts range from 120,000 to 600,000 per cubic millimeter.

The coagulation pathway consists of proteins, suspended in blood, that when activated form a web-like tangle of precipitated proteins. These proteins are called factors, and the most common congenital factor disorders are factor VIII deficiency (classic hemophilia), factor IX deficiency (Christmas disease), and von Willebrand's disease. It is possible to develop *acquired factor deficiencies* through autoimmune illnesses, but these are rare. Also, many

people have medically induced factor deficiencies because they take "blood thinners" such as the medicine Coumadin. Fortunately, medical anticoagulation very rarely causes spontaneous bleeding.

The general clinical manifestations of each of these bleeding disorder problems can be summarized as follows:

- Thrombocytopenia—petechial bleeding
- Hemophilia (hemarthrosis)—bleeding into joints with subsequent contractures, retroperitoneal bleeding
- von Willebrand's—prolonged bleeding after minor trauma, gastrointestinal bleeding
- Medical anticoagulation—easy bruisability, gastrointestinal bleeding

Effects on the Exercise Response

The major risks for exercise in persons with low platelet counts or coagulation factor deficiencies are bleeding from trauma and very high blood pressure. In sedentary persons, bleeding from a low platelet count is rarely a problem unless the count is well below 100,000 per cubic millimeter. Occasionally, intracranial (inside the skull) bleeds occur spontaneously when the platelet count is markedly low (< 20,000 per cubic millimeter). There are no controlled data on exercise in patients with low platelets, but vigorous exercise is probably contraindicated when platelet counts are below 50,000 per cubic millimeter. Use of elastic bands, stationary bicycles, range of motion exercises, and ambulation should be encouraged in persons with platelet counts higher than 20,000 per cubic millimeter.

A few circumstances deserve special mention. First, since lifting heavy weights dramatically increases blood and intracranial pressures, the risk of an intracranial bleed probably outweighs the benefits in persons with platelets between 50,000 and

100,000 per cubic millimeter. Second, in persons with hemophilia or von Willebrand's disease, the mode of testing should minimize joint trauma and weight bearing. Additional limitations may be imposed by preexisting joint contractures from prior bleeds. Of course, these contractures may be good targets for flexibility testing and stretching exercises.

Effects of Exercise Training

There is no known effect of exercise training on bleeding disorders. In theory, one may consume platelets and coagulation factors during exercise (as a result of minor trauma). Persons with hemophilia benefit from regular exercise, but at some risk of bleeding into joints and developing joint contractures as a consequence. Frequently, obesity is a co-morbid condition that adds further insult to the weight-bearing joints. Neither aerobic nor strength training alters the underlying disorder of hemophilia, but non-weight-bearing aerobic exercise, as well as strength and flexibility training, can be of immense functional and psychological benefit.

Management and Medications

The management of bleeding disorders is determined by whether the problem predisposes to bleeding or to clotting and also by the cause of the disease. Persons with platelet disorders, then those with coagulation factor disorders, and finally those with prosthetic heart valves will be considered in turn.

In persons with low platelets due to an overly rapid destruction of platelets (most often by the immune system), the treatment is to decrease the rate of platelet destruction. This is done with immunosuppressive medicines such as prednisone, and sometimes through removal of the spleen. Replacing platelets by transfusion works only for a very short while and is therefore limited to hospitalized persons. In people with high platelets resulting from overproduction of platelets, the treatment is to decrease the rate of platelet formation. This is usually achieved by chemotherapy.

In persons with coagulation factor deficiencies, a variety of medicines can be used to raise factor concentrations. Purified factor transfusions are available for some factor deficiencies. Mild von Willebrand's disease can be treated to increase the level of von Willebrand factor. Unfortunately, as with platelet disorders, treatment for coagulation factor deficiencies is temporary.

Persons at risk for inappropriate clot formation because of mechanical heart valves, dilated hearts, or deep vein thrombosis require some form of anticoagulation. These inappropriate clots are very dangerous because they can either grow in place and block blood flow, or break off and lodge downstream in blood vessels critical to vital organs such as the brain or lungs. For this reason, such individuals are given a "blood thinner," which is usually Coumadin or heparin.

Recommendations for Exercise Testing

- Persons with hemophilia should avoid weight-bearing exercise.

- Range-of-motion testing will help in managing flexibility exercises for persons with hemophilia.

- No high-resistance strength testing should be performed by persons with low platelet counts (risks intracranial bleed).

Recommendations for Exercise Programming

The goal of exercise training is to improve endurance, strength, and flexibility. Swimming or stationary cycling is recommended for persons with hemophilia. Outdoor cycling is non-weight-bearing on joints, but risks trauma and subsequent bleeding in a crash (sooner or later, virtually every cyclist falls). Flexibility exercises may help restore joint mobility in persons with hemophilia who are affected with contractures. The optimal frequency and duration of training are not known. Adaptability is not known, but is presumably normal.

Special Considerations

- Aspirin and other nonsteroidal anti-inflammatory drugs (e.g., ibuprofen) render platelets inactive, and their use is dangerous in individuals who have concomitant bleeding or platelet disorders.

- Persons who have any bleeding disorder or who are receiving medical anticoagulation should avoid collisions and contact sports (e.g., football, hockey, basketball).

- Persons with low platelet counts should avoid high-resistance strength training; lower resistance should not be a risk.
- Nonsteroidal anti-inflammatory drugs shouldn't be used either as analgesics or as thrombosis prophylaxis.

Suggested Reading

Gilbert, M., J. Schorr, T. Holbrook, and D. Tiberio. 1985. *Hemophilia and sports.* New York: National Hemophilia Foundation.

BLEEDING DISORDERS: EXERCISE TESTING

METHODS	MEASURES	ENDPOINTS	COMMENTS
Strength **Free weights, machines, elastic bands**			• Avoid high-intensity resistance in persons with platelets < 100,000/mm³ or hemophilia/ von Willebrand's disease.
Flexibility **Goniometry**		• Asymmetrical or limited range of motion	• Hemarthrosis or surgery may attenuate walking ability.
Functional capacity **Gait analysis**		• Asymmetric gait	• Hemarthrosis or surgery may attenuate walking ability.

MEDICATIONS	SPECIAL CONSIDERATIONS
• Anticoagulant therapy: Minor risk of hemarthrosis. • Aspirin and other nonsteroid anti-inflammatory drugs (e.g., ibuprofen): Contraindicated.	• Hemophilia/von Willebrand's disease patients may have decreased range of motion and secondary atrophy of shoulders, elbows, wrists, hips, knees, and ankles secondary to old hemarthroses. • Avoid high-impact activities. • If considered at risk for CAD, see table on testing in chapters 3, 4, and 5.

BLEEDING DISORDERS: EXERCISE PROGRAMMING

MODES	GOALS	INTENSITY/ FREQUENCY/DURATION	TIME TO GOAL
Strength • Circuit training	• Reverse secondary atrophy.	• Mix of high repetitions/low resistance and low repetitions/high resistance.	• 4-6 months
Flexibility • Stretching	• Normalize range of motion in hemarthritic joints.		

SPECIAL CONSIDERATIONS

• Avoid high-impact activities.
• Consider psychiatric counseling if patient exhibits self-destructive behavior and recurrent injury.
• See table on exercise testing.

CHAPTER 23

Acquired Immune Deficiency Syndrome

Arthur LaPerriere, PhD, FACSM
Nancy Klimas, MD
Patricia Major, MD
Arlette Perry, PhD, FACSM
University of Miami School of Medicine

Overview of the Pathophysiology

The acquired immune deficiency syndrome (AIDS) will continue to pose serious health problems well into the next century. In fact, current figures from the World Health Organization reflect over 5 million cases of AIDS worldwide. Furthermore, it is estimated that more than 12 million people throughout the world (1 in 250) may be infected with the immunodeficiency virus (HIV), the etiologic agent for AIDS. In recent years, remarkable gains have been made in the prevention, diagnosis, and treatment of HIV disease. However, a vaccine or a cure for HIV is still unavailable and is not expected in the near future. Therefore, complementary strategies for the management of HIV disease, including behavioral interventions such as exercise training, constitute important adjunctive therapeutic modalities. Significant quantities of scientific evidence exist to indicate that exercise training is not only appropriate but warranted for many people with HIV.

HIV disease is a very dynamic and progressive disease, occurring from the selective infection (by HIV) of the CD4 cell of the immune system. This lymphocyte, also called the T-helper cell, is crucial for the normal defensive mechanisms of the immune system. The CD4 cells along with the macrophages release cytokines, such as various interleukins and tumor necrosis factor (alpha), that will activate other cells as well as potentiate activation of each other. Therefore, the absence of these critical elements will decrease all immune function. Depletion of the CD4 cells, then, results in immunosuppression that leads to

- increased risk of opportunistic infections,
- decreased food consumption and lean body mass,
- further decreased immune system function and advanced body tissue wasting, and
- disease progression and eventual death.

The progressive clinical nature of HIV disease can be usefully viewed in three dissimilar stages. Important distinctions are made between each stage and are useful for exercise testing and training. These are the three stages of HIV disease:

- **Stage One**—asymptomatic HIV seropositive
- **Stage Two**—early symptomatic HIV
- **Stage Three**—AIDS

In **Stage One** the individual is infected with HIV and therefore is potentially infectious to others by sexual or blood-borne routes. The person remains relatively healthy and completely free of any symptomatology for HIV disease. Stage One may last 10 or more years, probably depending on the health habits maintained by the individual. During **Stage Two**, often referred to as AIDS-related complex (ARC), the number of CD4 cells is moderately diminished, resulting in the development of a variety of intermittent or persistent signs and symptoms to include fatigue, diarrhea, weight loss, fever, and lymphadenopathy. With appropriate management of these early symptoms, most individuals are able to retard further disease progression for several years. **Stage Three**, characterized immunologically as a severe depletion of CD4 cells in the presence of malignancy or opportunistic infection, is the most advanced and severe stage of HIV disease. Advances made in antiviral agents and other adjuvant therapies for AIDS-related problems have allowed many to live a relatively high quality of life for numerous years after an AIDS diagnosis.

Effects on the Exercise Response

For individuals who are asymptomatic, HIV infection in most cases does not alter the exercise-related physiological responses to a single session of exercise. However, at a more advance stage of immunodeficiency, a decrease in exercise performance and training response has been observed. It appears that a limited exercise response to a maximum graded exercise test measuring aerobic capacity will vary.

- **Stage One**
  - No limitations on maximum graded exercise test for most individuals
  - All metabolic parameters within normal limits for most individuals

- **Stage Two**
  - Reduced exercise capacity
  - Reduced $\dot{V}O_2$ max, $\dot{V}O_2$ at ventilatory threshold, and maximal oxygen pulse
  - Reduced heart rate reserve and breathing reserve

- **Stage Three**
  - Dramatically reduced exercise capacity (maximum graded exercise test may not be possible for all individuals)
  - More severe $\dot{V}O_2$ limitations than in stage two
  - Altered neuroendocrine responses

The reasons for a reduced exercise capacity are not fully understood, but such reduction may be the result of symptoms secondary to HIV infection. Many individuals who are HIV positive will terminate a graded exercise test because of physical exhaustion, muscular fatigue, or both.

Effects of Exercise Training

Exercise is safe and beneficial for most individuals infected with HIV, even though a full understanding of the risks and benefits of exercise training has not yet been reached. Several studies have shown that regular participation in moderate aerobic activities results in an increase in the number of CD4 cells. In addition, aerobic and progressive resistance exercise regimes can increase lean body mass, mood state, oxidative and endurance capacity, and cognitive and physical energy needed for daily living. For most HIV-positive individuals this will result in an improved quality of life. In addition, the following effects of routine moderate exercise regimens are specific to the different stages of HIV disease:

- **Stage One**
  - Increase in CD4 cells.
  - Possible delay in onset of symptoms.
  - Increase in muscle function and size.

- **Stage Two**
  - Increase in CD4 cells (lesser magnitude of change).
  - Possible diminished severity and frequency of some symptoms.

- **Stage Three**
  - Effects on CD4 cells are unknown.
  - Effects on symptoms are inconclusive.

Intense exercise temporarily depletes T-cell counts in healthy athletes who are not HIV infected. The effects of intense exercise on the immune systems of individuals infected with HIV are not known, but it is recommended that *intense exercise be avoided* because of its immunosuppressive activity.

Management and Medications

Exercise training is an excellent adjuvant therapy for most people infected with HIV, but it should be used in combination with nutritional therapy and psychologic interventions, not to mention primary medical treatments. The multitude of varied symptoms and opportunistic infections seen in HIV disease are usually managed with myriad medications including antivirals, antibacterials, and gastrointestinal medication as well as anti-cancer treatments that can have a variety of implications for exercise.

Recommendations for Exercise Testing

All people infected with HIV, regardless of age or stage of disease, and prior to beginning any type of training, should have a complete physical examination and obtain medical clearance to exercise. In addition, a *comprehensive* assessment of aerobic capacity, strength, neuromuscular ability, and flexibility is recommended. Measurement of the aerobic component should use symptom-limited tests and will vary depending upon the stage of disease.

- **Stages One and Two**
  - Maximal aerobic power

- **Stage Three**
  - Submaximal aerobic power

The primary objectives of the exercise evaluation are to determine

- functional capacity,
- appropriate intensity range for aerobic exercise training,
- appropriate mode of exercise training,
- potential hazards or contraindications to exercise training,
- perceived exertions and potential psychological stressors, and
- psychomotor skills for appropriate mode of exercise.

The use of a stationary bicycle ergometer is strongly encouraged because of neuromuscular complications that develop as the disease progresses, which preclude treadmill testing.

Recommendations for Exercise Programming

Individuals with HIV should begin to use exercise as an adjuvant therapy as early as possible during their disease, preferably while still asymptomatic and healthy. The exercise program should be individualized and should integrate the outcomes of the exercise evaluation with the stage of disease, immunological blood work profiles (CD4 count), and medical treatments.

Special Considerations

It should be remembered that HIV is a contagious disease, and **Universal Precautions** should be followed at all times. In addition, the individual with HIV is at an increased risk for infectious diseases, and care should be taken to minimize the risk. It is important that before each exercise session, particularly during the early weeks of training, one assess the individual's general health status (e.g., evaluate blood pressure, pulse rate, temperature, body composition, and psychomotor skills, and ask a few simple questions to determine whether it is OK to exercise). As an example, if an individual has had diarrhea for a few days, the exercise session should be postponed. In addition, the exercise program should be routinely reassessed and modified as the individual increases in aerobic capacity or progresses in the disease. It is also important to develop relapse prevention strategies to help people continue to exercise on a routine basis throughout their disease, even after acute illness.

Suggested Readings

Calabrese, L.H., and A. LaPerriere. 1993. Human immunodeficiency virus infection, exercise and athletics. *Sports Med.* 15 (1): 6-13.

Fauci, A.S. 1988. The human immunodeficiency virus: Infectivity and mechanisms of pathogenesis. *Science* 239: 627.

LaPerriere, A., ed. In press. *Handbook of exercise medicine.* New York: Gordon and Breach.

LaPerriere, A., M.H. Antoni, M.A. Fletcher, and N. Schneiderman. 1992. Exercise and health maintenance in HIV. In *Clinical assessment and treatment of HIV,* ed. M.L. Galantion, 65-76. Thorofare, NJ: Slack.

LaPerriere, A., M.H. Antoni, and N. Schneiderman. 1990. Exercise intervention attenuates emotional distress and natural killer cell decrements following notification of positive serologic status for HIV-1. *Biofeedback and Self-Regulation* 15: 229-42.

LaPerriere, A., M.A. Fletcher, and N. Klimas. 1991. Aerobic exercise training in an AIDS risk group. *Int. J. Sports Med.* 12: 53-57.

LaPerriere, A., N. Schneiderman, M.H. Antoni, and M.A. Fletcher. 1990. Aerobic exercise training and psychoneuroimmunology in AIDS. In *Psy-*

chological perspectives on AIDS, ed. A. Baum and L. Temoshok. Hillsdale, NJ: Erlbaum.

Pothoff, G., K. Wassermann, and H. Ostmann. 1994. Impairment of exercise capacity in various groups of HIV-infected patients. *Respiration* 61: 80-85.

Rigsby, L., R.K. Dishman, A.W. Jackson, G.S. Maclean, and P.B. Raven. 1992. Effects of exercise training on men seropositive for the human im-munodeficiency virus-1. *Med. Sci. Sports Exerc.* 24: 6-12.

Spence, D.W., M.A. Galantino, K.A. Mossberg, and S.O. Zimmerman. 1990. Progressive resistance exercise: Effect on muscle function and anthropometry of a select AIDS population. *Arch. Phys. Med. Rehabil.* 71: 644-48.

ACQUIRED IMMUNE DEFICIENCY SYNDROME: EXERCISE TESTING

METHODS	MEASURES	ENDPOINTS*	COMMENTS

Aerobic power
 	
Treadmill
   (1-2 METs/stage)
 	
Cycle
   Ramp protocol (5-50 watts/
   3 min stage)
	• 12-lead ECG, heart rate
	
	• Blood pressure
	
	• RPE
		• Serious dysrhythmias
		• > 2 mm ST-segment depression or elevation
		• Ischemic threshold
		• T-wave inversion with significant ST change
		
		• SBP > 260 mmHg or DBP > 115 mmHg
		
		• Volitional fatigue
			• Indicated for asymptomatic patients or those with early symptoms. Not indicated for those with severe symptoms.
			
			• Record time to exhaustion.

Endurance **1-mile walk** **6-minute walk**	• Time elapsed • Distance travelled	• 1 mile • 6 minutes	
Strength **Isotonic/isokinetic**	• 10-12 repetitions maximum • Maximal voluntary contraction		
Flexibility **Sit-and-reach**			
Neuromuscular **Gait analysis** **Reaction time** **Balance**			• Especially useful for severely symptomatic people.
Functional capacity **Daily living activity, performance-based tests**			

*Measurements of particular significance; do not *always* indicate test termination.

(continued)

ACQUIRED IMMUNE DEFICIENCY SYNDROME: EXERCISE TESTING *(continued)*

MEDICATIONS	SPECIAL CONSIDERATIONS
• Antibiotics: No direct effect on exercise, but opportunistic pneumonia risks desaturation. • AZT/DDI: Can cause anemia. • Inhaled bronchodilators: Tachycardia. • Theophylline: Tachycardia. • Thiazide diuretics: Reduced exercise tolerance. • Over-the-counter remedies: Include cardiovascular stimulants (tachycardia/hypertension).	• Fatigue is common and may signify progression of HIV/opportunistic disease or thyroid disease. • Anemia common. • Muscle wasting/weakness common. • Scarring from pneumocystis pneumonia is the most common clinical disorder. Upper respiratory tract infections occur frequently. • Chronic diarrhea can lead to hypovolemia, hyponatremia, and hypoglycemia. • HIV encephalopathy/neuropathy may lead to neuromuscular sequelae. • Strict infection control procedures must be followed as outlined by CDC/OSHA. • Body composition analysis may be desirable.

ACQUIRED IMMUNE DEFICIENCY SYNDROME: EXERCISE PROGRAMMING

MODES	GOALS	INTENSITY/ FREQUENCY/DURATION	TIME TO GOAL
Aerobic • Large muscle activities	• Increase aerobic capacity. • Increase work capacity.	• 50-85% peak HR • RPE 10-14 on Borg 6-20 scale • 3-5 days/week • 20-60 minutes/session	• 3-6 months
Strength • Free weights, weight machines	• Increase maximal number of repetitions.		• 3-6 months
Flexibility • Stretching/yoga • Massage therapy	• Increase range of motion. • Increase neuromuscular excitability. • Decrease joint soreness and risk of injury.		
Functional • Activity-specific exercise	• Increase daily living activities, prevent deterioration. • Restore vocational potential. • Improve quality of life. • Recreation/fun.		

MEDICATIONS	SPECIAL CONSIDERATIONS
• See table on exercise testing.	• See table on exercise testing.

CHAPTER 24

Organ Transplant

Patricia L. Painter, PhD, FACSM

University of California at San Francisco

Overview of the Pathophysiology

The most common organ transplants performed in the United States are kidney, liver, heart (see chapter 9), lung, and pancreas. Transplant surgery is performed on persons with end-stage organ failure with the exception of pancreas transplant, which is performed on individuals with type I diabetes. Some centers perform simultaneous multiple organ transplant (e.g., simultaneous kidney and pancreas or heart and lung) when indicated. The pathophysiology of each of the end-stage diseases requiring transplant differs. After successful transplantation, however, most concerns are related to side effects or complications of immunosuppression medications. Except for the case of primary nonfunction or rejection of the transplant, the pathology present after transplant is related primarily to side effects of medications with a major concern being infection. Other side effects will include hypertension, hyperlipidemia, corticosteroid-induced diabetes, corticosteroid-induced muscle weakness, and reduced bone density. Many individuals experience significant and often excessive weight gain that is frequently attributed to increased appetite related to corticosteroid use. However, accumulating evidence suggests that weight gain may be related to increased caloric intake—not necessarily due to increased appetite induced by the medication, but to increased feelings of well-being with no restrictions in diet.

Individuals presenting for organ transplant are typically deconditioned, since the progression of the disease prevents significant physical activity. Physical activity levels may, however, be higher in the dialysis patients.

Effects on the Exercise Response

Peak $\dot{V}O_2$ in kidney transplant recipients averages 30 ml·kg^{-1}·min^{-1} and is similar to normal sedentary values. These clients often exhibit exaggerated blood pressure responses to a single session of exercise. Generally, heart rate responses to exercise are normal.

Preliminary data indicate that one year after surgery, liver transplant recipients have peak $\dot{V}O_2$ levels below those measured for kidney transplant recipients (average in 10 recipients was 26 ml·kg^{-1}·min^{-1}). Normal exercise heart rate and blood pressure responses were reported for this group. Peak $\dot{V}O_2$ measured in another group of 18 subjects six months postsurgery was found to be similar to the pretransplant levels of 18 ml·kg^{-1}·min^{-1}. Six-minute walk distances and measures of muscle strength may increase after transplant. Lung transplant recipients initially show an increase in exercise capacity after three months; but measurements of exercise capacity one and two years after surgery do not show further increases, despite improved measures of pulmonary function. No studies exist in pancreas transplant recipients.

Effects of Exercise Training

Anecdotal information suggests that organ transplant recipients are able to achieve very high levels of functional capacity as evidenced by impressive showings in such events as the United States and

International Transplant Games. Presently, exercise training studies in various transplant populations are limited. Two exercise training studies with kidney transplant recipients indicated significant improvements in exercise capacity (magnitude of change was 25-28%). In addition, improved blood pressure control, indications of bone remodeling, and increased muscle strength have been reported. Although muscle weakness may continue to persist, specific resistance training programs increase muscle strength and reduce the fat-to-muscle ratio, presumably counteracting the muscle-wasting effects of glucocorticoid therapy.

Management and Medications

After organ transplant, virtually all persons are treated with immunosuppression therapy to prevent rejection. Medications include glucocorticoids (prednisone), cyclosporine, and azathioprine. Although new immunosuppressive medications are continually being developed, transplant recipients are always at risk for rejection of their transplant. In addition to the immunosuppression medications, many persons are on antihypertensive therapy and lipid-lowering medications (see chapters 10 and 17 and appendix A).

Recommendations for Exercise Testing

Standard exercise testing protocols are acceptable for transplant recipients. Low-level exercise protocols are indicated early after transplant. The high prevalence of cardiac risk factors and high incidence of cardiovascular disease after transplantation indicate that a 12-lead ECG should be used during exercise testing. Since skeletal muscle weakness is prevalent and may result in nonmaximal performances, exercise tests may be of limited diagnostic use.

Recommendations for Exercise Programming

Exercise training should begin soon after transplant and should incorporate activity and lifestyle into the "new life." Although gradual progression is essential, aerobic activities are tolerated well. Since transplant recipients present in a significantly deconditioned state, most will need strength training. Joint discomfort may be experienced by those on high doses of prednisone and during the "taper" phase of the immunosuppression management. Non-weight-bearing activities may be best tolerated while many recipients are able to progress to jogging and other sporting activities without difficulty. It is recommended that some low-level activities be continued during rejection episodes to maintain a pattern of activity and counteract muscle-wasting effects of the prednisone doses. Prednisone affects muscle metabolism so that a longer period is necessary for strength gain. Therefore, strength training programs may have to incorporate a slower rate of progression to allow for this longer adaptation time.

Suggested Readings

Kempeneers, G.L.G., T.D. Noakes, R. Van Zyl-Smit, K.H. Myburgh, M. Lambert, B. Adams, and T. Wiggins. 1990. Skeletal muscle limits the exercise tolerance of renal transplant recipients: Effects of a graded exercise program. *Am. J. Kidney Dis.* 16: 57-65.

Miller, T.D., R.W. Squires, G.T. Gau, D.M. Ilstrup, P.P. Frohnert, and S. Steriot. 1987. Graded exercise testing and training after renal transplantation: A preliminary study. *Mayo Clin. Proc.* 62: 773-77.

Painter, P.L. 1992. Exercise following organ transplantation. *J. Cardiovascular Physical Therapy* 3 (1): 4-8.

ORGAN TRANSPLANT: EXERCISE TESTING

METHODS	MEASURES	ENDPOINTS*	COMMENTS
Aerobic power **Treadmill** (0.5-2 METs/stage) **Cycle** (5-20 watts/min) ramp protocol (15-25 watts/3 min stage)	• 12-lead ECG, heart rate • Blood pressure • RPE • METs	• Serious dysrhythmias • > 2 mm ST-segment depression or elevation • Ischemic threshold • T-wave inversion with significant ST change • SBP > 260 mmHg or DBP > 115 mmHg • Leg fatigue	• Submaximal fitness testing may be appropriate for most clients since cardiac status is, in most cases, known prior to acceptance for transplant. • Leg fatigue is typically the reason for test termination.
Strength **Isotonic/isokinetic**	• Maximal number of repetitions • Isokinetic work/peak torque at fast speeds		• Be aware of prior long-standing bone disease in kidney transplant recipients and other persons who have been on long-term glucocorticoid therapy; 1 repetition maximum test may not be appropriate.
Flexibility **Sit-and-reach**			

*Measurements of particular significance; do not *always* indicate test termination.

MEDICATIONS	SPECIAL CONSIDERATIONS
• Prednisone: Causes muscle weakness and wasting, some joint discomfort; associated with excessive weight gain and truncal obesity. • Immunosuppressants (e.g., cyclosporine, azathioprine, FK506): Rare myopathies. • Antihypertensive agents: See exercise testing table in chapter 10 and appendix A. • Lipid-lowering agents: See exercise testing table in chapter 17 and appendix A.	• Persons typically present in a deconditioned state. • Most persons are limited by muscle weakness. • Be aware of steroid-induced diabetes that occurs after transplant in about 30% of persons.

ORGAN TRANSPLANT: EXERCISE PROGRAMMING

MODES	GOALS	INTENSITY/ FREQUENCY/DURATION	TIME TO GOAL
Aerobic • Large muscle activities	• Increase aerobic capacity. • Increase time to exhaustion. • Increase work capacity. • Improve blood pressure. • Assist with weight management. • Reduce risk of cardiovascular disease.	• 50-90% peak HR. • 50-85% peak $\dot{V}O_2$. • Monitor RPE. • 4-7 days/week. • 20-60 minutes/session.	• 3-6 months
Strength/Anaerobic • Free weights, weight machines, isokinetic machines • Interval training	• Increase maximal number of repetitions. • Reverse steroid-induced muscle wasting and weakness. • Improve performance for patients interested in competition.		• 4-6 months
Flexibility • Stretching/yoga	• Maintain/increase range of motion.		
Functional • Activity-specific exercise	• Increase daily living activities. • Recreation/fun.		

MEDICATIONS	SPECIAL CONSIDERATIONS
• See table on exercise testing.	• Vigorous training and training for competition are possible for those with a good baseline of regular activity. Gradual progression should be practiced. • Persons typically present in a deconditioned state. • Most persons are limited by muscle weakness. • Be aware of steroid-induced diabetes that accurs in about 30% of patients. • Low-impact activities may be most appropriate for persons on high doses of prednisone and/or those with joint disease. • Progression with resistance training may have to be slower due to the prednisone-induced muscle wasting. • Exercise intensity should be reduced to mild levels during rejection episodes until rejection therapy return measures of rejection back to baseline levels. • Caloric reduction must be a part of weight management strategy.

CHAPTER 25

Chronic Fatigue Syndrome

Kathy E. Sietsema, MD

Harbor - UCLA Medical Center

Overview of the Pathophysiology

Chronic fatigue syndrome (CFS) is the term currently used in the United States for a condition characterized by persistent debilitating fatigue, not relieved by rest and not accounted for by any specifically identified medical or psychiatric condition. Although it frequently appears to be a sequela of prior viral infection, the cause of this syndrome remains unknown. Considerable research effort is currently directed at identifying a possible immunologic, inflammatory, or neuroendocrine basis for CFS, yet no pathognomonic finding on physical or laboratory examination has been identified. The condition is therefore defined primarily by its symptoms, which in addition to fatigue may include frequent sore throats, painful lymph nodes, headache, difficulty with concentration and memory, low-grade fever, and others. Diffuse nonarticular soft tissue pain, often fitting the definition of a condition termed *fibromyalgia,* is also common in clients with CFS, and in some clients is the dominant complaint. Approximately 75% of clients with CFS are women.

In order to provide a basis for standardizing populations used in clinical research of this condition, the Centers for Disease Control (CDC) published a set of criteria for defining cases of CFS. To be designated as having CFS by these criteria, clients must meet both of the major criteria and have six to eight

of the symptoms and physical findings outlined in the minor criteria. These criteria are simply a description of the most typical features of the syndrome and are designed to identify relatively homogeneous client populations for research purposes. Thus there may be individuals who are judged by their physicians to have CFS even though they do not fully fit the CDC criteria. Conversely, since the symptoms are not specific for CFS, it is possible for a client with another condition causing the symptoms to be erroneously designated as having CFS. Therefore, it is important that other conditions that could account for the symptoms be excluded before a diagnosis of CFS is made. Criteria have been established by the CDC for case definition of CFS (adapted from Holmes et al. 1988).

- **Major Criteria***
  - New onset of persistent or relapsing fatigue, not resolving with bed rest, and severe enough to reduce or impair average daily activities below 50% of previous levels for at least six months.
  - Other clinical conditions that could cause similar symptoms must be excluded by appropriate medical evaluation. These other conditions include, but are not limited to, malignancy, autoimmune disease, localized infection, chronic bacterial or parasitic disease, endocrine disorder, and other chronic disease.

- **Minor Criteria***
- **Symptom Criteria***
  - Mild fever
  - Sore throat
  - Painful lymph nodes in the neck or underarm regions

- Generalized muscle weakness
- Muscle discomfort or myalgia
- Prolonged (24 hour or more) generalized fatigue after levels of exercise that were previously well tolerated
- Generalized headache
- Migratory arthralgia
- Neuropsychologic complaints
- Sleep disturbance
- History of symptom complex having begun acutely following viral infection
- **Physical Criteria***
  - Low-grade fever documented by a health care professional
  - Nonexudative pharyngitis
  - Palpable or tender lymph nodes in the neck

*To meet the case definition, clients must meet both *major* criteria and in addition must either meet eight *symptom* criteria, or meet six *symptom* criteria plus two *physical* criteria.

Effects on the Exercise Response

Exercise testing is not a routine part of establishing the diagnosis of CFS, as there are no unique diagnostic findings. When tested, clients with CFS are found on average to have mild reductions in both peak $\dot{V}O_2$ and ventilatory threshold compared to normal, but findings in individual clients vary considerably. It is not known whether a reduction in exercise capacity may be attributed in part to CFS itself or whether it is wholly due to the deconditioning that accompanies a reduction in activity level. Although there are occasional reports to the contrary, the consensus of findings from studies of clients with CFS is that cardiac, pulmonary, and muscular function remain essentially normal, and the symptom of fatigue is therefore viewed as being "central" (neurologic) in nature. While exercise testing does not establish a diagnosis of CFS, it may be requested as part of a client's evaluation for excluding other conditions, such as cardiovascular diseases, that could account for the same symptoms. Exercise testing may also be used for designing an individualized exercise program for clients who have a diagnosis of CFS.

Effects of Exercise Training

A common complaint among clients with CFS is that their fatigue and other symptoms are worsened in the days following any amount of physical exertion. The basis for this is not understood. Attempts at exercise conditioning may be frustrated by this circumstance, however, and a successful exercise prescription needs to respect the observation. Despite the initial aggravation of symptoms caused by exercise, some overall improvement in symptoms has been reported for clients with the diagnosis of fibromyalgia after moderate exercise training, and one other published study has reported similar success with exercise training in CFS clients. In both instances, clients were reported to demonstrate increased aerobic capacity and improved subjective sense of well-being after exercise conditioning.

Management and Medications

Because the pathogenesis of CFS is not understood, treatment is directed at reduction of symptoms rather than reversal of the underlying condition. Medications and other interventions therefore vary according to which symptoms are predominant, and may also vary with the experience and judgments of the primary physician.

Most commonly used medications include antidepressants, often taken at night to aid in initiation of sleep, and analgesics for clients with fibromyalgia or other pain symptoms. It may be anticipated that a variety of experimental treatments, both pharmacologic and nonpharmacologic, will continue to undergo evaluation for treatment of this condition in the coming years.

Recommendations for Exercise Testing

Incremental exercise testing with monitoring of standard cardiovascular and ventilatory responses (electrocardiogram, blood pressure, heart rate, respiratory gas exchange, and ventilation) may be indicated as a screening test for clients whose diagnosis is not yet established. If a myopathic disease is suspected as an alternative diagnosis, appropriate screening for metabolic intermediates in blood or muscle samples might also be incorporated into the study. Clients with long-standing symptoms are very likely to have had a low level of exercise activity and to have undergone deconditioning as a result. Work rate increments used in testing will therefore usually be low relative to the levels that would be predicted for age, size, and gender.

Recommendations for Exercise Programming

Little is known about the clinical effect of exercise training in this group of clients. Thus, general recommendations regarding exercise programming for all clients with CFS are difficult to make. Reports of clinical improvement resulting from exercise conditioning could reflect a systematic bias, in that clients who do not tolerate exercise may be underrepresented in such studies and therefore not be fully reflected in the outcome measurements. To date, however, there does not appear to be any evidence of adverse outcomes from prospectively studied exercise trials in clients with CFS.

For clients who wish to undertake an exercise program, the following general guidelines offer a conservative approach to exercise programming that takes into account some of the unique difficulties characteristic of this client population:

- The goal of exercise programming in this condition should be first and foremost to prevent further deconditioning that can compound the disability of chronic fatigue. Clients and trainers alike should resist the temptation to adopt a traditional method of training aimed at optimization of aerobic capacity, and should focus instead on modest goals of preventing progressive deconditioning.

- Clients should be warned that they may feel increased fatigue in the first few weeks of an exercise program.

- Exercise should generally be initiated at very low levels, based on the client's current activity tolerance.

- Aerobic exercise should utilize a familiar activity, such as walking, that can be started at a low level.

- Flexibility exercises may be prescribed to preserve normal range of motion.

- Strength training, if prescribed, should focus on preservation of levels of strength commensurate with daily living activities.

- The progression of exercise activity should focus primarily on increasing the duration of moderate-intensity activities in preference to increasing exercise intensity.

Special Considerations

Several psychological considerations are relevant to exercise in people with CFS:

- Chronic fatigue syndrome is often accompanied by depression, although it is not clear how much of the depression is the result of the change in lifestyle resulting from persistent symptoms and how much may be inherent to CFS itself.

- Because misunderstanding abounds concerning CFS, some clients may express frustration and disillusionment with both lay and medical communities, which may have been less than sympathetic to their problems.

- A supportive and understanding environment is important in evaluating and counseling clients with CFS.

It may also be useful to consider the following with these clients:

- Fibromyalgia or other soft tissue pain is sometimes a component of CFS symptomatology, most often affects the shoulder girdle and hip regions, and may necessitate individualizing of exercise testing postures and procedures.

- Clients with CFS cope with their symptoms in part by planning their activities so as to "budget" their energy. Providing advance information about what they can anticipate when referred for exercise testing or training will help them to do so.

Suggested Readings

Fukada, K., S.E. Straus, I. Hickie, M.C. Sharpe, J.C. Dobbins, and A. Komaroff. 1994. The chronic fatigue syndrome: A comprehensive approach to its definition and study. International Chronic Fatigue Study Group. *Ann. Intern. Med.* 121: 953-59.

Fulcher, K., K. Claery, and P. White. 1994. A placebo controlled study of a graded exercise programme in patients with the chronic fatigue syndrome *Eur. J. Appl. Physiol.* 69 (suppl.): S35.

Holmes, G.P., J.E. Kaplan, N.M. Gantz, A.L. Komaroff, L.B. Schonberger, S.E. Straus, J.F. Jones, R.E. Dubois, C. Cunningham-Rundles, S. Pahwa, G. Tosato, L.S. Zegans, D.T. Purilo, N. Brown, R.T. Schooley, and I. Brus. 1988. Chronic fatigue syndrome: A working case definition. *Ann. Intern. Med.* 108: 387-89.

McCain, G.A. 1986. Role of physical fitness training in the fibrositis/fibromyalgia syndrome. *Am. J. Med.* 81 (suppl. 3A): 73-77.

Riley, M.S., C.J. O'Brien, D.R. McClusky, N.P. Bell, and D.P. Nicholls. 1990. Aerobic work capacity in patients with chronic fatigue syndrome. *Br. Med. J.* 301: 953-56.

Shafran, S.D. 1991. The chronic fatigue syndrome. *Am. J. Med.* 90: 730-39.

Wilson, A., I. Hickie, A. Lloyd, and D. Wakefield. 1994. The treatment of chronic fatigue syndrome: Science and speculation. *Am. J. Med.* 96: 544-50.

CHRONIC FATIGUE SYNDROME: EXERCISE TESTING

METHODS	MEASURES	ENDPOINTS*	COMMENTS
Aerobic power **Cycle** (1-20 watts/min) ramp protocol (25-50 watts/3 min stage) **Treadmill** (1-2 METs/3 min stage)	• 12-lead ECG, heart rate • Blood pressure • RPE (Borg 6-20 scale) • METs • Other measures as clinically indicated	• Serious dysrhythmias • > 2 mm ST-segment depression or elevation • Ischemic threshold • T-wave inversion with significant ST change • SBP > 260 mmHg or DBP > 115 mmHg	• Maximal aerobic power test may be indicated for exclusion of other diagnoses.

*Measurements of particular significance; do not *always* indicate test termination.

MEDICATIONS	SPECIAL CONSIDERATIONS
• Most commonly used agents: Unlikely to interfere. Individual history should be obtained.	• Patients may have soft tissue pain syndromes that limit tolerance for standard testing postures. • Patients may be quite deconditioned. Low work rate increments are usually appropriate. • Schedule testing for a day that the client does not have other activities scheduled.

CHRONIC FATIGUE SYNDROME: EXERCISE PROGRAMMING

MODES	GOALS	INTENSITY/ FREQUENCY/DURATION	TIME TO GOAL
Aerobic • Large muscle activities (walking, rowing, cycling, swimming, etc.)	• Increase aerobic capacity. • Increase and maintain functional work capacity.	• RPE 9-12. • Exercise intensity is not main focus. • 3-5 days/week. • 5 minutes/session, progressing to 60 minutes/session as tolerated.	• Average of 3 months
Functional • Activity-specific exercise	• Increase ease of performing daily living activities.		

MEDICATIONS	SPECIAL CONSIDERATIONS
• Most commonly used agents: Unlikely to interfere. Individual history should be obtained.	• Optimal dosing for these patients is unknown. A prudent approach is to begin with an activity that the individual patient is known to tolerate and build duration slowly. • Symptoms may worsen initially when exercise training begins.

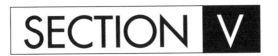

SECTION V

Orthopedic Diseases and Disabilities

Section Editor:

Kenneth H. Pitetti, PhD, FACSM
Wichita State University

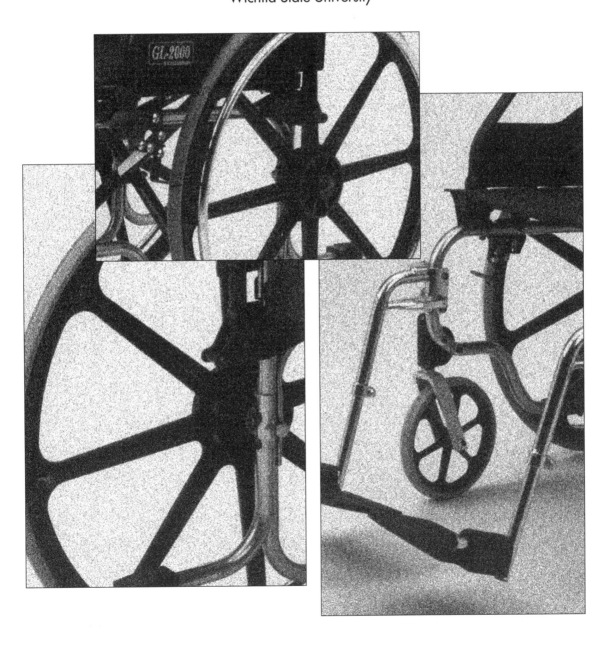

CHAPTER 26

Arthritis

Marian A. Minor, PT, PhD

Missouri Arthritis Rehabilitation Research and Training Center

Donald R. Kay, MD, FACP, FACR

University of Missouri Health Sciences Center

Overview of the Pathophysiology

There are more than 100 rheumatologic diseases, each having varying degrees of articular and systemic involvement. The two most common conditions are osteoarthritis (degenerative joint disease) and rheumatoid arthritis (an inflammatory, multi-joint, multi-system disease). Rheumatoid arthritis is an inflammatory disease arising from pathologic activity of the immune system against joint tissue. The inflammatory response may affect many joints and other organ systems. Degenerative joint disease is localized to the affected joint or joints and appears first as deficits in articular cartilage. Table 26.1 outlines the most common rheumatologic diseases.

Effects on the Exercise Response

The potential for inflammatory rheumatic diseases to affect cardiac and pulmonary function, as well as to cause widespread vasculitis, must be considered in the decision for anyone with a systemic rheumatic disease to perform vigorous exercise. Vigorous exercise is contraindicated in the presence of

Table 26.1	MOST COMMON RHEUMATOLOGIC DISEASES WITH JOINT INVOLVEMENT		
DIAGNOSIS	**DISEASE TYPE**	**COMMONLY AFFECTED JOINTS**	**FEATURES RELATED TO EXERCISE**
Osteoarthritis	Local degeneration	Hands, spine, hips, knees	Joint pain, stiffness Osteophyte Cartilage destruction
Rheumatoid arthritis	Inflammatory, systemic	Wrist, hands, knees, feet, cervical spine	Morning stiffness > 30 min Acute and chronic inflammation Chronic pain & loss of joint integrity
Lupus	Inflammatory, systemic	Hands, knees, elbows, feet	Arthralgia Fatigue
Ankylosing spondylitis Psoriatic arthritis	Inflammatory, systemic	Spine, hip/shoulder girdle, knees	Pain Joint fusion Enthesopathy
Gout Pseudogout	Crystal deposition	Great toe, ankles, knees, wrists	Acute joint inflammation Pain Tophi

acute joint inflammation (red, hot, swollen, painful) or uncontrolled systemic disease. However, the more common presentation of a person with inflammatory rheumatic disease is subacute or chronic joint symptoms and possible sequelae of previous systemic inflammation. In the absence of acute flare-ups in persons with systemic forms of arthritis (e.g., rheumatoid, lupus), the musculoskeletal, biomechanical, and cardiovascular effects of degenerative and inflammatory joint disease on exercise testing are similar. There is not much difference among the various systemic forms of arthritis in terms of effects on the exercise response. In persons having an acute flare-up of systemic illness, the exercise response can be quite blunted.

- Persons with joint involvement tend to be less active and less fit (cardiovascular and musculoskeletal) than their unaffected peers.

- Pain, stiffness, biomechanical inefficiency, and gait abnormalities can increase the metabolic cost of physical activity by as much as 50%.

- Joint range of motion may be restricted by stiffness, swelling, pain, bony changes, fibrosis, and ankylosis.

- Inability to perform rapid, repetitive movements affects exercise performance in terms of walking speed and bicycle revolutions per minute.

- Site and severity of joint involvement determine exercise mode for aerobic and strength tests.

- Deconditioned and poorly supported joints are at high risk for injury from high-impact or poorly controlled movement.

Effects of Exercise Training

Persons with either inflammatory or degenerative joint disease are able to participate in regular, conditioning exercise to improve cardiovascular status, muscular fitness, flexibility, and general health status. Improved aerobic capacity, endurance, strength, and flexibility are associated with improved function, decreased joint swelling and pain, increased social and physical activity in daily life, and lessened depression and anxiety. Disease-specific patterns of joint involvement should be considered during exercise prescription, monitoring, and follow-up assessments.

The most immediate benefit of conditioning exercise in this population may be to diminish effects of inactivity. Loss of flexibility, muscle atrophy, weakness, osteoporosis, elevated pain threshold, depression, and fatigue, which are problems common to both inflammatory and degenerative conditions, respond favorably to a low to moderate, gradually progressed exercise program. The potential for conditioning exercise to have a therapeutic effect on the disease process itself has yet to be determined.

Management and Medications

Joint protection, exercise, and education for self-management are essential components of comprehensive management. The goals are to decrease impairment, maintain or restore function, protect joint structures from further damage, and maintain healthful levels of physical activity. Ideally, care is coordinated in a multidisciplinary setting that offers preventive and rehabilitative care as well as medical management. To meet individual needs in an integrated program, the exercise component should incorporate joint protection and therapeutic exercise as needed. Health, safety, and successful exercise experiences for persons with joint disease can best be achieved by ongoing consultation with health care providers experienced in rheumatologic care and rehabilitation.

The major therapeutic goal in treatment of inflammatory rheumatic disease is to control the destructive inflammatory process. Medications prescribed to achieve this goal range from aspirin and other nonsteroidal anti-inflammatory drugs (NSAIDs) to disease-modifying drugs (DMARDs), oral and injectable gold therapy, and newer immunosuppressive agents. Oral corticosteroids may be used when other drugs do not control inflammation. Combination therapy with two or more slower-acting DMARDs is common to provide maximum inflammation and disease suppression. Drug therapy is usually continued indefinitely except when all signs of disease activity/progression disappear. In osteoarthritis, NSAIDs or acetaminophen is prescribed to manage symptoms of pain and stiffness. Local corticosteroid injections may be effective in both inflammatory and noninflammatory diseases to alleviate inflammation within specific joints or at other specific sites. Intra-articular injections should be given no more often than every four to six months, as frequent injections can cause tissue destruction. The need to restrict activity following an injection is debated; however, vigorous weight-bearing activities should be avoided for at least one week.

Recommendations for Exercise Testing

In spite of the challenges presented by joint pain and dysfunction in arthritis, safe and clinically meaningful exercise testing can be performed. Submaximal and subjective symptom-limited treadmill tests requiring less than 3 mph walking speed are well tolerated and are informative of aerobic capacity. Early-onset muscle fatigue may limit information regarding cardiopulmonary disease. If a client is suspected of having coronary artery disease, the recommendations outlined in chapter 3 should be followed. Range-of-motion measurements (goniometry) are useful for persons who have limited flexibility and need stretching programs. Gait analysis may be necessary for people who have severe disease, altered biomechanics, and a need for orthotics.

Recommendations for Exercise Programming

The major impact of joint disease on exercise programming is the need for joint protection:

- Select low-impact activities.
- Avoid stair climbing, jogging, and running in persons in whom the hip or knee is involved with the arthritic condition.
- Condition muscles prior to more vigorous activity.
- Include flexibility and joint range of motion as key exercise components.
- Avoid overstretching and hypermobility.
- Reduce load on joint (exercise in a pool, or use biking or rowing).
- Select shoes and insoles for maximum shock attenuation during weight-bearing activities.
- Evaluate for rigid/semirigid orthotics for biomechanical correction at ankles and knees.

Table 26.2 lists complications related to exercise programming for people with various forms of arthritis.

One should also design programs with an individualized progression of intensity and duration:

- Use low intensity and duration during initial phase of programming.

Table 26.2 COMPLICATIONS IN EXERCISE PROGRAMMING

OSTEOARTHRITIS	
Spinal stenosis	Localized and radiating back pain; spinal cord compression; neurologic deficits; claudication-like symptoms; worsens with spinal extension and weight bearing
Spondylosis	Localized and/or radiating back pain
RHEUMATOID ARTHRITIS	
Cervical spine subluxation	Cervical instability; spinal cord compression; neurologic deficits– numbness, tingling, weakness Life-threatening
Foot disease	Metatarsalgia; subluxation of metatarsal heads; mid-foot pain/instability; calcaneal valgus; overpronation on weight bearing; gait deviation
Wrist/hand disease	Joint pain/instability, loss of grip strength Avoid power grip, ulnar deviation, joint stress at wrist
SYSTEMIC LUPUS ERYTHEMATOSUS	
Necrosis of femoral head	Hip pain (also associated with long-term corticosteroid use)
ANKYLOSING & PSORIATIC SPONDYLITIS	
Enthesopathy	Acute and chronic plantar fasciitis, Achilles tendinitis, costochondritis

- If necessary, accumulate exercise dose in several sessions throughout the day.

- Use modified *"interval training"* of brisk/rest exercise session.

- Set time goals, rather than distance goals, to encourage a controlled pace of activity.

Choose an appropriate exercise/fitness goal, and recommend that the person not exceed intensity, duration, and frequency guidelines for training.

Encourage exercise as a component of a fitness routine that is part of self-management:

- Stretching/warm-up should be used daily, even on days when the disease flares and vigorous activity is undesirable.

- Use aerobic activities that incorporate alternative forms of exercise (weight-bearing, partial weight-bearing, and non-weight-bearing) to allow for migrating joint symptoms and changes in disease activity.

- Recommend that the person learn a strengthening routine.

- Avoid activities that cause increased joint pain lasting more than an hour or two after exercise.

- Some postexercise soft tissue discomfort may be expected.

Suggested Readings

Boulware, D.W., and S.L. Byrd. 1993. Optimizing exercise programs for arthritis patients. *Physician Sportsmed.* 21 (4): 104-20.

Bunning, R.D., and R.S. Materson. 1991. A rational program of exercise for patients with osteoarthritis. *Semin. Arthritis Rheum.* 21 (3) suppl. 2: 33-43.

Gordon, N.F. 1993. *Arthritis: Your complete exercise guide.* Champaign, IL: Human Kinetics.

Kelley, W.N., E.D. Harris, S. Ruddy, and C.B. Sledge, eds. 1993. *Textbook of rheumatology.* 4th ed. Philadelphia: Saunders.

Minor, M.A. 1991. Physical activity and management of arthritis. *Ann. Behavioral Med.* 13 (3): 117-24.

Minor, M.A. 1994. Exercise considerations in osteoarthritis. *Arthritis Care Res.* 7 (4): 198-204.

Schumacher, H.R., ed. 1993. *Primer on the rheumatic diseases.* 10th ed. Atlanta: Arthritis Foundation.

Semble, E.L., R.F. Loeser, and C.M. Wise. 1990. Therapeutic exercise for rheumatoid arthritis and osteoarthritis. *Semin. Arthritis Rheum.* 20 (1): 32-40.

Stenstrom, C.H. 1994. Therapeutic exercise in rheumatoid arthritis. *Arthritis Care Res.* 7 (4): 190-97.

ARTHRITIS: EXERCISE TESTING

METHODS	MEASURES	ENDPOINTS*	COMMENTS
Strength **Isokinetic machines at 90-120°/sec** **Isometric knee extension**		• Ability to exceed 20-30% body weight for knee extension • 70 kg force	• Mode depends on specific joint involvement and pain.
Endurance **6-minute walk** **Time to exhaustion** **Maximum repetitions (iso-kinetic)**	• Walk: Heart rate, RPE • Time to exhaustion: Use 75% of maximal voluntary contraction/peak torque	• 6 minutes • Fatigue	• Mode depends on specific joint involvment and pain.
Flexibility **Goniometry**	• Assess asymmetry		• Physical/occupational therapist consultation may help clarify goals.
Neuromuscular **Gait analysis** **Balance**			
Functional capacity **50-foot walk** **Sit-to-stand** **Timed stands** **Arthritis Impact Measurement Scale/Health Assessment Questionnaire**	• Walk: Observe for symmetry • Stands: Use if patient is weak and/or unstable		• Assess vocational potential.

*Measurements of particular significance; do not *always* indicate test termination.

MEDICATIONS	SPECIAL CONSIDERATIONS
• Nonsteroidal anti-inflammatory drugs: May cause anemia from GI bleeding. • Rheumatoid arthritis-remitting drugs: May cause secondary organ disease, including myopathy. • Oral corticosteroids: May cause skeletal myopathy, truncal obesity, osteoporosis, and anemia from GI bleeding.	• Pain/swelling may reduce performance. • Vigorous, highly repetitive exercise should not be performed with unstable joints. • Some arthritides involve cardiopulmonary systems, which may decrease performance. • Spinal involvement may cause radiculopathy. • Avoid morning exercise in rheumatoid arthritis clients because of morning stiffness. • Variable-speed protocols should be available. Cycle ergometers should have loose-fitting toe straps to accommodate genu valgum. • If at risk for CAD, see table on exercise testing in chapter 3.

ARTHRITIS: EXERCISE PROGRAMMING

MODES	GOALS	INTENSITY/ FREQUENCY/DURATION	TIME TO GOAL
Aerobic • Large muscle activities (e.g., walking, cycling, rowing, swimming, water aerobics, dance)	• Increase $\dot{V}O_2$ max, peak work, and endurance.	• 60-80% peak HR or 40-60% $\dot{V}O_2$ max. • RPE 11-16. • 3-5 days/week. • 5 minutes/session building to 30 minutes/session. • Emphasize progression of duration over intensity.	• 4-6 months
Strength • Circuit training with free weights, weight machines, isometric exercises, or elastic bands	• Increase maximal voluntary contraction (MVC), peak torque, or power.	• Use pain tolerance to set %MVC. • 2-3 repetitions initially, build to 10-12. • 2-3 days/week.	
Flexibility • Stretching	• Increase/maintain pain-free range. • Decrease stiffness.	• 1-2 sessions/day.	
Neuromuscular • Any appropriate	• Improve gait, balance.		
Functional • Activity-specific exercises	• Increase/maintain daily living activities. • Return to work. • Improve quality of life.		

MEDICATIONS	SPECIAL CONSIDERATIONS
• Steroids: Predispose to stress fractures. • See table on exercise testing.	• Avoid overstretching unstable joints. Avoid medial/lateral forces. • High-repetition, high-resistance, and high-impact exercise not recommended. • Depression may be an obstacle to lifestyle change.

CHAPTER 27

Low Back Pain Syndrome

N.B. Oldridge, PhD, FACSM
J.E. Stoll, MD
University of Wisconsin

Overview of the Pathophysiology

Two recently published documents, a report by the Quebec Task Force on Spinal Disorders (1987) and the AHCPR (Agency for Health Care Policy and Research) Clinical Practice Guideline for Acute Low Back Pain in Adults (Bigos et al. 1994), provide important and valuable information on the effectiveness of clinical care methods in clients with low back problems. Acute low back pain (less than three months' duration) and associated low back problems, most commonly presenting as activity intolerance, are frequently associated with either back-related leg pain (sciatica) or nonspecific lower back symptoms that suggest neither nerve root compromise nor serious underlying spinal conditions (e.g., fracture, tumor, infection, or cauda equina syndrome). Back symptoms are the most common cause of disability for persons under the age of 45 years. Although the duration of absence from work is less than four weeks for about 75% of clients with an episode of acute low back pain, the single major factor in the high cost associated with low back pain appears to be the number of persons affected by low back disorders. The 1987 Quebec Task Force concluded that although "biologic effects provide the rationale for the use of most treatments . . . few have been validated in scientifically admissible clinical or epidemiological investigations [and that] in general, the symptoms of acute pain in the lumbar, dorsal and cervical regions tend to *resolve spontaneously*" (S30). The 1994 AHCPR Clinical Practice Guidelines support these conclusions about treatment effectiveness and in addition clearly point out that "treatment of persons who have chronic low back problems (with symptoms lasting over three months) may be quite different than for patients with acute problems" (1).

Effects on the Exercise Response

Lower back pain usually does not alter the exercise response to a single session of exercise unless the client has a secondary illness (e.g., coronary artery disease). In such a case, attention must be given to the exercise response in light of this other condition. Additionally, since either the standing or the sitting position may exacerbate pain and in many cases might *prevent* the client from obtaining a *maximal effort*, the choice of exercise modality is important.

Effects of Exercise Training

Although extended bed rest is contraindicated, there is little information regarding the specific therapeutic value of physical exercise in the treatment of low back pain. The following is a summary of the evidence for the effectiveness of the therapeutic exercise modalities considered in the Quebec Task Force report:

- Exercise to increase strength is not common practice and has no scientific support for clients who have had low back pain for less than seven days; for clients with low back pain of greater than seven days but less than seven weeks, strength exercises are common practice but without scientific support; in clients with back pain of greater than seven weeks there is scientific support of usefulness from nonrandomized controlled trials.

- Exercise to increase range of motion is common practice, but without scientific support, for clients with low back pain.

- Exercise to increase endurance is not in common practice, and there is no scientific support for clients with low back pain of less than seven days; for clients with pain of greater than seven days, endurance exercises are common practice but with no scientific support.

- Structural intervention programs to increase functional and physical work capacity include physical exercises as part of the program. Back school has been shown to be useful by randomized trial in clients who have had low back pain for less than seven weeks and who have not yet returned to work; functional training programs have been demonstrated to be useful by nonrandomized trial in clients who have not returned to work for more than seven weeks and who are deconditioned.

The findings and recommendations statements in the 1994 AHCPR Clinical Practice Guidelines on clinical care methods for clients with acute low back problems (duration less than three months) are based on evidence that is either "A = strong" (multiple relevant and high-quality scientific studies), "B = moderate" (one relevant, high-quality study or multiple adequate scientific studies), "C = limited" (at least one adequate scientific study), or "D = panel interpretation of information that did not meet inclusion criteria as research-based evidence" (13). None of the findings and recommendations for exercise in the care of acute low back problems received more than a limited evidence rating, and include the following:

- Low-stress aerobic exercise can prevent debilitation and may help return clients to the highest level of functioning appropriate to their circumstances (strength of evidence = C).

- Conditioning exercises for trunk muscles (especially back extensors) are helpful for clients with acute low back problems, especially if symptoms persist. During the first two weeks, these exercises may aggravate symptoms since they mechanically stress the back more than endurance exercise (strength of evidence = C).

*Recommended exercise programs that are gradually increased result in better outcomes than telling clients to stop exercising if pain occurs (strength of evidence = C).

The other three exercise recommendations and findings in the AHCPR Clinical Practice Guidelines were given a strength of evidence = D; that is, they represented the panel's interpretation of information that did not meet the inclusion criteria as research-based evidence:

- Aerobic (endurance) exercise that minimally stresses the back (walking, biking, or swimming) can be started during the first two weeks for most clients with acute low back problems.

- Back-specific exercise machines provide no apparent benefit over traditional exercise in the treatment of clients with acute low back problems.

- Evidence does not support stretching of the back muscles in the treatment of clients with acute low back problems.

The role of exercise in the prevention of low back problems is, if anything, even more unclear, with few well-designed studies available. However, there are limited data to suggest that behavioral factors including "unhealthy lifestyles" (e.g., smoking, obesity, and inactivity) are independent risks for low back pain. On the other hand, recent reviews of exercise to strengthen back or abdominal muscles, and to improve overall fitness in the prevention of low back pain, suggest that there is limited evidence from epidemiological studies and randomized trials for a lower incidence and duration of low back pain episodes in asymptomatic persons who perform these exercises. Most studies demonstrate only weak correlations between poor aerobic fitness, poor endurance, poor back or abdominal strength, and a greater incidence of low back pain; it may equally be that the low back pain is responsible for the poor aerobic fitness, back and abdominal strength, and endurance.

Management and Medications

The 1994 Clinical Practice Guidelines panel suggests that oral pharmaceuticals are a primary method of symptom control and recommend the following to control the discomfort associated with low back pain problems: 1) Acetaminophen is recommended as reasonably safe and acceptable; 2) non steroidal anti-inflammatory drugs, including aspirin, are acceptable although there is the potential for side effects such as gastrointestinal irritation; and 3) muscle relaxants, which induce drowsiness in as many as 30% of patients, are no more effective than non-steroidal anti-inflammatory drugs. The panel recommended that opiods, if needed, should be used for only a short time and recommended against the use of oral steroids, colchine, and anti-depressant medications for acute low back problems.

A large number of therapeutic modalities, with a large range of therapeutic objectives, are available for the treatment of low back pain. Therapeutic modalities include, among others, reduced physical activity and bed rest, medication, surgery, chemonucleolysis, thermotherapy, psychotherapy, biofeedback, manipulation, postural retraining, and various types of exercise, and, if therapy fails, surgery. Therapeutic objectives include, among others, reducing pain, diminishing spasm, altering mechanical and neurological structure, providing treatment adapted to the psychological aspects of the problem, and increasing strength, range of motion, endurance, functional, and physical work capacity.

Recommendations for Exercise Testing

An accurate history is essential in evaluation of a client with low back pain. Knowing whether the onset of pain is sudden and associated with a specific physical task or activity, knowing whether it is associated with a slow onset or with mild recurrence, and identifying physical activities associated with exacerbation or relief of pain will help define the origin of the pain. An occupational and recreational history will provide useful information about degree of disability. Exercise testing of clients with acute low back problems is not helpful during the first four weeks of low back symptoms. An initial assessment of muscle strength and range of motion of the back as well as straight leg raising is helpful in differentiating the origin of the low back pain.

Clinical experience suggests that exercise testing in clients who have low back pain but have been referred for other reasons (e.g., evaluation of coronary heart disease) may not be useful, as the exercise frequently is limited by symptoms associated with low back pain and not those associated with coronary heart disease. If exercise testing must be carried out, the choice of exercise testing equipment is

important, as low back pain may be exacerbated in either the standing or the sitting position.

Assessment of lower limb muscle strength (hamstrings, gluteals, and particularly the lumbar extensors) and aerobic exercise tolerance, in addition to range of motion of the back and straight leg raising, may be useful in documenting intervention effectiveness. Leg and trunk dynamometers, iso-machines, roman chair, and weights can be used to assess trunk and lower and upper limb muscle strength. Ambulation (treadmill or a six-minute walk test) or stationary cycle ergometry can be used to assess aerobic exercise tolerance. The use of iso-machines to measure trunk strength for preemployment screening, routine clinical assessment, or medico-legal evaluation is not supported by adequate scientific evidence.

Recommendations for Exercise Programming

The AHCPR Clinical Practice Guidelines point out that there is insufficient evidence to allow as much specificity about exercise programming for the client with low back problems as, for example, for the client with coronary artery disease. On the basis of available information, it is difficult to provide specific exercise program recommendations for clients with acute low back pain. However, it is clear that the program of exercise for clients with low back pain must be highly individualized and that it will depend on a number of factors such as origin, duration, and severity of the pain. It is important that the physician and the client agree on the level of pain that can be tolerated, and the client needs to be assured that some pain is normal and not dangerous. Although few clients will exercise to a level that will produce unacceptable pain levels, people should be advised against exercising at a level that might produce unacceptable levels of low back pain.

- The goal of exercise programs for clients with acute low back problems is to prevent debilitation due to inactivity and to improve exercise tolerance so that clients may by their own efforts regain their optimal level of functioning as soon as possible. Aerobic exercise that minimally stresses the back (walking, cycling, swimming) can be started during the first two weeks of acute low back problems for most clients.

- The progression of the level of physical activity must be individualized and is largely determined by the amount of pain produced by the activity. Clients may improve faster when they are given a specific prescription than when told to stop exercise when pain occurs.

- Aerobic (endurance) conditioning such as walking, stationary cycling, swimming, and even slow jogging may be recommended within the limitations already described to minimize debilitation from activity.

- Conditioning exercises for trunk muscles, when gradually increased, are helpful for most clients with symptomatic acute low back problems. These exercises are commonly delayed at least two weeks after onset of low back pain.

In carefully monitored exercise programs, appropriately prescribed high-dose exercise, even over short periods of time, tends to produce more benefit than low-dose exercise in clients with chronic low back pain. However, this is not true for acute low back pain, particularly in those with sedentary occupations.

Both isometric and dynamic back exercise appear to be useful in clients with chronic, but not acute, low back pain. In general, the progression of exercise to strengthen the muscles of the back and abdomen in clients with low back pain should be in the number of repetitions, not the resistance to be overcome. Exercises to develop strength and endurance may include those requiring gravitational forces to provide resistance (calisthenics or free exercises), those requiring the use of weights or barbells to provide resistance, and those requiring the use of specific machines to provide resistance (iso-machines). The effectiveness of iso-machines over traditional modalities has not been demonstrated, although there is little concern about their safety. Evidence does not support stretching of the back muscles in clients with acute low back problems.

It is clear that prolonged bed rest is contraindicated. Submaximal exercise such as walking, cycling, and swimming may be useful in improving exercise tolerance; but the degree to which an improvement in exercise tolerance is associated with a decrease in pain, or whether a decrease in pain results in an improvement in exercise tolerance, is not clear. The same observation is true for improvement in strength and flexibility.

In conclusion, the goal of exercise programs for clients with acute low back problems is to prevent debilitation due to inactivity and to improve endurance exercise tolerance, strength, and flexibility so that clients may by their own efforts regain their optimal level of functioning as soon as possible.

However, it is clear that there are few definitive recommendations that can be made about the role of exercise in the treatment and prevention of low back pain. Exercise to improve general endurance, muscular strength, and flexibility may be of benefit to some clients with acute low back problems. The usefulness of exercise testing in the assessment of clients with low back problems is not clear, although the assessment of sciatic tension (straight leg raise) and lower limb strength in the evaluation of treatment effect may be helpful. The assessment of range of motion and straight leg raising is useful in the clinical assessment of low back pain.

Special Considerations

The AHCPR Clinical Practice Guideline recommendations for the modification of occupational activity are as follows (both with D strength of recommendation, i.e., panel interpretation of information that did not meet inclusion criteria as research-based evidence):

- Clients with acute low back problems may be more comfortable if they temporarily limit or avoid specific activities known to increase mechanical stress on the spine, especially prolonged unsupported sitting, heavy lifting, and bending or twisting the back while lifting.

- Activity recommendations for the employed client with acute low back problems should reflect the client's age and general health as well as the physical demands of the required job tasks.

Suggested Readings

Biering-Sørensen, F., T. Bendix, K. Jørgensen, C. Manniche, and H. Nielsen. 1994. Physical activity, fitness, and back pain. In *Physical activity, fitness, and health*, ed. C. Bouchard, R.J. Shephard, and T. Stephens, 737-48. 2nd ed. Champaign, IL: Human Kinetics.

Bigos, S., O. Bower, G. Braen, K. Brown, R. Deyo, S. Haldeman, J.L. Hart, E.W. Johnson, R. Keller, D. Kido, M.H. Liang, R.M. Nelson, M. Nordin, B.D. Owen, M.H. Pope, R.K. Schwartz, D.H. Stewart, J. Susman, J.J. Triano, L.C. Tripp, D.C. Turk, C. Watts, and J.N. Weinstein. December 1994. *Acute low back pain in adults*. U.S. Department of Health and Human Services. Public Health Service.

Agency for Health Care Policy and Research. Guideline No. 14. AHCPR Publication No. 95-0642. Rockville, MD.

Faas, A., A.W. Chavannes, J.T.M. van Eijk, and J.W. Gubbles. 1993. A randomized, placebo-controlled trial of exercise therapy in patients with acute low back pain. *Spine* 18: 1388-95.

Frymoyer, H.W. 1993. Quality: An international challenge to the diagnosis and treatment of disorders of the lumbar spine. *Spine* 18: 2147-52.

Hansen, F.R., T. Bendix, P. Skov, C.V. Jensen, J.H. Kristensen, L. Krohn, and H. Schioeler. 1993. Intensive dynamic back-muscle exercises, conventional physiotherapy, or placebo-control treatment of low-back pain. *Spine* 18: 98-107.

Koes, B.W., L.M. Bouter, H. Beckerman, G.J.M.G. van der Heijden, and P.G. Knipschild. 1991. Phys-

iotherapy exercises and back pain: A blinded review. *Br. Med. J.* 302: 1572-76.

Lahad, A., A.D. Maler, A.O. Berg, and R.A. Deyo. 1994. The effectiveness of four interventions for the prevention of low back pain. *JAMA* 272: 1286-91.

Quebec Task Force on Spinal Disorders. 1987. Scientific approach to the assessment and management of activity-related spinal disorders. A monograph for clinicians. *Spine* 12: S1-S59.

Sachs, B.L., S.S. Ahmad, M. LaCroix, D. Olimpio, R. Heath, J-A. David, and A.D. Scala. 1994. Objective assessment for exercise treatment on the B-200 isostation as part of work tolerance rehabilitation. A random prospective blind evaluation with comparison control population. *Spine* 19: 49-52.

LOW BACK PAIN SYNDROME: EXERCISE TESTING

METHODS	MEASURES	ENDPOINTS	COMMENTS
Aerobic power Maximal and submaximal testing unnecessary			• Testing may be warranted if risk factors/symptoms of CAD are present (see table on testing in chapter 3).
Strength Isokinetic trunk testing			• Check for smoothness of motion and peak torque. • Jerky movement may suggest pain.
Flexibility Sit-and-reach Straight leg stretch			

SPECIAL CONSIDERATIONS

• Testing is not helpful during the first 4 weeks of low back symptoms.
• Avoid high-impact exercise such as running.

LOW BACK PAIN SYNDROME: EXERCISE PROGRAMMING

MODES	GOALS	INTENSITY/ FREQUENCY/DURATION	TIME TO GOAL
Strength • Sit-ups • Back extensions	• Increase muscular strength cof trunk.	• 8-12 repetitions/day • Minimum of 2 days/week	• 2-4 weeks
Flexibility • Sit-and-reach	• Increase trunk flexibility.		

SPECIAL CONSIDERATIONS

• Avoid high-impact exercise such as running.
• On the basis of the Quebec Task Force report (1987) and the AHCPR Clinical Practice Guidelines (1994), there is little evidence to suggest that exercise has any direct impact on reducing low back pain. However, there are proponents of exercise who suggest that factors such as increased submaximal endurance, improved strength, and greater flexibility and range of motion may be beneficial to the general health of some patients with low back pain. Whether or not these will potentially result in increased daily living activities and prevent deterioration, will improve quality of life, or will restore ability to work in patients with low back pain is unclear.
• Low-stress aerobic activities can be safely started in the first 2 weeks following onset of low back symptoms. Trunk exercises should be delayed at least 2 weeks.

CHAPTER 28

Osteoporosis

Susan A. Bloomfield, PhD

Texas A & M University

Overview of the Pathophysiology

Because of declining activity of bone-forming cells after the age of 35 years, all humans incur some minute loss of bone mass every year. This phenomenon has been observed in multiple races, geographical locations, and historical epochs. Dietary habits and physical activity patterns over the life span may alter the timing or rate of bone loss, but nearly all elderly men and women in industrialized countries have some degree of *osteopenia*, or lowered bone mass. This is of concern because bone strength and resistance to fracture, key functional attributes of bone, are determined in large part by bone mass. Once osteopenia becomes severe enough to result in fractures from minimal trauma, such as a fall to the floor, it is clinically defined as *osteoporosis*. Bone status for most individuals over the age of 60 years is somewhere on the continuum between benign age-related osteopenia and bone loss severe enough to make fracture imminent.

Women tend to start losing bone early in life and may experience a three- to five-year acceleration of bone loss after menopause because the effects of estrogen withdrawal are temporarily superimposed on age-related loss. This fact, in addition to a lower peak bone mass in young adulthood, explains the greater incidence of osteoporotic fractures in women as compared to men. Two types of osteoporosis generally recognized are shown in table 28.1.

The presumed mechanism for type I osteoporosis (in women) is estrogen deficiency, and is the result of an increased activity of bone-resorbing cells and an acceleration of bone resorption. Males less frequently experience clinically significant bone loss before the age of 70, but various diseases, medications (e.g., chronic glucocorticoid therapy), or lifestyle factors (e.g., alcoholism) can produce early loss of bone mass and strength. Type II osteoporosis is thought to be related to vitamin D deficiency and secondary hyperparathyroidism; the severe osteopenia observed in this group, and the resulting hip fractures, make it less likely that these individuals can safely engage in regular exercise routines. Most of the commonly cited risk factors for osteoporosis are related either to estrogen deficiency or to the other exogenous factors affecting bone metabolism:

- Female gender
- Advanced age
- Caucasian/Asian race
- Positive family history
- Low body weight
- Premature menopause

Table 28.1 TYPES OF OSTEOPOROSIS	TYPE I OSTEOPOROSIS	TYPE II OSTEOPOROSIS
Age at onset (years)	50-75	70+
Type of bone loss	Trabecular	Trabecular + cortical
Typical fracture sites	Vertebrae, wrist	Vertebrae, hip

- Prolonged premenopausal amenorrhea
- Nulliparity (condition of a woman who has borne no children)
- Lack of physical activity
- Chronic smoking
- Excessive alcohol consumption
- Low dietary calcium intake

Compression or wedge fractures of the vertebrae are common in older individuals with osteoporosis. Several may accumulate without obvious symptoms before they are detected, often as a chance finding with a chest x-ray done for other purposes. A significant functional limitation imposed by multiple vertebral fractures is the severe kyphosis that can result. In extreme cases, this spinal deformity can impede normal ventilatory function by altering respiratory muscle function and decreasing vital capacity. It can also produce a forward shift in the center of gravity, increasing the risk of falls. About one-third of individuals with vertebral fractures experience significant back pain in the acute phase of recovery. If pain persists for a longer period, weakness of the back extensor muscles may be a causative factor. It should be noted that the loss of lean body mass over the decades with chronic inactivity may be a strong contributor to the development of osteoporosis; individuals with low muscle mass and strength are more likely to have lower bone mass.

Effects on the Exercise Response

The primary consideration relative to this clinical group is the degree of orthopedic limitation imposed by bony fractures. It is unlikely that people suffering a hip fracture will be referred for exercise testing for the purpose of starting a regular exercise program; the primary clinical goals for this group tend to be appropriate physical therapy to maximize mobility and prevent further falls. Exercise testing can proceed as usual for individuals with diagnosed vertebral fractures (once physician approval has been obtained) unless severe kyphosis is present. In many cases, the fear of falling often leads to reduced physical activity in elderly populations; this further exacerbates their risk of developing coronary artery disease (CAD). Therefore, ECG monitoring for ischemic responses to exercise is always advised.

Effects on Exercise Training

There are two primary interactions of established osteoporosis with exercise training effects. First, many of these individuals are likely to be more unfit than the average population because of the decreased mobility common in persons with diagnosed osteoporosis, mandating a low-intensity program at the outset. Second, orthopedic limitations may slow progress or mandate the use of additional supports during walking. There is no evidence in the literature that osteoporosis, in and of itself, should alter the usual beneficial cardiovascular and skeletal muscle adaptations with chronic exercise. One exception might be the mechanical limitations imposed on respiratory muscle function in individuals with severe kyphosis. Whether regular participation in physical activity by itself can reverse the primary defect with osteoporosis and provide a significant anabolic stimulus for increased bone mass appears doubtful. Better evidence suggests that regular exercise can slow or perhaps halt the age-related decline in bone mass and could delay the time point at which osteopenia progresses to clinically significant osteoporosis. There is no support for the concept that exercise can provide an effective alternative to hormone replacement therapy (HRT) in preventing bone loss in the early menopausal years.

Management and Medications

Once osteoporosis has been diagnosed, with confirmation of low bone mineral density and fractures incurred with little or no trauma, the primary form of treatment is the use of medications to slow bone resorption or, more rarely, to increase bone formation. Should significant spinal deformities develop, bracing of the torso may be recommended to prevent worsening of the deformity, along with appropriate physical therapy to symptomatically treat back pain and improve back extensor muscle strength.

Hormone replacement therapy is the most commonly prescribed of all medical regimens. Estrogens with or without progestogen components are prescribed in relatively low doses in an effort to replace the endogenous hormone levels lost at menopause or after surgical removal of the ovaries. Estrogen's benefits derive from its inhibitory effect on bone remodeling; in its absence, remodeling activity accelerates. There is limited evidence that estrogen therapy may increase the frequency of ST-segment depression. Therefore, ST-segment changes observed during a graded exercise test should be interpreted with caution in these individuals. A very small number of individuals on HRT experience an increase in resting blood pressure; it is doubtful that exercise blood pressures are affected. A positive effect of estrogen replacement therapy (when taken without progesterone) on high-density lipoprotein cholesterol, and hence on lowering risk of CAD in postmenopausal women, has been documented. If engaging in exercise training while on HRT, a postmenopausal woman is more likely to experience absolute gains in bone mass. Preliminary evidence indicates that estrogen-deficient women do not develop increases in ventricular volumes with endurance training; HRT may allow for the usual myocardial adaptations that in young women are seen to occur with training. Other medications currently used to treat osteoporosis include the following:

- **Calcitonin** is used in pharmacological doses and inhibits bone resorption at cancellous bone sites; its effects on cortical bone are uncertain. Until clinical trials on intranasal forms are complete, calcitonin must be administered via subcutaneous injection.

- **Bisphosphonates** are administered intermittently, in alternation with intervals of calcium administration. They inhibit bone resorption and may have an anabolic effect on vertebral cancellous bone. Common side effects include nausea and diarrhea. Late in 1995, the FDA approved one particular bisphosphonate, Alendronate (tradename Fosamax) for clinical treatment of osteoporosis.

- **Sodium fluoride, vitamin D, and parathyroid hormone (PTH)** all promote bone formation when given in appropriate doses and have been shown to increase bone mass in some cases, but are not yet FDA approved. There are also reports of increased fracture incidence after fluoride therapy, which may promote the rapid formation of mechanically weak bone at some sites.

Recommendations for Exercise Testing

The usual exercise testing protocols employed with older individuals at risk for CAD are appropriate for people with diagnosed osteoporosis. For those with severe kyphosis, treadmill exercise is likely to be unsafe if forward vision is limited or if the neck is affected; a significant shift in the center of gravity may occur that could affect balance. Stationary bicycle ergometry, if it does not compress the anterior aspect of the spine, provides a safer alternative.

Additional testing beyond the standard graded exercise test would be extremely beneficial for this population (see table on testing). Assessment of muscle strength, to identify particularly weak muscle groups, would also assist in exercise prescription. Tests of neuromuscular function such as dynamic balance, assessed by a timed backward walk over 20 feet, are appropriate, as are functional tests such as time to rise from a chair without use of the arms.

Recommendations for Exercise Programming

Definitive training studies have yet to be done, but our current knowledge indicates that a well-balanced exercise program focusing on both aerobic and strength training activities should be emphasized for the person with osteoporosis. The individual's physician, ideally in consultation with a physical therapist experienced with the limitations of persons with osteoporosis, needs to make the initial judgment about the safety of the proposed exercise program for this specific individual. There is little information in the literature about the safety of various forms of exercise for osteopenic individuals.

Strength helps to conserve bone mass and improve dynamic balance. Best results are obtained when exercisers can progress to using relatively high intensities (> 75% of 1 repetition maximum) and fewer repetitions. Adaptations in bone are site-specific to the limbs used; any program should include exercise for upper and lower body and trunk muscles, particularly the extensors. Floor calisthenics and some lifting activities need to be modified to avoid forward flexion of the spine, particularly in combination with stooping. Regular performance of flexion exercises increases the risk of causing new vertebral fractures in the person with established osteoporosis. If multiple vertebral fractures, severe osteopenia, or back pain limit an individual's participation in weight-bearing exercise, shift to swimming, walking in the water, water aerobics programs, or chair exercises. Although not as optimal for impacting on bone as strength training, these programs are likely to improve muscle strength and balance and contribute to a lowered risk of CAD.

Special Considerations

One special consideration that exercise professionals must be aware of in working with people with osteoporosis relates to the justifiable anxiety many may have about falling. Careful attention must be paid to making the exercise environment free of hazards such as loose floor tiles or mats and exercise equipment strewn over the floor. Wall railings in exercise areas would be helpful for exercises done while standing. Close monitoring by staff, particularly if balance training is used (e.g., heel-to-toe walks, balancing on a single foot), should help prevent unintended injuries suffered during exercise sessions.

Suggested Readings

American College of Sports Medicine. ACSM position stand on osteoporosis and exercise. 1995. *Med. Sci. Sports Exerc.* 27 (4): i-vii.

Bloomfield, S.A. 1995. Bone, ligament, and tendon. In *Perspectives in exercise science and sports medicine, exercise in older adults,* ed. C.V. Gisolfi, E.R. Nadel, and D.R. Lamb, 175-227, vol. 8. Carmel, IN: Cooper Publishing Group.

Dalsky, G.P. 1990. Effect of exercise on bone: Permissive influence of estrogen and calcium. *Med. Sci. Sports Exerc.* 22 (3): 281-85.

Forwood, M.R., and D.B. Burr. 1993. Physical activity and bone mass: Exercise in futility? *Bone Miner.* 21: 89-112.

Gutin, B., and M.J. Kasper. 1992. Can vigorous exercise play a role in osteoporosis prevention? A review. *Osteoporosis Int.* 2: 55-69.

McClung, M.R. 1994. Nonpharmacologic management of osteoporosis. In *Osteoporosis,* ed. R. Marcus, 336-53. Boston: Blackwell Scientific.

Sinaki, M. 1988. Exercise and physical therapy. In *Osteoporosis: Etiology, diagnosis, and management,* ed. B.L. Riggs and L.J. Melton III, 457-79. New York: Raven Press.

Sinaki, M. 1989. Exercise and osteoporosis. *Arch. Phys. Med. Rehabil.* 70: 220-29.

Snow-Harter, C., and R. Marcus. 1991. Exercise, bone mineral density, and osteoporosis. *Exerc. Sport Sci. Rev.* 19: 351-88.

OSTEOPOROSIS: EXERCISE TESTING

METHODS	MEASURES	ENDPOINTS*	COMMENTS
Aerobic power **Treadmill** (1-2 METs/stage) **Cycle** (5-20 watts/min) ramp protocol (10-25 watts/3 min stage)	• 12-lead ECG	• Serious dysrhythmias • > 2 mm ST-segment depression or elevation • Ischemic threshold • T-wave inversion with significant ST change	• Most clients will be at high risk for CAD.
	• Blood pressure	• SBP > 260 mmHg or DBP > 115 mmHg	• To determine if hypertensive.
	• RPE	• Volitional fatigue	• Useful for clients who have difficulty with HR measurements.
	• Heart rate, METs		• Helpful in determining exercise program.
Strength **Weight machines**	• 1 repetition maximum • 3 repetitions maximum (for more frail subjects)		• Used to determine intensity of resistance training. • Decline in muscle strength in postmenopausal women elderly men is a common finding in those with osteoporosis.
Neuromuscular **Gait analysis** **Balance**			• Especially useful for severely symptomatic patient.
Functional capacity **6-meter walk** **Tandem gait speed** **Sit-to-stand**	• Distance • Speed • Try to perform without use of arms		• Sit-to-stand provides good practical evaluation of strength. Requirement of arms for assistance individual for strength improvement of hip extensors.

*Measurements of particular significance; do not *always* indicate test termination.

MEDICATIONS	SPECIAL CONSIDERATIONS
• See table on testing in chapter 19.	• Neuromuscular and functional performance testing is best performed by skilled physical therapists familiar with standardized. • Orthopedic: Extreme kyphosis in advanced cases alters center of gravity and can affect gait and balance. • Pulmonary: Severe kyphosis may result in increased fatiguability due to impaired pulmonary function (i.e., decreased vital ca impaired function of the pulmonary muscles). • Sensory: Severe kyphosis may make seeing the front of the treadmill difficult. • Muscular: Chronic back pain with multiple vertebral fractures is an issue in some individuals; may be muscular in origin due to extensive weakness of the back extensors. • Psychological: Anxiety about falling during a treadmill test may be an impediment to testing and, therefore, mode of choice in ergometer.

OSTEOPOROSIS: EXERCISE PROGRAMMING

MODES	GOALS	INTENSITY/ FREQUENCY/DURATION	TIME TO GOAL
Aerobic • Walking, cycling, swimming	• Improve/maintain work capacity.	• 40-70% peak HR, METs. • 3-5 days/week. • 20-30 minutes/session.	• 2-3 months
Strength • Dumbbells, weight machines, floor calisthenics	• Improve strength of arms, shoulders, legs, and hips. Emphasize hip flexors/extensors and back extensors.	• 50% of 1 repetition maximum or 70% of 3 repetitions maximum. • 2-3 sets of 8 repetitions. • 2 days/week for 20-40 minutes.	• 2-3 months
Flexibility • Stretching • Chair exercises	• Increase/maintain range of motion, especially in pectoral muscles.	• 5-7 days/week	
Functional • Activity-specific exercises	• Increase/maintain daily living activities.		

MEDICATIONS	SPECIAL CONSIDERATIONS
• Estrogen and bisphosphonates: Will affect exercise only if nausea or diarrhea is experienced; can interfere with motivation to exercise.	• Aerobic power: All modes of exercise (walking, cycling, swimming) are possible as long as *forward flexion* is minimized. •Time frame: Any long-term effect on conservation of bone mass will require at least 9-12 months of effort before change (or lack of change) can be ascertained. • Orthopedic: Clients with extreme kyphosis will be limited to stationary equipment or walking with support. Avoid *flexion* of spine and stooping with forward flexion; can increase incidence of vertebral fractures. • Cardiac: Since most individuals with osteoporosis are > 50 years old, many have latent or overt CAD; thus staff must be alert to signs of myocardial ischemia. • Muscular: Many patients with vertebral fractures are likely to have reduced strength of the back extensor muscles and, therefore, must start with *low* workloads and progress slowly. • Psychological: Assure a safe exercise environment with a minimum of obstacles on the floor to reduce anxiety and the possibility of falling.

SECTION VI

Neuromuscular Disorders

Section Editor:

Stephen F. Figoni, PhD, RKT, FACSM
University of Kansas Medical Center

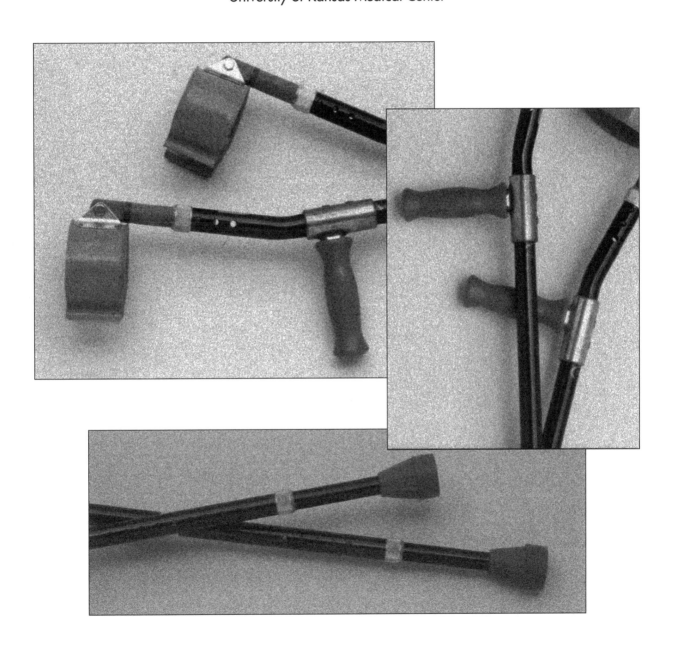

CHAPTER 29

Stroke and Head Injury

Karen Palmer-McLean, PhD, PT

University of Wisconsin, LaCrosse

Jack E. Wilberger, MD

Tri-State Neurosurgical Assoc., Inc.

Overview of the Pathophysiology

The pathophysiology of stroke and head injury is often similar, with a few exceptions noted below.

Stroke

A cerebral vascular accident (CVA), commonly referred to as a *"stroke,"* occurs secondary to vascular insufficiency in the brain. Common causes include thrombosis, embolism, or hemorrhage secondary to aneurysm. Cell death follows and results in an impairment of central nervous system function.

In North America, the following factors put one at risk of developing a CVA: systolic and diastolic hypertension, diabetes mellitus, cigarette smoking, alcoholism, and coronary artery disease. Other factors may also increase the risk of stroke, but their roles are less well defined. They include obesity, platelet hyperaggregability, and elevated blood lipid levels. Although 20% of strokes occur in individuals less than 65 years of age, the majority of strokes affect the elderly with the incidence increasing during the sixth, seventh, and eighth decades of life.

The resulting neurological impairment depends on both the size and the location of the ischemic area, as well as the availability of collateral blood flow. Following a CVA, persons may present with

- impairment of motor and sensory function in the upper or lower extremity, or in both extremities, on the involved side,

- visual field deficits,

- expressive and receptive aphasia (impaired ability to communicate through speech),

- mental confusion, and

- apraxia (impaired learning and performance of voluntary movements).

Head Injury

Traumatic head injuries occur at the rate of approximately 500,000 new cases per year in the United States and are generally classified as mild, moderate, or severe, depending on the extent of injury and the ultimate disability produced. While similar to stroke with respect to the extensive structural brain damage that may result, head injury occurs predominantly in young people without underlying medical problems. Most head injuries occur as a result of motor vehicle accidents, although gunshot wounds are being seen with increasing frequency. It has been predicted that by the year 2000, gunshot wounds may be the primary cause.

The sequelae from head injury may occur as a result of primary or secondary insults. Primary insults refer to the structural brain injury that occurs at the time of injury, while secondary insults include events such as edema, ischemia, and metabolic derangements that may be superimposed on the initial trauma. These secondary insults may result in increasing the degree and extent of permanent brain damage.

While physical disabilities are prominent after the more severe head injuries, cognitive disturbances may be preeminent and can be significant even after a mild head injury. Agitation, confusion, compulsiveness, inattention, memory disturbances, and learning deficits may all occur acutely and chronically after head injury.

Effects on the Exercise Response

Exercise responses of persons with stroke or head injury depend upon the pathophysiology of the individual.

Stroke

The ability to exercise depends on the severity of neurological involvement. The following are some examples:

- Flaccidity or developing spasticity of the lower extremity and/or impairment of sensory function on the involved side may preclude independent ambulation after a CVA.
- Lack of adequate trunk balance may interfere with the ability to perform sitting arm crank or leg cycle ergometry.
- Spasticity or weakness of the involved upper or lower extremity may also interfere with the ability to maintain crank rates during ergometry.
- Since the majority of strokes occur in elderly individuals, participation in aerobic exercise may be further complicated by the arthritic, orthopedic, and cardiovascular problems common in elderly populations.
- Receptive aphasia and mental confusion may interfere with the ability to follow directions during exercise testing or training sessions.

Ambulatory persons with stroke may be able to perform about 70% of the peak power output that can be achieved by age-matched persons without a history of CVA.

Head Injury

As with stroke, the ability to exercise depends on the severity of the neurological impairment. Cognitive disturbances, however, must also be taken into account in planning and implementing an exercise regimen.

While most individuals with head injuries are young, their general physical capacities and endurance may be severely limited secondary to orthopedic and other injuries incurred at the time of the accident. Additionally, a severe head injury is associated with a marked catabolic response with nitrogen and subsequent muscle wasting. This relative state of malnutrition may persist for a number of months after the injury.

A person with a head injury and a known history of seizures may be at some increased risk for seizures during exercise testing that induces hyperventilation. If such concerns arise, ensuring adequate therapeutic anticonvulsant levels before testing is appropriate.

Effects of Exercise Training

Exercise training may have different impacts on people who have had a stroke and those who have suffered a head injury.

Stroke

Most individuals with a recent history of CVA are very deconditioned, exhibiting a peak $\dot{V}O_2$ that is about half of that achieved by age-matched individuals without CVA. This very deconditioned state leaves tremendous room for improvement. If a person with CVA recovers enough motor function to take part in a leg cycle exercise program, the few aerobic training studies that have included persons with stroke suggest that 60% increases in $\dot{V}O_2$ peak might be expected. Endurance training for eight weeks has been found to increase self-selected walking speeds by 100% to 150%. In one case an assistive device for ambulation was no longer required, and other subjects had greater mobility and less dependence on assistive devices.

Head Injury

Patients who sustain a head injury will also have very low oxidative capacities. In addition, neurological deficits secondary to the head injury result in above-average energy cost for locomotion. Exercise training programs can significantly improve $\dot{V}O_2$ peak and muscle strength. As a result, clients can become more independent in their daily activities and more efficient in their locomotion.

Management and Medications

Medical management for people after CVA depends on the type of stroke, the degree of neurologic deficit, and the condition of the individual. For those who have incurred a head injury, several medical issues may require medical management following acute treatment of the injury.

Stroke

Medical treatment for persons who have experienced CVA may include

- short-term use of anticoagulants and long-term use of platelet-inhibiting agents,

- vasodilators if vasospasm of the cerebral arteries is suspected, and

- antihypertensive medication for those with hemorrhagic stroke requiring strict control of blood pressure.

The use of some medications may affect acute physiologic response during graded exercise tests:

- Individuals on vasodilators will require a longer cool-down period after a single session of exercise in order to prevent postexercise hypotension.

- Lower peak heart rates will be achieved by persons receiving medication that limits cardiac output by reducing heart rate.

- Use of diuretics to reduce fluid volume may alter electrolyte balance, causing dysrhythmias.

Head Injury

It is unusual for persons with a head injury to require intensive medical management after the acute treatment of their injury. Many, however, may have a tendency toward seizures and require long-term anticonvulsant medication. Clients that survive traumatic head injury are at risk for sustaining permanent cognitive and behavioral sequelae that might interfere with their ability to follow directions for exercise testing and training. Cognitive deficits might include memory loss and decreased rate of information processing, while behavioral problems might include loss of impulse control, increased agitation, and mood lability. Depression and apathy are also common and might interfere with long-term adherence to an endurance training program. It should be noted that many of these deficits can be cumulated with cognitive retraining, behavioral management, and medication.

Recommendations for Exercise Testing

Since most strokes occur secondary to atherosclerotic lesions, many persons who experience CVA either have coexisting coronary artery disease or are at risk for developing coronary artery disease. Thus, testing of clients with stroke should be supervised by a physician, and clients should be monitored with a 12-lead ECG. The mode of exercise testing depends on the severity of neurological involvement.

Treadmill Walking

Treadmill testing may be appropriate in individuals with minimal motor impairment who have good standing balance and are able to ambulate independently without the use of an assistive device such as a cane or walker. Preferred walking speeds will be much slower, and energy expenditure at a specific work rate will be about 55% to 64% greater than in the individual without a stroke. Exercise protocols with a very gradual increase in exercise intensity, such as the Naughton-Balke or Modified Balke, should be used. The treadmill speed in these protocols may have to be decreased to accommodate the slower walking speeds in this population.

Leg Cycle Ergometry

A standard leg cycle ergometer could be used if the individual can safely maintain sitting balance on the bike. The affected lower extremity may have to be secured on the pedal with straps if the person is unable to keep it secure independently. Test protocols may have to be individually determined on the basis of the person's strength. A pedaling rate of 50 rpm and a starting power output of 20 watts with 20-watt increments per stage are suggested as general guidelines.

Combined Arm and Leg Ergometry

If spasticity or muscle weakness in the affected extremity interferes with the ability to maintain pedal cadence during leg cycle testing, the subject should use only the unaffected lower extremity. However, it is very difficult to achieve a work rate that can stress the heart when using only one extremity. In such cases, a combination arm and leg ergometer, such as the Schwinn Air-Dyne, is particularly useful. Subjects can use just the unaffected upper and lower extremity, or can assist with the affected upper and/or lower extremity, if spasticity or weakness does not interfere with cadence. Because of muscle fatigue of the upper extremities, an intermittent protocol is suggested.

Other Adaptations

For individuals with poor sitting balance, both the leg cycle ergometer and combined arm and leg cycle ergometer can be pedaled from a wheelchair or stationary chair placed behind the leg cycle ergometer. Extensions can be added to the arm cranks of the combined arm and leg ergometer to allow the subject to crank with arms as well as with legs from a wheelchair. The person with poor sitting balance may also be tested in a supine position with use of a cycle ergometer.

Lack of motor function may interfere with exercise performance. In previous studies, only 20% to 34% of individuals with stroke were able to achieve 85% of predicted maximal heart rate.

Recommendations for Exercise Programming

As indicated earlier, hypertension is one of the primary risk factors for stroke. Exercise training programs for individuals with stroke should be aimed not only at increasing the level of physical fitness, but also at reducing risk factors such as hypertension. Tipton (1991) has reviewed 99 longitudinal aerobic exercise training studies utilizing hypertensive human and animal subjects and suggests that hypertension can be reduced when exercise intensities of 40% to 70% $\dot{V}O_2$ peak are employed. Results of animal studies suggest that intensities greater than this level will result in further increases in blood pressure.

Training mode depends on the individual's ability, but the various modes described for exercise testing could be employed for exercise training. Suggested frequency is three to five times per week. Duration of training sessions depends on the subject's initial level of fitness. Intermittent training protocols may be needed during the initial weeks of training because of the extremely deconditioned level of many subjects with CVA.

Special Considerations

Persons who have experienced a CVA are at increased risk for subsequent CVA. Theoretically, a reduction of risk factors should decrease the incidence of secondary strokes. An aerobic conditioning program can alter several of the risk factors associated with the incidence of CVA. Exercise can

- reduce hypertension,
- enhance glucose regulation,
- improve blood lipid profile, and
- reduce body fat.

Large-scale clinical trials are needed to evaluate the impact of aerobic exercise on the incidence of secondary stroke.

There is a paucity of published studies addressing methods of exercise testing for individuals with stroke. Even less information is available on aerobic training programs for this population. Directions for future research include evaluating other modes of exercise testing and training. Intensity of exercise can be altered by changing the rate of stepping and the length of the lever arm on the pedals. The position of the person can also be progressed from a sitting to a more upright weight-bearing position.

Suggested Readings

Brinkman, J.R., and T.A. Hoskins. 1979. Physical conditioning and altered self-concept in rehabilitated hemiplegic patients. *Physical Therapy* 59: 859-65.

Fisher, S.V. 1978. Energy cost of ambulation in health and disability: A literature review. *Arch. Phys. Med. Rehabil.* 59: 124-33.

Goldberg, G., and G.G. Berger. 1988. Secondary prevention in stroke: A primary rehabilitation concern. *Arch. Phys. Med. Rehabil.* 69: 32-40.

Gordon, N.F. 1993. *Stroke: Your complete exercise guide.* Champaign, IL: Human Kinetics.

Gresham, G.E., P.W. Duncan, W.B. Stason, H.P. Adams, A.M. Adelman, D.N. Alexander, D.S. Bishop, L. Diller, N.E. Donaldson, C.V. Granger, A.L. Holland, M. Kelley-Hayes, F.H. McDowell, L. Myers, M.A. Phipps, E.J. Roth, H.C. Siebens, G.A. Tarvin, and C.A. Trombly. May 1995. *Clinical practice guideline number 16: Post-stroke rehabilitation.* U.S. Department of Health and Human Services. Public Health Service. Agency for Health Care Policy and Research. AHCPR Publication No. 95-0662. Rockville, MD.

King, M.L., M. Guarracini, L. Lennihan, D. Freeman, B. Gagas, A. Boston, B. Bates, and N. Subhadra. 1989. Adaptive exercise testing for patients with hemiplegia. *J. Cardiopulmonary Rehabil.* 9: 237-42.

Moldover, J.R., M.C. Daum, and J.A. Downey. 1984. Cardiac stress testing of hemiparetic patients with a supine bicycle ergometer: Preliminary study. *Arch. Phys. Med. Rehabil.* 65: 470-73.

Monga, T.N., D.A. Deforge, J. Williams, and L.A. Wolfe. 1988. Cardiovascular responses to acute exercise in patients with cerebrovascular accidents. *Arch. Phys. Med. Rehabil.* 69: 937-40.

O'Sullivan, S.B. 1989. Stroke. In *Physical rehabilitation: Assessment and treatment,* ed. S.B. O'Sullivan and T.J. Schmitz. 2nd ed. Philadelphia: Davis.

Tipton, C. 1991. Exercise, training, and hypertension: An update. *Exerc. Sport Sci. Rev.* 19: 447-506.

World Health Organization. 1989. Stroke-1989: Recommendations on stroke prevention, diagnosis, and therapy. *Stroke* 18: 830-36.

STROKE AND HEAD INJURY: EXERCISE TESTING

METHODS	MEASURES	ENDPOINTS*	COMMENTS
Aerobic power **Treadmill** (1-2 METs/stage) **Cycle** (20 watts/min) ramp protocol (20 watts/3 min stage) **Schwinn Air-Dyne (or any other upper/lower-body ergometer)** **Arm ergometer**	• 12-lead ECG • Blood pressure • RPE, heart rate, METs • $\dot{V}O_2$peak	• Serious dysrhythmias • > 2 mm ST-segment depression or elevation • Ischemic threshold • T-wave inversion with significant ST change • SBP > 260 mmHg or DBP > 115 mmHg • Volitional fatigue	• CAD is a major risk factor with stroke patients. • Hypertension is a major risk factor with stroke patients. • Useful in prescribing exercise intensity. • Necessary only if conducting research
Endurance **6- or 12-minute walk**	• Distance walked	• Time	• Use with ambulatory persons (with or without assistive devices). Also, use to document improvement and endurance or to prescribe exercise.
Strength **Isotonic/isokinetic**	• Peak torque/force, maximal voluntary contraction		• Monitor and document changes due to treatment intervention or neurological recovery.
Flexibility **Goniometer**	• Range of motion of shoulder, elbow, wrist, knee, ankle, and other joints of affected limbs		• Can be used to document change due to treatment intervention.
Neuromuscular **Gait analysis Balance Sit-and-stand Hand-eye coordination**			• Monitor and document changes due to treatment intervention.

*Measurements of particular significance; do not *always* indicate test termination.

(continued)

STROKE AND HEAD INJURY: EXERCISE TESTING (continued)

MEDICATIONS	SPECIAL CONSIDERATIONS
• A large percentage of stroke patients are on hypertensive and cardiovascular medications. See appendix A. • Anticonvulsants are usually indicated for seizure-prone patients.	• Arthritis, particularly osteoarthritis, in shoulder, hip, and knee is common with stroke patients. Mode of exercise may have to be modified (e.g., cycle ergometry rather than treadmill or walking for testing and training). • Stroke patients are at risk for CAD, so close monitoring of ECG is essential. • Stroke patients may also have peripheral arterial disease, which may impair their ability to ambulate or cycle. • Sensation may be impaired, so careful observation is necessary to prevent injury. • Reduced motor control of limb may necessitate using only the uninvolved limb in arm, leg, or arm/leg ergometry.

STROKE AND HEAD INJURY: EXERCISE PROGRAMMING

MODES	GOALS	INTENSITY/ FREQUENCY/DURATION	TIME TO GOAL
Aerobic • Schwinn Air-Dyne (or any upper/lower-body ergometer) • Cycle ergometer • Treadmill • Arm ergometer	• Increase daily living activities.	• 40-70% $\dot{V}O_2$ peak . • 3 days/week. • 20-60 minutes/session.	• 4-6 months
Strength • Isometric exercise • Weight machine	• Increase daily living activities. • Increase strength for both involved and uninvolved limbs.	• 3 sets of 8-12 repetitions. • 2 days/week.	• 4-6 months
Flexibility • Stretching	• Increase range of motion of involved side. • Prevent contractures.	• Before and after either aerobic or strength exercise.	• 4-6 months
Neuromuscular • Coordination and balance exercises	• Increase daily living activities.	• Perform on same day as strength program.	• 4-6 months

$\dot{V}O_2$ max is undefined in stroke, head injury, and all major disabilities.

MEDICATIONS	SPECIAL CONSIDERATIONS
• See table on exercise testing.	• See table on exercise testing.

CHAPTER 30

Spinal Cord Injury

Stephen F. Figoni, PhD, RKT, FACSM

University of Kansas Medical Center

Overview of the Pathophysiology

Spinal cord injury (SCI) results in impairment or loss of motor or sensory function (or both) in the trunk and/or extremities due to damage to the neural elements within the spinal canal. Injury to the cervical segments (C1-C8) or the highest thoracic segment (T1) causes *quadriplegia* or *tetraplegia*, with impairment of the arms, trunk, legs, and pelvic organs (bladder, bowels, and sexual organs). Injury to thoracic segments T2-T12 causes paraplegia, with impairment to the trunk, legs, and/or pelvic organs. Injury to the lumbar or sacral segments of the cauda equina (L1-5, S1-4) results in impairment to the legs or pelvic organs, or both. The neurological level and completeness of injury determine the degree of impairment.

Physiologic impairment may include extensive muscular paralysis and sympathetic nervous system impairment. These frequently result in two major exercise-related problems:

- Reduced ability to voluntarily perform large muscle group aerobic exercise (i.e., without electrical stimulation of paralyzed muscles)

- Inability to stimulate the cardiovascular system to support higher rates of aerobic metabolism

Therefore, catecholamine production by the adrenal medullae, skeletal muscle venous pump, and thermoregulation may be impaired, restricting exercise cardiac output to subnormal levels. Common secondary complications during exercise, especially in persons with quadriplegia, may include limited positive cardiac chronotropic and inotropic states, excessive venous pooling, orthostatic and exercise hypotension, exercise intolerance, autonomic dysreflexia (a syndrome resulting from mass activation of autonomic reflexes causing extreme hypertension [BP > 200/100 mmHg]), headache, bradycardia, flushing, gooseflesh, unusual sweating, shivering, and nasal congestion.

Effects on the Exercise Response

In persons with paraplegia, the primary pathologic effects are usually limited to paralysis of the lower body, precluding exercise modes such as walking, running, and voluntary leg cycling. Therefore, the upper body must be used for all voluntary activities of daily living and exercise: arm cranking, wheelchair propulsion, and/or ambulation with orthotic devices and crutches. The proportionally smaller active upper body muscle mass typically restricts peak values of power output, oxygen consumption ($\dot{V}O_2$), and cardiac output to approximately one-half of those expected for maximal leg exercise in individuals without SCI.

In persons with quadriplegia, the pathologic effects are more extensive than with paraplegia. The active upper body muscle mass will be partially paralyzed, and the sympathetic nervous system may be completely separated from control by the brain. Upper body power output and $\dot{V}O_2$ and cardiac output are typically reduced to approximately one-half to one-third of the levels seen in individuals with paraplegia. Furthermore, strenuous exercise may not be tolerated because of orthostatic and exercise hypotension, which may produce symptoms of dizziness or nausea and others. Peak heart rates for persons with quadriplegia typically do not exceed 130 beats per minute.

Effects of Exercise Training

Arm exercise training adaptations are believed to be primarily peripheral (muscular) in nature, and may include increased muscular strength and endurance of the arm musculature in the exercise modes used. These may result in 10% to 20% improvements in peak power output and $\dot{V}O_2$ max, as well as enhanced sense of well-being. Central cardiovascular adaptations to exercise training, such as increased maximal stroke volume or cardiac output, have not yet been documented.

Management and Medications

Management of persons with SCI is complex because of the multitude of associated complications.

- **Skin**. People with SCI should avoid sitting for long periods without pressure relief; avoid abrasion/bumping of bony weight-bearing areas of hips, especially ischial tuberosities, sacrum, and coccyx; sit on a cushion.

- **Bones**. Those working with persons with SCI should avoid dropping during transfers or allowing the person to fall from wheelchair or exercise equipment. Persons with SCI have an increased risk for fractures secondary to osteoporosis.

- **Stabilization**. Because of loss of trunk control and balance, sufficient strapping and seat belts should be used during upright exercise.

- **Handgrip**. The hands of persons with weak/absent handgrip should be secured to ergometer handles with elastic bandages, gloves with Velcro straps, and the like.

- **Bladder**. The person should empty bladder or leg bag just before exercise test to avoid bladder overdistension or overfilling of the leg bag during exercise, as this may induce autonomic dysreflexia (with hypertension) in persons with paraplegia above T6 or with quadriplegia.

- **Bowels**. A regular bowel maintenance program is useful in order to avoid autonomic dysreflexic symptoms in persons with quadriplegia or accidental bowel movement during exercise.

- **Illness**. Postpone test if person is ill (i.e., has such conditions as bladder infection, pressure ulcer, cold, flu, allergy, unusual spasticity, autonomic dysreflexia, constipation).

- **Hypotension**. If resting BP before test is < 80/50 mmHg, the person should wear elastic support stockings and an abdominal binder, or both, to elevate resting BP. Exercise should be avoided within three hours of eating a large meal, as meals may induce hypotension. Monitor BP and symptoms of hypotension regularly (dizziness, light-headedness, nausea, pallor, cyanosis, extreme or sudden weakness, mental confusion, visual disturbances, inability to respond to questions or instructions).

- **Hypertension**. Autonomic dysreflexia is possible in persons with paraplegia above T6 or quadriplegia. Preventive measures include proper bowel and bladder management. Monitor BP regularly, and check for dysreflexic signs and symptoms. Discourage "boosting" (i.e., induction of autonomic dysreflexia to improve exercise tolerance).

- **Pain**. Discontinue arm exercise that aggravates chronic shoulder joint pain, as overuse syndromes are common in people who use their arms to propel wheelchairs.

- **Orthopedic**. Bone or joint swelling, discomfort, or deformity may indicate fracture or sprain.

Allow the person to take normal prescription medications. However, beware of medications that either induce hypotension (e.g., Ditropan/oxybutinin chloride, Dibenzyline/phenoxybenzamine hydrochloride) or induce diuresis (e.g., alcohol, diuretics).

Recommendations for Exercise Testing

- Consult a medical or allied health professional with specific training in exercise testing of persons with chronic disability such as SCI.

- Utilize exercise modes such as arm crank ergometry, arm cranking, seated aerobics, wheelchair ergometry, wheelchair propulsion on treadmill, electrical stimulation–induced leg cycle ergometry (ESLCE), or ESLCE combined with arm cranking.

- Adapt the exercise equipment as needed, and provide for special needs in terms of trunk stabilization (straps), securing hands on crank handles (holding gloves), skin protection (seat cushion and padding), prevention of bladder overdistension (i.e., emptying bladder or using urinary collection device immediately before test), and vascular support to help maintain BP and improve exercise tolerance (elastic stockings and abdominal binder).

- Use an environmentally controlled thermo-neutral or cool laboratory or clinic to compensate for impaired thermoregulation.

- Design a discontinuous incremental testing protocol that allows monitoring of heart rate, BP, rating of perceived exertion, and exercise tolerance at each stage. Power output increments may range from 5 to 20 watts depending on exercise mode, level and completeness of injury, and training status.

- Expect peak power outputs for persons with quadriplegia to range from 0 to 50 watts, and to range from 50 to 120 watts for persons with paraplegia. Treat postexercise hypotension and exhaustion with recumbency, leg elevation, rest, and fluid ingestion.

Recommendations for Exercise Programming

- Cardiopulmonary training modes may include arm cranking, wheelchair ergometry, wheelchair propulsion on treadmill or rollers, and free wheeling; swimming; vigorous sports such as wheelchair basketball, quad rugby, and racing; arm-powered cycling; vigorous activities of daily living such as ambulation with crutches and braces; seated aerobic exercises; and ESLCE, or ESLCE combined with arm cranking.

- To prevent upper-extremity overuse syndromes, (1) vary exercise modes from week to week; (2) strengthen muscles of the upper back and posterior shoulder, especially external shoulder rotators; and (3) stretch muscles of anterior shoulder and chest.

- Use an environmentally controlled, thermo-neutral gym, lab, or clinic for persons with quadriplegia. Individuals with thermoregulatory abilities can exercise outdoors if provisions are made for extreme conditions. Emptying the bladder or urinary collection device immediately before exercise may prevent dysreflexic symptoms during exercise. The person should drink plenty of fluids after exercise.

- The greater the exercising muscle mass, the greater the expected improvements in all physi-ologic and performance parameters. Arm training will probably induce training effects in the arm muscles only; combined arm and leg exercise may induce both muscular and cardiopulmonary training effects.

- Remember such training principles as specificity, overload, progression, and regularity.

Special Considerations

- **Psychologic.** Be supportive and set realistic goals.

- **Progression.** Expect small absolute improvements—5% per week.

- **Personnel.** Always supervise persons with quadriplegia. If they are not exercising in their own wheelchair, two people may be needed for manual transfer of large individuals to and from exercise equipment.

- **Safety.** Follow the precautions outlined concerning skin, bones, stabilization, handgrip, bladder, bowels, illness, hypotension, hypertension, pain, orthopedic complications, and medications. If necessary, hypotensive individuals should use supine posture and wear support stockings and abdominal binder to help maintain BP.

- **Supervision and monitoring.** Never leave a person with quadriplegia unsupervised. Monitor BP and symptoms regularly during exposure to orthostatic or exercise stress.

- **Follow-up.** Consult physician and appropriate allied health personnel to answer specific questions concerning medical complications to which subject may be susceptible.

- **Environmental.** Exercise should take place only in thermally neutral environments, such as a laboratory or clinic with air conditioning to control temperature and humidity, especially for persons with quadriplegia.

- **Cautions/comments.** In many conditions, little research is available to support specific guidelines. Thus, for some conditions the exercise professional may want to emphasize this point and suggest some innovative recommendations.

Suggested Readings

Davis, G., and R. Glaser. 1990. Cardiorespiratory fitness following spinal cord injury. In *Key issues in neurological physiotherapy,* ed. L. Ada and C. Canning, 155-96. London: Butterworth-Heinemann.

Davis, G.M. 1993. Exercise capacity of individuals with paraplegia. *Med. Sci. Sports Exerc.* 25: 423-32.

Ditunno, J.F., W. Young, W.H. Donovan, and G. Creasey. 1994. The international standards booklet for neurological and functional classification of spinal injury patients. *Paraplegia* 32: 70-80.

Figoni, S.F. 1993. Exercise responses and quadriplegia. *Med. Sci. Sports Exerc.* 25: 433-41.

Hoffman, M.D. 1986. Cardiorespiratory fitness and training in quadriplegics and paraplegics. *Sports Med.* 3: 312-30.

Glaser, R.M. 1987. Exercise and locomotion for the spinal cord injured. *Exerc. Sport Sci. Rev.* 13: 263-303.

Glaser, R.M., and G.M. Davis. 1989. Wheelchair-dependent individuals. In *Exercise in modern medicine,* ed. B.A. Franklin, S. Gordon, and G.C. Timmis, 237-67. Baltimore: Williams & Wilkins.

Miller, P. 1994. *Fitness programming and physical disability.* Champaign, IL: Human Kinetics.

Rimmer, J.H. 1994. *Fitness and rehabilitation programs for special populations.* Madison, WI: Brown.

Shephard, R.J. 1990. *Fitness in special populations.* Champaign, IL: Human Kinetics.

SPINAL CORD INJURY: EXERCISE TESTING

METHODS	MEASURES	ENDPOINTS*	COMMENTS
Aerobic power **Arm ergometer** **Wheelchair ergometer** **Wheelchair treadmill** **"Pushing" on track or** **treadmill**	• Heart rate, METs, or $\dot{V}O_2$ max	• Serious dysrhythmias • > 2 mm ST-segment depression or elevation • Ischemic threshold • T-wave inversion with significant ST change	• Adjust incremental power levels to subject's capacity. • Peak HR will be low (110-125 contractions/minute) in quadriplgia (above T-1) due to sympathetic impairment. • Persons working with quadriple gics will need gloves or wrap pings (see Special Considerations below).
	• Blood pressure	• SBP > 260 mmHg or DBP > 115 mmHg • Quadriplegics: SBP > 200mmHg	• Take between stages (i.e., stop exercise). Watch for hypertension due to autonomic dysreflexia or hypotension due to orthostasis and exertion.
	• RPE	• Volitional fatigue	• Indicates basic exercise tolerance and effort.
Flexibility **Goniometer** **Stretching tests**	• Flexibility of shoulders, elbow, wrist, hip, and knee		• To prevent contractures and injury.

*Measurements of particular significance; do not *always* indicate test termination.

SPECIAL CONSIDERATIONS

• Osteoporosis may exist in leg bones; possible contractures.
• Persons working with quadriplegics will usually display bradycardia and have peak HR limited to approximately 120 beats/minute. They do not adapt acutely to stressors such as heat or cold (i.e., blood shunting, shivering, and sweating may be profoundly impaired or abolished) or to exercise due to sympathetic dysfunction including

SPECIAL CONSIDERATIONS

vasomotor paralysis, cardiac sympathetic blockade, and adrenal denervation. Orthostatic and exercise hypotension is common. Persons with quadriplegia are also at risk for deep venous thrombosis leading to pulmonary embolism.
- Depending on level of injury, forced expiration can be limited or absent.
- Skeletal muscle paralysis depends on the level and completeness of injury, with upper motor neuron injury producing spastic paralysis and lower motor neuron injury producing flaccid paralysis. Spastic paralyzed muscles can be electrically stimulated to produce movements for functional or therapeutic purposes; flaccid paralyzed muscles do not respond to electrical stimulation techniques. Paralyzed leg muscles are also aggravated by venous pooling secondary to loss of the venous muscle pump.
- Sensory loss depends on level and completeness of injury according to dermatome maps. Insensate weight-bearing areas are at risk for pressure ulceration and need periodic pressure relief.
- In some settings, electrically stimulated muscle contractions can recruit sufficient muscle mass to significantly increase $\dot{V}O_2$ peak.
- $\dot{V}O_2$ peak depends on total active muscle mass.
- Each subject has his/her own bladder program. Be sure bladder is empty prior to testing.
- Voluntary anal sphincter control is often lost along with abdominal muscle denervation, necessitating special bowel care programs.

SPINAL CORD INJURY: EXERCISE PROGRAMMING

MODES	GOALS	INTENSITY/ FREQUENCY/DURATION	TIME TO GOAL
Aerobic • Arm ergometer • Wheelchair ergometer • Wheelchair treadmill • Free wheeling • Arm power cycling • Seated aerobics • Swimming • Wheelchair sports • Electrical stimulation leg cycle ergometry, with or without arm cranking	• Increase active muscle mass and strength. • Maximize overall strength for functional independence. • Improve efficiency of manual wheelchair propulsion.	• 50-80% peak HR. • 3-5 days/week. • 20-60 minutes/session.	• 4-6 months
Strength • Weight machines or dumbbells/wrist weights	• Increase active muscle mass and strength. • Maximize overall strength for functional independence. • Improve efficiency of manual wheelchair propulsion.	• 3 sets of 8-12 repetitions. • 2 days/week.	• 4-6 months
Flexibility • Stretching	• Avoid joint contracture.	• Before aerobic or strength exercise.	• 4-6 months

SPECIAL CONSIDERATIONS

- See table on exercise testing.

CHAPTER 31

Muscular Dystrophy

Oded Bar-Or, MD, FACSM

McMaster University
Chedoke Hospital
Children's Exercise Nutrition Center

Overview of the Pathophysiology

Muscular dystrophy (MD) is a family of hereditary diseases in which the primary pathology is within the muscle cell. The diseases vary in the rate of progression and the anatomic distribution of the pathology, but all are manifested by a progressive deterioration of muscle strength, power, and endurance. This section will highlight Duchenne MD (DMD), which has the highest incidence (20-30 boys out of 100,000 live births) among the MDs. Some mention will be made also of Becker MD (BMD) and facioscapulohumeral dystrophy (FSHD). These are characterized by loss of dystrophia in muscle cells. Duchenne MD and Becker MD are inherited through an X-linked recessive gene and affect males, although they can affect carrier females to a mild degree. Facioscapulohumeral MD is transmitted through an autosomal dominant gene and affects both sexes. Duchenne MD progresses rapidly and is fatal. Seldom does a patient with DMD reach the third decade of life. In addition to muscle dysfunction, the child slowly develops joint contracture secondary to the paralysis and resulting inactivity, usually during the wheelchair stage. At the early stage of DMD, persons still can walk. They subsequently become wheelchair-dependent and eventually bedridden. Becker MD is also progressive and fatal, but it advances at a slower pace. Individuals with BMD often maintain ambulation throughout the second decade. Persons with DMD or BMD often die from cardiac complications, as the disease affects the heart muscle, or from pulmonary compli-

cations. Facioscapulohumeral MD, which affects mostly the face and limb girdles, is the most benign among the three and does not have cardiac muscle involvement.

Effects on the Exercise Response

During the first three to four years of life, isometric strength (even in DMD) may be still within normal limits, but beyond age six it usually drops below the fifth percentile of healthy boys. There are no normative data on muscle endurance and peak power at these young ages, but the pattern of functional loss in persons with MD follows that of loss of strength. The ability to exercise is limited more by muscle weakness than by the oxygen transport system. Indeed, even during an "all-out" effort, peak heart rate in DMD and BMD seldom exceeds 120 to 140 beats/minute, suggesting a low metabolic drive. Rating of perceived exertion is very high for a given power in patients with DMD and BMD, but it becomes normal when calculated as percentage peak power. Because of a distorted gait pattern, oxygen cost of ambulation is likely to be excessive. However, the clinical utility of testing submaximal oxygen uptake during walking has not been reported. Muscular dystrophy is sometimes accompanied by obesity, which may further limit exercise ability.

Effects of Exercise Training

There are no published long-term, randomly controlled training studies of persons with MD. It is therefore premature to state categorically whether or not a certain physiologic function improves with training. On the basis of scant literature and anecdotal information from the author's laboratory, resistance training can slow down, and for a while even slightly reverse, the deterioration in muscle function. Improvement has been documented in the more benign dystrophies, particularly in the person who is slowly progressing. There are no data on the effects of training on maximal oxygen uptake or oxygen cost of locomotion. The drop in muscle function after a brief period of bed rest (discussed in the next section) is further, albeit indirect, evidence for the importance of physical activity.

Management and Medications

There is no cure available for MD. Medications such as corticosteroids have been used, and they can retard muscle weakness and prolong ambulation. However, their efficacy in slowing the long-term deterioration in muscle function is questionable. Rehabilitation therapy is aimed mostly at maintenance of activities of daily living (e.g., by prevention of contracture). Assistive devices (e.g., ankle-foot orthoses) may possibly prolong the ambulation phase in the more benign forms. Surgery is sometimes used (e.g., for release of an Achilles tendon and stabilization of the spine). There is no evidence that any surgery helps to improve the child's response to exercise. However, it can help prevent contracture if combined with orthoses and regular exercise to maintain range of motion. Bed rest that accompanies surgery, even if it lasts as little as two to three weeks, is often accompanied by a precipitous decline in muscle performance. Therefore, individuals should be mobilized for exercise within 24 to 48 hours of any surgical procedure.

Recommendations for Exercise Testing

- Focus on muscle endurance, peak power, and strength rather than on maximal aerobic power.

- Although subjective muscle testing is a common practice in a clinical setting and is useful to document deterioration, functional grading of gait and other skills is also useful for follow-up purposes.

- Measure muscle strength with a hand-held dynamometer or with a more sophisticated dynamometer.

- The Wingate anaerobic test, which assesses muscle endurance and peak power, has been found to be feasible and highly reliable for persons with DMD and BMD. It seems to be sensitive to changes in anaerobic performance

due to training or natural deterioration. Use the test for either the upper or lower limbs.

- Monitor the person's pulmonary functions (to detect a restrictive pattern) and body composition (to detect any tendency for excessive fat gain). When using aerobic protocols, monitor heart rate, ECG, and rating of perceived exertion.

- Frequency of testing will depend on the specific objective and the rate of disease progression. A person with DMD will require more frequent evaluations (e.g., three times per year) than the person with BMD.

- Some individuals will require deviations from routine testing protocols. Keep an open mind as to such needs.

Recommendations for Exercise Programming

- Provide realistic short-term goals to the individual and parents.

- The program should focus on maintaining (or reducing the rate of deterioration of) muscle endurance, peak power, and strength, as well as on prevention of contracture and enhanced overall caloric expenditure. For most cases, only submaximal resistance exercises should be used.

- If a client complains of exercise-induced cramps or excessive fatigue, reduce the intensity. Overwork weakness may occur, as dystrophic muscles do *not* respond well to overload.

- Because of the young age of these individuals, include as many game-like "fun" situations as possible.

- To prevent the person's becoming overweight, provide nutritional counseling in conjunction with physical training.

Special Considerations

Special issues to consider while working with people who have MD involve safety, exercise intensity, requirements relating to the use of ergometers, and psychological aspects.

Safety

At advanced stages, DMD may be accompanied by congestive heart failure and other cardiac abnormalities. Conceptually, maximal efforts should be contraindicated in these individuals. It is highly unlikely, however, that a person with such an advanced disease will be able to perform exercise of more than minimal intensity. Traditionally, clinicians have objected to training clients with DMD because exercise may induce a marked increase in their plasma creatine kinase (CK) concentration, suggesting damage to muscle cell membranes. The CK leaks out of cells in DMD because of the loss of dystrophin in the membrane. More recent observations, however, suggest that there is no clear relationship between plasma CK level and prior exercise, particularly at low-to-moderate exercise intensities. Some persons complain of limb pain and muscle cramps following exertion. These are usually eliminated by reducing exercise intensity.

In conclusion, it seems that exercise at low-to-moderate intensities is safe for persons with milder forms of MD, but of questionable benefit in individuals with DMD. As a general rule, muscles with manual muscle testing grades of 3 or less will not benefit from active or resistive exercises.

Ergometry

Ergometers must be suitable for arm cranking and leg cycling alike. Most persons with MD generate extremely low peak muscle power; values as low as 10 to 20 watts are common in DMD. Therefore, one needs ergometers with braking forces that yield power outputs as low as 5 to 10 watts. Furthermore, the ergometer must allow for very small increments in power (e.g., 2 to 3 watts). These considerations are important because various commercially available ergometers require muscle power of more than 10 watts even at "zero" resistance. Another consideration is the length of the pedal shaft: some persons can arm crank by using only their triceps, with very little contribution of the elbow flexors. Such individuals can arm crank only if the radius of pedal excursion is small (e.g., 10 instead of the standard 17.5 centimeters).

Psychologic Aspects

Enhanced physical activity is virtually the only therapeutic modality through which a person with a debilitating disease such as MD can *actively* participate and "take charge" (rather than be treated by others). Individuals with MD often like to take up such a challenge, even when they know that exercise and sport will not reverse the inevitable outcome of their disease. Such an effect on the person's self-esteem outweighs, in this author's opinion, any potentially deleterious effect of exercise. The individual should seek advice from a competent medical expert before undertaking such activities.

Suggested Readings

Bar-Or, O. 1983. *Pediatric sports medicine for the practitioner.* New York: Springer-Verlag.

Bar-Or, O. 1993. Noncardiopulmonary pediatric exercise test. In *Pediatric laboratory exercise testing,* ed. T.W. Rowland, 165-85. Champaign, IL: Human Kinetics.

Bar-Or, O., and S.L. Reed. 1987. Rating of perceived exertion in adolescents with neuromuscular disease. In *Perception of exertion in physical work,* ed. G. Borg, 137-48. Stockholm: Wenner-Gre.

Brooke, M.H. 1986. *A clinician's view of neuromuscular diseases.* 2nd ed. Baltimore: Williams & Wilkins.

Edwards, R.H.T. 1980. Studies of muscular performance in normal and dystrophic subjects. *Br. Med. Bull.* 35: 159-65.

Florence, J.M., and J.M. Hagberg. 1984. Effect of training on the exercise responses of neuromuscular disease patients. *Med. Sci. Sports Exerc.* 16: 460-65.

Fowler, W.M., Jr. 1988. Management of musculoskeletal complications in neuromuscular disease: Weakness and the role of exercise. *Arch. Phys. Med. Rehabil.* 2: 489-507.

Jackson, M.J., J.M. Round, D.J. Newham, and R.H.T. Edwards. 1987. An examination of some factors influencing creatine kinase in blood in patients with muscular dystrophy. *Muscle and Nerve* 10: 15-21.

McCarthy, N., D. Moroz, S.H. Garner, and A.J. McComas. 1988. The effects of strength training in patients with selected neuromuscular disorders. *Med. Sci. Sports Exerc.* 20: 362-68.

Milner-Brown, H.S., and R.G. Miller. 1988. Muscle strengthening through high-resistance with training in patients with neuromuscular disorders. *Arch. Phys. Med. Rehabil.* 69: 14-19.

Scott, O.M., S.A. Hyde, C. Goddard, R. Jones, and V. Dubowitz. 1981. Effect of exercise in Duchenne muscular dystrophy. *Physiotherapy* 67: 174-176.

Tirosh, E., O. Bar-Or, and P. Rosenbaum. 1990. New muscle power test in neuromuscular disease: Feasibility and reliability. *Am. J. Dis. Child.* 144: 1083-87.

MUSCULAR DYSTROPHY: EXERCISE TESTING

METHODS	MEASURES	ENDPOINTS*	COMMENTS
Aerobic power **Treadmill** (0.5-1 METs/stage) **Cycle** (5-10 watts/min) ramp protocol (2-3 watts/3 min stage) **Arm ergometer**	• 12-lead ECG • Heart rate, blood pressure • RPE	• Serious dysrhythmias • > 2 mm ST-segment depression or elevation • Ischemic threshold • T-wave inversion with significant ST change • SBP > 260 mmHg or DBP > 115 mmHg • Hypotensive response • Perceived shortness of breath and fatigue	• Use if cardiac involvement is suspected. • HR helpful in developing exercise program and detecting deterioration of metabolic drive. • Helpful in developing exercise program.
Muscular endurance and power **20-30-minute walking tests** **Wingate test** **Maximum repetitions at 60% maximal voluntary contraction**	• Distance • Anaerobic power	• Time • Fatigue	
Strength **Weight machine or dynamometer**	• 1 repetition maximum or maximal voluntary contraction		• Test arm, shoulder, leg, and hip strength.
Flexibility **Goniometry**	• Range of motion of major joints		
Neuromuscular **Gait/balance analysis** **Gross motor fitness evaluation**	• Comfort of walking • Speed, balance, stability, reaction time		• Important to follow progression or regression of program or disease, respectively.
Functional capacity **Lifestyle-specific tests**	• Performance related to daily living activities, especially dressing and personal hygiene		• Can be used as an indication of functional capacity in involved clients.

*Measurements of particular significance; do not *always* indicate test termination.

(continued)

MUSCULAR DYSTROPHY: EXERCISE TESTING *(continued)*

SPECIAL CONSIDERATIONS

- All of the tests listed should be performed every 4-6 weeks to determine progress of disease/treatment.
- Orthopedic: Contractures and muscle imbalance may affect client's ability to exercise.
- Cardiac: Congestive heart failure and other cardiac anomalies have been reported in advanced cases, but it is doubtful whether these patients can perform exercise.
- Pulmonary: Vital capacity and inspiratory and expiratory reserve volumes will indicate a restrictive pattern at advanced stages due to weakness of respiratory muscles.
- Muscular: Extreme and progressive muscle weakness will affect performances in all tests.
- Since most available ergometers require muscle power of more than 10 watts when at "zero" resistance, ergometers and dynamometers need adapting to the *very low* power that can be generated by people with MD.

MUSCULAR DYSTROPHY: EXERCISE PROGRAMMING

MODES	GOALS	INTENSITY/ FREQUENCY/DURATION	TIME TO GOAL
Aerobic • Arm and leg ergometry	• Maintain work capacity.	• 50-85% HR reserve. • Daily. • Exercise until fatigued.	
Muscular endurance and power • Short walking sessions (20-30 meters)	• Increase work capacity.	• As fast as possible. • 4-6 sessions daily.	
Strength • Weight machines or dynamometer	• Maintain strength of arms, shoulders, legs, and hips.	• Use light weights or no resistance. • 3 sets of 8-12 repetitions. • 3 sessions/week.	
Flexibility • Stretching	• Increase or maintain range of motion.	• 5-7 sessions/week.	
Functional • Activity-specific exercise	• Maintain capacity to perform as many daily living activities as possible (useful when "traditional" exercise program is no longer possible).	• To tolerance.	

SPECIAL CONSIDERATIONS

- Expectations of "improvement" in any of the above functions should be moderate; it is more realistic to aim for *slowing down the progress of the disease.*
- See table on testing.

CHAPTER 32

Epilepsy

Ronald H. Spiegel, MD
John R. Gates, MD
The University Epilepsy Group, P.A.

Overview of the Pathophysiology

Epilepsy is defined as recurring seizures. A seizure is an abnormal electrical discharge within the brain resulting in involuntary change in movement, sensation, perception, behavior, and/or level of consciousness. Although the revised international classification of epilepsies defines many types of seizures, generalized tonic-clonic, complex partial, and absence seizures account for over 90%. Approximately 10% of the population will have at least one seizure during his or her lifetime, and 3% will develop epilepsy.

Dramatic physiologic changes may take place during a seizure, depending on its type and duration. During a generalized tonic-clonic seizure, autonomic changes can produce cyanosis, diaphoresis (sweating), pallor, vomiting, and loss of bladder control. Arterial pH may fall below 7.0 with a mixed metabolic and respiratory acidosis. Hypoxemia may occur along with hyperglycemia during brief seizures, and hypoglycemia may occur during status epilepticus (seizures longer than 30 minutes). Recovery varies with duration and intensity of seizure, with a period of fatigue lasting from seconds to several hours. Multiple seizures in a day may leave the person persistently in either an ictal or a postictal state.

Effects on the Exercise Response

Most studies have focused on the possibility of exercise precipitating seizures, and in particular, of seizures leading to an injury. Studies of exercise in general note few seizures occurring during or in the aftermath of physical activity. In one study, 5 of 250 individuals reported a seizure during sport participation. Exercise has consistently produced a trend toward normalization of the interictal electroencephalogram. Seizure frequency is typically less during exercise than in resting states; mental activity also tends to diminish seizure frequency. Although hypoglycemia, hypoxia, hyperventilation, extreme fatigue, and hyperthermia may precipitate seizures, there have been no reports of the seizures actually precipitated by those conditions resulting from exercise. Certain activities have potential risk, such as hang gliding and scuba diving, but there has been no documented morbidity or mortality related to seizures during sport activities.

Exercise does not directly affect antiepileptic drug metabolism. However, a 10% change in weight may affect antiepileptic drug blood levels.

Effects of Exercise Training

Individuals with epilepsy generally have a lower physical work capacity than individuals without epilepsy, probably as a reflection of a sedentary lifestyle. However, exercise capacity appears not to be markedly different from that of the general population.

Management and Medications

A graduated and comprehensive approach to fitness development is recommended. When a person with epilepsy is in the ictal state, it is helpful for professionals involved with exercise testing and training to have knowledge of seizure first aid. During the postictal state, observation of the seizing person is warranted until he or she is fully reoriented. After the seizure, the person with epilepsy may resume exercise as tolerated but be aware of impaired alertness, balance, coordination, and fatigue. Resumption of exercise should be evaluated on an individual basis.

Be aware of possible side effects such as ataxia and decreased alertness, especially with changes in medications. A physician should reevaluate antiepileptic drug dosage if a 10% weight loss or gain occurs.

Recommendations for Exercise Testing

Recognize that work capacity and baseline fitness may be below values for the general population. Although exercise usually does not cause seizures, be prepared for seizures during maximal exercise testing.

- Avoid testing in the immediate postictal state, as these persons may overestimate their abilities.
- Be aware of possible drug side effects such as lethargy and ataxia.
- The exercise professional should know seizure first aid.

Recommendations for Exercise Programming

Follow standard guidelines for exercise testing and prescription as for persons without epilepsy, with the precautions already discussed. There is evidence that exercise and sport participation may improve self-esteem for the person with epilepsy. Not only should exercise not be restricted, it should be encouraged. Taken as a whole, the data on risks and benefits of exercise for the person with epilepsy strongly favor participation with few, if any, restrictions. The evidence is ample enough to recommend that the burden of proof rest on establishing that a certain exercise or sport should be restricted. In the absence of such data, participation would be accepted, if not encouraged. This attitude is reflected in changes of opinion regarding sport participation, both by the American Medical Association and by the American Academy of Physicians.

Suggested Readings

Cordova, F. 1993. Epilepsy and sport. *Aust. Fam. Physician* 22: 558-62.

Ellertsen, B., H.R. Eriksen, R. Hege, D.I. Mostofsky, and H. Ursin. 1993. Exercise and epilepsy. In *The neurobehavioral treatment of epilepsy*, ed. D.I. Mostofsky and Y. Loyning, 107-122. Hillsdale, NJ: Erlbaum.

Gates, J.R. 1991. Epilepsy and sports participation. *Physician Sportsmed.* 19: 98-104.

Gates, J.R., and R.H. Spiegel. 1993. Epilepsy, sports and exercise. *Sports Med.* 15: 1-5.

Roth, D.L., K.T. Goode, V.L. Williams, and E. Faught. 1994. Physical exercise, stressful life experience, and depression in adults with epilepsy. *Epilepsia* 35: 1248-55.

Schmitt, B., L. Thun-Hohenstein, H. Vontobel, and E. Boltshauser. 1994. Seizures induced by physical exercise: Report of two cases. *Neuropediatrics* 25: 51-53.

van Linschoten, R., F.J. Backx, O.G. Mulder, and H. Meinardi. 1990. Epilepsy and sports. *Sports Med.* 10: 9-19.

EPILEPSY: EXERCISE TESTING

METHODS	MEASURES	ENDPOINTS*	COMMENTS
Aerobic power **Treadmill** (1-2 METs/stage) **Bike** (17 watts/min) ramp protocol (25 watts/3 min stage)	• 12-lead ECG • Heart rate, blood pressure • RPE	• Serious dysrhythmias • > 2 mm ST-segment depression or elevation • Ischemia • T-wave inversion with significant ST change • SBP > 260 mmHg or DBP > 115 mmHg • Volitional fatigue	• Testing and screening may be warranted if risk factors/symptoms of CAD are present (see exercise testing table in chapter 3).
Muscular endurance and power **6-12-minute walk**	• Distance	• Time	• Useful for measurement of improvement throughout conditioning program.
Strength **Free weights, machines**	• 1 repetition maximum or maximal voluntary contraction		

*Measurements of particular significance; do not *always* indicate test termination.

MEDICATIONS	SPECIAL CONSIDERATIONS
• Following are the possible side effects of epilepsy medications: lethargy, ataxia, decreased alertness, and weight loss or gain.	• Know seizure first aid. • Avoid exercise immediately after seizure.

EPILEPSY: EXERCISE PROGRAMMING

MODES	GOALS	INTENSITY/FREQUENCY/DURATION	TIME TO GOAL
Aerobic endurance • Large muscle activities (e.g., walking, biking, rowing, swimming, jogging—whatever participant enjoys most)	• Increase peak $\dot{V}O_2$, peak work rate, and endurance.	• 60-90% peak work rate. • 3-5 days/week. • 20-40 minutes/session. • Progressively increase intensity and duration.	• 4-6 months
Strength • Isotonic/isokinetic exercises	• Improve general fitness. • Prevent muscle atrophy.	• Start with low resistance, high repetitions.	

MEDICATIONS	SPECIAL CONSIDERATIONS
• See table on exercise testing.	• See table on exercise testing.

CHAPTER 33

Multiple Sclerosis

Janet A. Mulcare, PhD, FACSM

Andrews University

Overview of the Pathophysiology

Multiple sclerosis (MS) is a demyelinating disease affecting the central nervous system (CNS). The pathological definition of MS includes the demonstration of areas of specific demyelination that are disseminated in both time and space in the white matter of the CNS. The loss of myelin, the fatty material that insulates nerves, adversely affects rapid, smooth conduction along the neural pathways in the CNS. This loss of myelin reduces the speed of conduction, subsequently interfering with smooth, rapid, coordinated movement. As a result, MS-associated problems range from minimal effects to severe disability.

Effects on the Exercise Response

Depending on the level and nature of impairment associated with the disease, individuals may experience a variety of symptoms that may have a direct effect on their responses to a single session of exercise. Symptoms that may affect a single session of exercise responses are

- spasticity,
- incoordination,
- impaired balance,
- fatigue,

- muscle weakness, paresis (partial paralysis), and paralysis,
- sensory loss and numbness,
- cardiovascular dysautonomia (dysfunction of the autonomic nervous system causing possible problem with cardioacceleration and reduction in blood pressure response),
- tremor, and
- heat sensitivity.

Effects of Exercise Training

Exercise training has no effect on the prognosis or progression of MS. However, exercise may improve short-term physical fitness and functional performance (e.g., strength, endurance, and aerobic fitness).

- Fatigue can reduce exercise tolerance.
- Impaired balance may affect the choice of exercise mode.
- Heat intolerance may affect intensity, duration, mode, and environmental demands.
- Spasticity may require special foot strapping and may cause hip adduction and abduction.
- Sensory loss may preclude upright activities such as walking or running.
- Muscle paresis can reduce exercise intensity and duration.

Management and Medications

Several medications are commonly prescribed to persons with MS to manage the symptoms associated with the disease (see table on exercise testing at the end of this chapter).

Recommendations for Exercise Testing

Common symptoms that affect ambulation (lower-extremity sensory decrement/loss, foot drop, balance difficulty, muscle spasticity, tremor) often make treadmill testing impractical for this population. Therefore, the preferred mode of clinical exercise testing is either upright or recumbent leg cycle ergometry. If a combination arm and leg ergometer is available, the increase in activated muscle mass may improve test results by eliciting greater cardiopulmonary stress. In both types of ergometry, toe clips and heel straps are recommended to ensure foot stability and counteract spasticity, tremor, and weakness in the lower extremities. However, it is recommended that arm and leg movements be mechanically linked to reduce the need for motor coordination. Individuals who are more severely impaired with significant lower-extremity paresis or paralysis may use arm cranking as a viable alternative to leg cycling. However, the primary problem associated with arm cranking is arm muscle fatigue occurring before a true cardiopulmonary maximum is elicited.

Other recommendations for performing exercise testing with this population include the following:

- Use a continuous or discontinuous protocol of three- to five-minute stages.

- Begin with a warm-up of unloaded pedaling or cranking.

- Increase the work rate for each stage by approximately 12-25 watts and 8-12 watts for legs and arms, respectively.

- Monitor heart rate and blood pressure.

- Typical test termination criteria are volitional fatigue, achievement of maximal heart rate, or decrease/plateau in $\dot{V}O_2$ with increasing work rate.

Research has shown that peak $\dot{V}O_2$ varies greatly among individuals with MS and is to some extent related to the individual's impairment of the lower extremities. Since very little data are available that can be reported by gender, age, and impairment level, it is difficult to provide standard values as guidelines. In the absence of cardiovascular dysautonomia or severe muscle paresis, research has shown that most individuals are able to reach 85% to 90% of their age-predicted maximal heart rate. Therefore, this may be a viable means for gauging maximal exercise capacity in the absence of supportive metabolic data.

Recommendations for Exercise Programming

Exercise prescription for individuals with MS should focus upon maintenance and, when possible, improvement of their current level of joint flexibility, muscular strength and endurance, and cardiopulmonary endurance. Since fatigue is a common complaint, any intervention that can increase energy by improving efficiency should be incorporated into a well-balanced exercise program. This might include activities related to the areas already mentioned as well as activities that focus on weight control or reduction. Recommendations for exercise training are found in the table on exercise programming at the end of this chapter.

Special Considerations

When working with a person who has MS, exercise personnel need to keep in mind possible psychological dimensions as well as the variability of progression of the disease itself. There are also considerations relating to safety and the exercise environment.

Psychological

Many individuals with MS have some level of cognitive deficit that will affect their understanding of testing and training instructions and/or have memory loss sufficient to require written instructions to supplement verbal cues. These individuals may require additional time for information processing as well as multiple forms of information presentation to ensure understanding.

Progression

It is common for the symptoms of MS to recur, resulting in progressive impairment. For some people, this progression is slow and may take years, while in others the disease may progress significantly within weeks or months. Therefore, the manner in which an exercise program progresses or regresses will vary among individuals. During a period of complete remission, persons with MS should be encouraged to follow the guidelines outlined in the table on programming. With use of a given target heart rate as a means for tracking physiologic responses, work rate can be increased to match training adaptations.

Personnel

Exercise professionals should be aware of the various symptoms experienced by persons with this disease and should recognize the effects such symptoms may have on exercise performance. The exercise professional should also be sensitive to daily variation in symptoms that can be influenced by changes in medications, sleep disorders, and increases in environmental or circadian temperature. Daily training expectations should be flexible to accommodate these factors. Personnel should be knowledgeable regarding transfers, lifting, and assistance techniques for individuals with physical disabilities.

Supervision and Monitoring

Resting heart rate and blood pressure should be obtained before aerobic exercise is begun. Heart rate should be monitored throughout an exercise session to assure that the target level is maintained. Ratings of perceived exertion may be beneficial; however, these ratings may not be valid in the presence of cognitive deficits.

Appropriate Follow-Up

The fitness of persons with MS should be reevaluated at least every six months. However, an annual assessment is acceptable. If individuals experience an exacerbation, they should not be encouraged to exercise until the disease status returns to full remission. Full remission means that the symptoms that have been manifested during the exacerbation have diminished or disappeared. When possible, this should be confirmed by the client's neurologist. Once it is determined that the person is in remission, a new baseline of exercise performance should be established and goals should be adjusted. For the client whose disease is progressing slowly, increased impairment may be very subtle, and distinct improvement may not be as obvious. In cases of the progressive nonremitting type of MS, the goal of the

exercise program may be simply to slow any further physical deterioration and optimize remaining function.

Environmental

Some persons with MS have either attenuated or absent sudomotor (sweating) responses. This impairment can further compound the already heightened sensitivity to increases in internal and external temperature that adversely affects these individuals. Therefore, even for moderate-intensity aerobic exercise, room temperature should be kept neutral (72-76 °F). Fans should be provided upon request. Persons with MS should be encouraged to drink water before, during, and following each exercise session. For moderate-intensity aquatic exercise, water temperature between 89 and 91 °F is comfortable and offers significant heat-dissipating potential.

Cautions and Comments

The general lack of research in this area and the variability in aerobic exercise capacity among persons with MS make it difficult to develop absolute standards for comparison among individuals with MS. Therefore, expected outcomes from training are often less evident. Preliminary data show that after a six-month program of moderate aerobic exercise, individuals with MS may show an average aerobic fitness gain of 30%; however, the variability among individuals is extremely high (2% to 54%).

Suggested Readings

Ponichtera-Mulcare, J.A. 1993. Exercise and multiple sclerosis. *Med. Sci. Sports Exerc.* 25: 451-65.

Ponichtera-Mulcare, J.A., and R.M. Glaser. 1993. Evaluation of muscle performance and cardiopulmonary fitness in patients with multiple sclerosis: Implications for rehabilitation. *Neurorehabil.* 3 (4): 17-29.

Schapiro, R.T. 1987. *Symptom management in multiple sclerosis.* New York: Demos.

Waksman, B.H., S.C. Reingold, and W.E. Reynolds. 1987. *Research on multiple sclerosis.* New York: Demos.

MULTIPLE SCLEROSIS: EXERCISE TESTING

METHODS	MEASURES	ENDPOINTS*	COMMENTS

Aerobic power
 	
Schwinn Air-Dyne
 	
Recumbent or Semirecumbent Cycle
    (17 watts/min) ramp
    protocol
    (12-25 watts/3 min stage)
	• Expired gas analysis
	
	• Heart rate
	
	• RPE
	
	• Blood pressure
		• Peak $\dot{V}O_2$, METs
		
		• Peak HR
		
		• Volitional fatigue
		
		• SBP > 200 mmHg or DBP > 115 mmHg
		• Hypotensive response
			• Peak $\dot{V}O_2$, METs, and RPE are the best predictors for developing an exercise program because of possible abnormal cardioacceleration responses.
			
			• Attenuated BP response may occur.

Endurance **Air-Dyne or cycle ergometer** **Walking (limited)**	• Distance	• Time	• Also a good indicator for developing an exercise program.
Strength **Isokinetic**	• Peak power output and peak torque of major muscle groups		• Has been shown to have moderate correlation with aerobic power.
Flexibility **Goniometry**	• Joint angles		• Helpful in explaining gait abnormalities.
Neuromuscular **Gait analysis**			• Use to determine and quantify asymmetry, muscle weakness or paresis, and functional changes.

*Measurements of particular significance; do not *always* indicate test termination.

MEDICATIONS	SPECIAL CONSIDERATIONS
• Amantadine HCl: May temporarily reduce fatigue. • Baclofen: High dosage may cause muscle weakness. • Amitriptyline HCl, fluoxetine HCl, hyoscyamine sulfate: May cause muscle weakness. • Prednisone: May cause muscle weakness, reduced sweating, hypertension, diabetes, and/or osteoporosis.	• Prediction of peak $\dot{V}O_2$ from submaximal performance has been shown to result in > 15% error in this population. • Patients may experience foot drop, affecting exercise capacity. • Reduced sensation is variable over the extremities; may be symmetrical or asymmetrical. Sensations of numbness and tingling are also common. • Paresis and paralysis are more prevalent in lower extremities and anti-gravity muscles. • Muscle imbalance may exist between agonist and antagonist muscles. • Some patients may have significant cognitive deficit. This may require careful instructions and cuing during testing. RPE scale may be difficult for them to understand. • Because of difficulty to adjust to temperature changes, the testing room should be kept cool or thermo-neutral.

MEDICATIONS	SPECIAL CONSIDERATIONS
	• Incontinence is common. Opportunities for voiding before and during testing should be planned. • Morning is usually the optimal time to test. • If possible, recumbent cycling is desirable over upright cycling due to balance problems. Toe clips or heel straps are needed because of ankle/foot clonus or leg spasticity.

MULTIPLE SCLEROSIS: EXERCISE PROGRAMMING

MODES	GOALS	INTENSITY/ FREQUENCY/DURATION	TIME TO GOAL
Aerobic and endurance • Cycling • Walking • Swimming	• Increase cardiovascular function.	• 60-85% peak HR/50-70% peak VO_2. • 3 sessions/week. • 30 minutes/session.	• 4-6 months
Strength • Weight machines • Free weights • Isokinetic machines	• Increase functional capacity.	• Perform on non-endurance training days.	
Flexibility • Stretching	• Increase or maintain range of motion.	• Perform before strength or endurance training. • 5-7 sessions/week.	

MEDICATIONS	SPECIAL CONSIDERATIONS
• See table on exercise testing.	• May experience attenuated HR or BP response during exercise. May have attenuated or absent sudomotor response. • Maintaining hydration is critical. • Secondary medical problems are common, with hypertension and obesity being common CAD risk factors. • Much of the disability incurred is also related to secondary deterioration from sedentary lifestyle. • Non-weight-bearing activities should be relegated to clients having balance problems, orthopedic complications, or sensory loss to the lower extremities. • Muscle weakness in the lower extremities often causes premature fatigue. Symptoms may change over the course of the exercise program and may require adjustments of intensity and duration. • Depression may affect adherence, so constant reinforcement and counseling are necessary for some clients.

CHAPTER 34

Polio and Post-Polio Syndrome

Thomas J. Birk, PhD, FACSM
Medical College of Ohio

Overview of the Pathophysiology

Poliomyelitis is an acute viral disease that attacks the anterior horn cells of lower motor neurons. This results in a flaccid paresis/paralysis and atrophy in affected muscle groups. Recovery from the self-terminating disease is generally good, and most individuals with polio lead active and productive lives. However, almost 40 years after contracting acute poliomyelitis during peak epidemic periods, approximately one-fourth of the affected population have developed symptoms similar to those of the initial onset of the disease. Common symptoms include fatigue, weakness, and muscle and joint pain. Other symptoms include sleep disorders and intolerance of cold. The return of these symptoms has been collectively called *post-polio syndrome (PPS)*.

Apparently the muscle weakness is secondary to chronic overload and eventual loss of motor units through the aging process. When a critical level of less than 50% of the original total number of motor units is reached, symptoms of fatigue, weakness, and pain become apparent. Other factors contributing to weakness, fatigue, and pain include excessive body fat (overloading already weakened leg muscles) and repetitive physical tasks (overloading a smaller muscle mass).

Effects on the Exercise Response

The majority of persons with PPS whose lower extremities have been affected will have altered acute responses to exercise. They can be expected to exhibit significantly diminished leg strength and aerobic capacity when compared with asymptomatic post-polio individuals of similar age. This appears secondary to a loss of motor units whereby fewer motor units can be activated to generate muscle tension, resulting in diminished strength and endurance. Thus, an additional burden is placed on the remaining motor units, and this can cause more rapid onset of fatigue. Aerobic power is diminished in many persons with PPS and appears to be related to muscle weakness and deconditioning.

Labile exercise blood pressures are potential risks that should be initially monitored. Secondary to premature peripheral fatigue, maximal heart rates are usually 20 to 30 beats/minute less than what would be expected for asymptomatic post-polio persons of similar age. Concomitantly, maximal oxygen consumption is typically up to 20% lower than what would be seen for similarly aged counterparts.

Effects of Exercise Training

Although there are few well-controlled prospective studies, the literature suggests that lower-extremity strength and aerobic capacity can be significantly increased in persons with PPS. The relative improvements in aerobic capacity have equaled those for asymptomatic post-polio persons of similar age.

However, inherent with prolonged high-intensity exercise are joint edema, possible deformity, and general muscle discomfort. Documented beneficial changes include:

- increases of 15% to 20% in aerobic capacity with the use of moderate-intensity exercise after eight weeks of training, and
- increases in quadriceps and hamstring muscle strength after six weeks of resistive training.

Management and Medications

Primary means of managing and treating PPS have included energy conservation, bracing/splinting, and antidepressant medications. Strength and moderate-intensity aerobic exercise training have been used as adjunctive therapy. For conservation of energy, it is advisable to

- perform exercise testing and training in the morning of relatively unstressful days, and
- avoid physically overstressing and overextending effort.

Some guidelines for bracing and splinting are the following:

- Support the joint around which muscles have significantly weakened.
- Fitting and braces/splints should allow for sufficient range of motion during exercise.
- Braces and splints increase muscular efficiency during activities of daily living, not during exercise.
- Fasten one or more limbs to ergometer pedals or cranks when necessary.

Medications are prescribed by a physician for chronic fatigue and sleep disorders. Antidepressants (such as Elavil, Pamelor, Sinequan, Prozac, Zoloft) inhibit neurotransmitters (serotonin, norepinephrine), decreasing fatigue and improving sleep. These medications may increase heart rate and decrease blood pressure during rest and exercise. Electrocardiogram abnormalities have included false positive and false negative exercise test results, as well as possible T-wave changes and dysrhythmias, especially in persons with a cardiac history. Exercise may help alleviate some of the prevalent anticholinergic side effects such as constipation and

lethargy. The therapeutic effect of these medications may be delayed from two to four weeks after the beginning of therapy.

Recommendations for Exercise Testing

Exercise testing of persons with PPS should incorporate the following principles:

- Optimal utilization of available muscle mass
- Avoidance of use of a painful limb during an exercise test
- Utilization of equipment that does not require complex motor coordination
- Use of submaximal intensity for testing

Four-limb ergometry is preferred, but for persons with severe lower limb involvement, an arm crank ergometer is recommended. Four-limb ergometry activates the greatest possible muscle mass, and if necessary the use of a painful limb can be minimized while the other limbs are still allowed to exercise. Because it increases the active muscle mass, use of a four-limb ergometer presents a greater challenge for the cardiopulmonary system. The four-limb ergometer should include a cycling mechanism for the legs and either a cycling or push/pull mechanism for the arms. Work rate should be measurable, accurate, and repeatable.

Although the treadmill is most commonly used by those without PPS, it is less preferred as a means of graded exercise testing for people with PPS even though the majority are ambulatory. Typically, a symptomatic and weakened lower extremity will fatigue locally before cardiopulmonary systems are challenged.

The testing protocol should deviate from standard procedures by using a submaximal intensity over an increased period of time. Although some persons with PPS can be maximally tested, excessive residual fatigue and possible further reduction of motor units could result from excessive maximal testing.

A submaximal intensity eliciting at least a "somewhat hard" rating of perceived exertion, performed continuously for at least six minutes, facilitates an accurate estimation of aerobic fitness while minimizing possible motor unit damage. Terminating the test at a "hard" or "strong" rating of perceived exertion should enable the tester to challenge the cardiopulmonary system to reach 85% of age-predicted maximum heart rate. If 85% is not reached and coronary artery disease is not suspected, an additional stage of higher intensity can be used and should not unduly debilitate the subject.

Exercise MET values may range from 2 to 9 METs, depending upon the limitation of skeletal muscle. Heart rate responses to acute maximal exercise may range from 120 beats per minute (for elderly persons using only the arms) to 175 to 180 beats per minute (for middle-aged persons using all four limbs). Both exercise systolic and diastolic blood pressures are generally similar to those observed for post-polio persons without PPS. Blood lactate concentration responses may range from 2 to 8 mmol/L during exercise testing. Ventilatory responses during exercise are approximately 10% to 20% lower than those observed in asymptomatic post-polio persons of similar age. Ratings of perceived exertion tend to focus on the peripheral component reflecting peripheral muscular fatigue. Consequently, the most limiting factors appear to be peripheral fatigue and pain as opposed to central cues such as dyspnea. Premature muscle fatigue and low maximal oxygen consumption explain the lower maximal ventilation. Peak external power outputs during four-limb ergometry range from 15 to 200 watts.

Exercise testing considerations may include utilization of stirrups for pedals and straps/gloves for hands on the handlebars or arm crank handles. These adaptations will secure weakened limbs to equipment, thus providing more efficient application of force and protection of impaired limbs. Discontinuous protocols are advised for individuals with weakened muscles, since this facilitates higher central physiologic responses while delaying fatigue of exercising muscles.

Recommendations for Exercise Programming

The primary purpose of an exercise program for individuals with PPS is similar to that for their asymptomatic counterparts: to prevent premature onset of hypokinetic diseases and maintain adequate muscle strength for occupational and leisure pursuits. However, individuals without PPS can usually perform a wider range of intensities and durations without long-lasting residual complications, whereas the person with PPS usually has a narrower range of acceptable exercise intensities. If persons with PPS overestimate their minimum intensity, they may risk premature acceleration of motor unit loss. The following principles of exercise prescription should be applied.

- *Intensity.* An exercise intensity of 60% to 70% of maximal oxygen consumption, or "moderate-to-somewhat hard" ratings of perceived exertion, is recommended.

- *Duration.* If the client is deconditioned or has been sedentary for more than one year, a total exercise duration of 20 minutes per session in 2- to 4-minute intervals is recommended. If the client is an irregular exerciser, use less than 25 minutes per session and divide the session into 5-minute intervals or less. If the client is an active regular exerciser, use 30 to 40 minutes continuously.

- *Frequency.* A frequency of three sessions per week is recommended. An alternate-day basis would be optimal to attain beneficial physiological changes without overtaxing the reduced number of motor units.

- *Mode.* Exercise involving as much musculature as possible is preferred. This should include four-limb ergometry, therapeutic aquatics, and other non-weight-bearing activities. Conventional weight-bearing activities such as walking and running may be appropriate for some less involved individuals who have PPS.

Routine exercise is appropriate in most cases of PPS. Furthermore, some individuals with a history of ventilator use or of four-limb involvement should have a thorough preparticipation medical examination and be supervised for two months to ensure safety. Any questions about exercise prescription should be directed to a physician and appropriately trained health professional.

Increased fatigue, weakness, or pain in a particular area should alert the individual to decrease intensity or duration of exercise, or both. If symptoms continue for more than two weeks and are exacerbated by exercise, then exercise should be terminated and appropriate medical follow-up is suggested.

Special Considerations

Most sedentary individuals with PPS are encouraged to consult a physician or appropriately trained health professional before beginning an exercise program. These professionals can supervise and monitor exercise responses to exercise over a two-month period. This will facilitate beneficial physical and psychological tolerance to exercise. Depression has a higher incidence in persons with PPS than in the asymptomatic post-polio population. Appropriate supervision should help the person with PPS not only with the physical but also with the mental obstacles of beginning and continuing an exercise program.

After the initial two-month period of supervision and perhaps follow-up with a health professional, persons with PPS should be able to self-monitor and adjust their exercise program. However, it is recommended that exercisers with PPS perform a submaximal evaluation every three to six months. This would allow a comparison of responses and help ensure fitness improvement and maintenance. If questions or concerns arise, an appropriately trained health professional should be consulted. The exerciser's own physician and an ACSM-certified rehabilitation therapist would be appropriate.

Suggested Readings

Agre, J.C., and A.A. Rodriquez. 1990. Neuromuscular function: Comparison of symptomatic and asymptomatic polio patients to control subjects. *Arch. Phys. Med. Rehabil.* 71: 545-51.

Birk, T.J. 1993. Poliomyelitis and the post-polio syndrome: Exercise capacities and adaptations - current research, future directions, and widespread applicability. *Med. Sci. Sports Exerc.* 25: 466-72.

Dalakas, M.C. 1987. New neuromuscular symptoms after old polio ("post-polio syndrome"): Clinical studies and pathogenic mechanisms. *Birth Defects* 23: 241-64.

Dean, E., and J. Ross. 1988. Modified aerobic walking program: Effect on patients with post-polio syndrome symptoms. *Arch. Phys. Med. Rehabil.* 69: 1033-38.

Edwards, R.H.T. 1983. Biochemical basis of exercise performance: Catastrophe theory of muscle fatigue. In *Biochemistry of exercise,* ed. H.G. Knuttgen, J.A. Vogel, and J. Poortmans, 3-28. Champaign, IL: Human Kinetics.

Einarsson, G. 1991. Muscle conditioning in late poliomyelitis. *Arch. Phys. Med. Rehabil.* 72: 11-13.

Grimby, G., G. Einarsson, M. Medberg, and A. Aniansson. 1989. Muscle adaptive changes in post-polio subjects. *Scand. J. Rehabil. Med.* 21: 19-26.

Gross, N.D., and C.P. Schuch. 1989. Exercise programs for patients of post-polio syndrome: A case report. *Phys. Ther.* 69: 72-76.

Jones, D.R., J. Speier, J. Canine, R. Owen, and G.A. Stull. 1989. Cardiorespiratory responses to aerobic training by patients with post-poliomyelitis sequelae. *JAMA* 261: 3255-58.

Jubelt, B., and N.R. Cashman. 1987. Neurological manifestation of the post-polio syndrome. *CRC Critical Reviews in Neurobiology* 3: 199-220.

Salazar-Gruesoe, F., I. Siegel, and R.P. Roos. 1990. The post-polio syndrome: Evaluation and treatment. *Compr. Ther.* 16: 24-30.

POLIO AND POST-POLIO SYNDROME: EXERCISE TESTING

METHODS	MEASURES	ENDPOINTS*	COMMENTS
Aerobic power **Schwinn Air-Dyne (or any upper/lower limb ergometer)** **Arm ergometer**	• Peak $\dot{V}O_2$, physical work capacity, 12-lead ECG	• Serious dysrhythmias • > 2 mm ST-segment depression or elevation • Ischemic threshold • T-wave inversion with significant ST change	• Use only if diagnosed CAD or related symptoms are present.
	• Blood pressure, heart rate	• SBP > 260 mmHg or DBP > 115 mmHg	• Calculate efficiency index.
	• RPE	• Volitional fatigue	• Acquire values for both involved and uninvolved limbs.
	• METs		• Estimates functional capacity and predicts type or amount of daily living and occupational tasks possible.
Endurance **6-12-minute walk** **1-mile walk**	• Distance or time	• Time or distance	• Can be adopted as a fitness indicator. • Mile walk is too long in most cases.
Strength **Weight machines** **Dynamometers**	• Submaximal endurance of involved and uninvolved limbs • Maximal voluntary contraction	• Fatigue	• Dynamometer: Hip and knee flexion/extension and ankle dorsi- and plantar-flexion should be measured, no more than a 6-second effort at 45° angle. Monitor and document changes due to intervention or neuromuscular changes.
Flexibility **Sit-and-reach** **Goniometry**			• Sit-and-reach measures middle and lower back flexibility which is important for static and dynamic balance. • Goniometry measures flexibility of specific range-of-motion joints.
Neuromuscular **Gait and balance analyses** **Nerve conduction studies**			• Gait and balance analyses are useful in determining static and dynamic balance and locomotion if ambulatory. • Nerve conduction studies along with electromyography are useful in prognosis of available motor units and their readiness.

METHODS	MEASURES	ENDPOINTS*	COMMENTS
Functional performance **Sit-to-stand, lifting**	• Balance and symmetry		• Use for daily living activities and occupational task assessment and prognosis.

*Measurements of particular significance; do not *always* indicate test termination.

MEDICATIONS	SPECIAL CONSIDERATIONS
• Tricyclic antidepressants: Can affect motivation. • Antidepressants (e.g., Elavil, Pamelor, Sinequan, Prozac, Zoloft) inhibit neurotransmitters (i.e., serotonin, norepinephrine).	• Weakness and pain may be present in the lower limbs of patients with braces or orthotic appliances. • Full or partial loss of sensation as well as fasciculations and paresthesia may be present in lower limbs. • A four-limb ergometer (e.g., Schwinn Air-Dyne) with foot straps and/or pegs to rest inactive or nonfunctional limbs should be used.

POLIO AND POST-POLIO SYNDROME: EXERCISE PROGRAMMING

MODES	GOALS	INTENSITY/ FREQUENCY/DURATION	TIME TO GOAL
Aerobic and endurance • Schwinn Air-Dyne (or any upper/lower limb ergometer) • Arm ergometer	• Increase cardiovascular condition and endurance of uninvolved and involved limbs. • Increase efficiency of daily living activities and ambulation.	• 40-70% peak METs. • 3 sessions/week. • 20-40 minutes/session.	
Strength • Isotonic exercises (weight machines) • Isometric exercises	• Increase strength of uninvolved and involved limbs. • Increase efficiency of daily living activities and ambulation.	• 3 sets of 8-12 repetitions. • 2-3 maximal contractions at 20°, 40°, and 60° angles of involved joints. • 3 sessions/week.	
Flexibility • Stretching	• Increase range of motion, prevent contractures.	• Perform with both involved and uninvolved joints. • 5-7 sessions/week.	

MEDICATIONS	SPECIAL CONSIDERATIONS
• See table on exercise testing.	• Spasms and fasciculations (involuntary twitching of muscle fibers) indicate a decrease in work period and an increase in recovery period. • Progressive sudden fatigue indicates high intensity. • Patients may lack motivation and/or compliance secondary to clinical depression. • Rest periods during the day may be necessary during the initial stages of the exercise program.

CHAPTER 35

Amyotrophic Lateral Sclerosis

Karen L. Nau, PhD, PT

University of Kansas Medical Center

Overview of the Pathophysiology

Amyotrophic lateral sclerosis (ALS) is the most common form of motor neuron disease in adults. The primary feature of this progressive disease is degeneration of lower and upper motor neurons. Degeneration of the lower motor neurons results in progressive muscular atrophy and weakness, while degeneration of the upper motor neurons results in spasticity and hyperreflexia. The average age at diagnosis of ALS is 55 years. The mean survival time is 2.5 to 3 years after onset of symptoms, with a range of six months to 30 years. While 50% of persons with ALS live less than 3 years after diagnosis, 20% live more than 5 years, and 10% live longer than 10 years. Factors that signify a better prognosis include a younger age and a slower progression of symptoms prior to diagnosis.

The major factor contributing to disability is the muscular weakness consequent to lower motor neuron degeneration. Weakness can occur in any of the skeletal muscles, although the ocular and sphincter muscles are generally spared. Initial signs and symptoms of weakness are typically asymmetric and localized, and typically occur in the muscles of the distal upper or lower extremities, trunk, or bulbar musculature. If weakness is present in one extremity, generally the contralateral side will become affected next. Individuals who present with initial symptoms in the bulbar region (difficulty enunciating words, chewing, and swallowing) may not have significant extremity weakness until fairly late in their disease progression. Others have significant extremity weakness but never develop bulbar weakness. Problems that occur secondary to the weakness include decreased coordination, endurance, functional ability, and breathing capacity.

Amyotrophic lateral sclerosis is a progressive disease occurring at a steady rate without periods of remission. While an individual's rate of muscular weakness remains fairly constant over time, that rate of decline is highly variable among individuals, with some people losing strength very quickly and others changing so slowly that they remain at a high functional capacity for many years. In addition to differences in the rate of muscle weakness, there is a high degree of variability among individuals with respect to which muscles become affected and in what order they become affected.

Spasticity is a second ALS-related factor that can lead to disability. The increased tone can interfere with coordinated movements and range of motion. It may also lead to increased energy expenditure during activity.

A third factor affecting functional ability is diminished pulmonary function secondary to weakness of the diaphragm and trunk musculature. Among individuals with ALS, pulmonary function is one of the best indicators of prognosis and survival time, since death typically occurs secondary to a complication of respiratory failure.

During the early phases of ALS, it has been shown that denervated muscle fibers can become reinnervated by neighboring motor units. This process is important in maintaining muscular function for prolonged periods of time, and may be a key element in the preservation of function among individuals with slow disease progression. However, one characteristic of the immature neuromuscular junction of the newly reinnervated muscle fiber is that it can experience transmission failure, a problem that does not occur in healthy neuromuscular junctions. This failure causes individuals with ALS to fatigue more quickly than persons without ALS. This is a transient process that repairs itself after a short rest period and results in no permanent damage to the motor neuron. In contrast, there is anecdotal evidence of permanent motor neuron death in severely overexercised muscle groups. This is an extreme and rare phenomenon that may occur because the surviving lower motor neurons become metabolically overtaxed from the severe overuse, causing premature death. For these reasons, individuals with ALS are encouraged to keep active but to rest frequently and avoid extreme overexertion.

Effects on the Exercise Response

When exercise testing an individual with ALS, typically the limiting factor will be that person's muscular strength and endurance, and muscular fatigue will occur before the cardiovascular system reaches its maximal capacity. Persons early in the disease process may still be functioning at near-normal levels and may be able to reach their maximal aerobic capacity, but these individuals are the exception. People who have pulmonary deficits may find breathing to be their limiting factor, and symptoms of dyspnea should be monitored closely. Persons with spasticity are limited by their decreased coordination; they may not be able to exercise at speeds fast enough to elicit a cardiovascular response or fatigue their muscles. Decreased coordination and balance secondary to muscular weakness also make many modes of exercise testing unsafe or impractical.

Effects of Exercise Training

There is no evidence that exercise reverses or even slows the progressive denervation caused by ALS. However, anecdotal evidence suggests that a portion of the weakness and atrophy associated with ALS is due to disuse, and that this weakness (in innervated muscle fibers) can be minimized. Although the disease process cannot be reversed and the individual with ALS will lose function despite his/her efforts, exercise will strengthen the healthy muscle fibers; this may temporarily lead to a stronger muscle and may permit an individual to maintain strength and a higher functional level for a longer time. Strengthening the muscles of respiration should likewise optimize the

functional ability of the intact fibers and prolong the time before pulmonary impairments become restrictive. Improving or maintaining aerobic endurance may also have a positive impact on functional ability by maximizing the efficiency of the innervated muscle fibers. Maintaining full range of motion in joints that are too weak to be moved actively, or in joints affected by spastic muscles, will minimize pain associated with joint stiffness (e.g., a frozen shoulder) and make it easier for someone else to provide care (e.g., dressing, positioning, transfers) for individuals who can no longer take care of themselves.

Management and Medications

At this time, there are no therapeutic regimens that have been proven effective in stopping or slowing the denervation process. Medical management revolves around controlling secondary symptoms. Medications are available to decrease muscle spasticity, decrease excessive saliva production, minimize emotional swings, and control the discomfort of joint stiffness. Other therapeutic interventions may include

- recommendations for adaptive equipment and assistive devices,
- nutritional supplementation and the placement of a feeding tube for those with bulbar involvement,
- a ventilator for those with severe respiratory muscle weakness,
- emotional support and counseling for the individual and the family,
- arrangements for home health personnel to assist with care-giving, and
- discussion of issues related to dying (i.e., hospice, use of a ventilator, taking a patient off a ventilator, the use of life-saving techniques, and the like).

None of the medications or medical management techniques commonly used by individuals with ALS should alter the results or negatively impact a person's ability to exercise.

Recommendations for Exercise Testing

Participant safety is one of the key elements to consider when exercise testing individuals with

ALS. If the person has diminished balance or coordination, an exercise mode that will maximize safety and functional ability should be used. Equipment may have to be modified to increase support. For more involved individuals, assessing their ability to complete functional tasks may be the most useful mode of exercise testing. As a matter of fact, functional assessment is one of the primary tools for monitoring ALS progression. Results from exercise testing will be highly variable, depending on the phase of disease progression—from near normal to severely compromised. Before beginning a test, ask the individual about his/her daily activities to develop an estimation of functional capacity. This will help determine an appropriate exercise test protocol.

Recommendations for Exercise Programming

The purpose of an exercise program for people with ALS is to maximize the functional capacity of the innervated muscle fibers, to prevent limitations in range of motion, and to maximize aerobic capacity, endurance, and functional level for as long as possible. Modest improvements may occur in these parameters at the onset of an exercise program, but it is more realistic to expect all parameters to decline slowly in spite of the exercise program. Since disease progression cannot be stopped and functional capacity will decline, the overall goal of an exercise program is to maintain a higher functional level than the person would have otherwise. Specific goals must be constantly modified to adapt to the progressive nature of the disease. Individuals with ALS will become weaker and more limited despite any type of exercise program. That must be understood and accepted by both the health professional and the individual with ALS. Exercise is only beneficial when it does not cause excessive fatigue in the participant. Once exercise becomes so tiring or so difficult that it prevents someone from completing activities of daily living, it is no longer appropriate. Excessive fatigue may be detrimental to individuals with ALS; therefore, they need to be active enough to minimize disuse atrophy but cautious enough to avoid overexertion.

Special Considerations

Little research is available on the effects of regular exercise in individuals with ALS. Therefore, specific exercise recommendations are not possible; however, common sense and moderation will be key elements of any exercise program. Goals should be practical, intensity and duration should be moderate, rest periods should be frequent, and expectations should be kept realistic. Disease progression cannot be stopped or even slowed down; exercise will affect only innervated muscle fibers. Exercise is not appropriate for all people with ALS, and eventually all with the disease will come to the point where they should stop exercising. The people who will benefit the most from an exercise program are those in the early phases of the disease and those with a slow rate of disease progression.

Suggested Readings

Amyotrophic Lateral Sclerosis Association. 1986. *Managing amyotrophic lateral sclerosis manual II: Managing muscle weakness.* Woodland Hills, CA: Amyotrophic Lateral Sclerosis Association.

Bohannon, R.W. 1983. Results of resistance exercise on a patient with amyotrophic lateral sclerosis. *Phys. Ther.* 63: 965-68.

Carroll, J.E., J.M. Hagberg, M.H. Brooks, and J.B. Shumate. 1979. Bicycle ergometry and gas exchange measurements in neuromuscular diseases. *Arch. Neurol.* 36: 457-61.

Nau, K.L. 1994. Changes in body composition, strength and metabolism during the progression of amyotrophic lateral sclerosis. Ph.D. diss., Department of Kinesiology, University of Michigan, 1994.

Nau, K.L., M.B. Bromberg, B.L. Eakin, and V.L. Katch. 1994. Peak exercise performance declines in men with ALS. *Med. Sci. Sports Exerc.* 26: S30.

Pradas, J., L. Finison, P.L. Andres, B. Thornell, D. Hollander, and T.L. Munsat. 1993. The natural history of amyotrophic lateral sclerosis and the use of natural history controls in therapeutic trials. *Neurol.* 43: 751-55.

Sanjak, M., D. Paulsen, R. Sufit, W. Reddan, D. Beaulieu, L. Erickson, A. Shug, and B.R. Brooks. 1987. Physiologic and metabolic response to progressive and prolonged exercise in amyotrophic lateral sclerosis. *Neurol.* 37: 1217-20.

Schiffman, P.L., and J.M. Belsh. 1993. Pulmonary function at diagnosis of amyotrophic lateral sclerosis. *Chest* 103: 508-13.

Sinaki, M., and D.M. Mulder. 1978. Rehabilitation techniques for patients with amyotrophic lateral sclerosis. *Mayo Clin. Proc.* 53: 173-78.

Tandan, R., and W.G. Bradley. 1985. Amyotrophic lateral sclerosis: Part 1. Clinical features, pathol- ogy, and ethical issues in management. *Ann. Neurol.* 18: 271-80.

AMYOTROPHIC LATERAL SCLEROSIS: EXERCISE TESTING

METHODS	MEASURES	ENDPOINTS	COMMENTS
Aerobic power **Recumbent cycle ergometer** **All-extremity ergometer**	• Heart rate • RPE • Blood pressure • METs • $\dot{V}_E$		• Maximal testing would be appropriate only for individuals at a high functional level; submaximal or functional tests are sufficient. • Heart rate and RPE are useful in determining exercise prescription. • Blood pressure measurement is useful to screen for hypertension. • METs can be used to estimate functional capacity and to predict the type and amount of daily living activities possible. • $\dot{V}_E$ is useful in indicating whether dyspnea will be a limiting factor. • Choose a mode that involves all extremities or the extremities with the greatest function. • Provide trunk support to maximize safety.
Endurance **6-minute walk**	• Distance	• Time	• Use to determine safety and whether assistive devices are necessary.
Strength **Weight machines** **Active range of motion with light resistance**	• Number of repetitions • Maximal voluntary contraction		• Expect strength to decrease as the disease progresses. • Test both upper and lower limbs. • Spasticity may influence results.
Flexibility **Goniometer**	• Range of motion of major joints		• Especially useful for persons with spasticity to indicate which joints need stretching.
Neuromuscular **Gait analysis**			• Use to determine safety and whether assistive devices are necessary.
Functional performance **Sit-and-stand** **Daily living activities**	• Level of assistance needed		• Use to determine whether assistive devices are necessary. • Use to determine functional capacity, especially dressing and personal hygiene.

(continued)

AMYOTROPHIC LATERAL SCLEROSIS: EXERCISE TESTING *(continued)*

MEDICATIONS	SPECIAL CONSIDERATIONS
• Pyridostigmine (Mestinon): Blocks acetylcholinesterase; may improve endurance. • Baclofen: Reduces spasticity. Patient may feel weaker. • Amitriptyline: For emotional stability; can cause sleepiness and decrease motivation.	• Orthopedic: Risk of injury due to flaccid limbs (caught, bumped, etc.) with joint discomfort (especially in shoulders), laxity, or stiffness. Constant vigilance is necessary during exercise testing because of muscle weakness and poor balance. • Pulmonary: Decreased pulmonary function (restrictive in nature) secondary to respiratory muscle weakness; decreased vital capacity, inspiratory and expiratory pressures, and reserve volumes. Some positions can limit function. Some clients become very dependent. • Psychological: Clients may be emotionally labile, frustrated, and/or depressed. Decreased motivation may be due to lack of improvement despite efforts. • Gastrointestinal: Clients may have difficulty chewing and swallowing if bulbar area is affected. Presence of a feeding tube may affect exercise capacity immediately after insertion. • Urological: Expect occasional urinary urgency.

AMYOTROPHIC LATERAL SCLEROSIS: EXERCISE PROGRAMMING

MODES	GOALS	INTENSITY/ FREQUENCY/DURATION	TIME TO GOAL
Aerobic and endurance • Recumbent cycling and walking	• Maintain work capacity.	• 30-50%. • Daily. • Continue as long as possible without excessive fatigue. • Goals should be very short-term.	
Strength • Weight machines • Active range-of-motion exercises with light weights	• Maintain strength of arms, legs, and trunk.	• 1 set of 8-12 repetitions. • Use light weights or no resistance. • 3-5 sessions/week. • Reduce resistance and repetitions as weakness progresses.	
Flexibility • Stretching • Active and passive range-of-motion exercises	• Increase or maintain range of motion.	• Once or twice daily.	
Functional performance • Daily living activities	• Maintain capacity to perform as many activities as possible.	• Useful when "traditional" exercise program is no longer possible.	

MEDICATIONS	SPECIAL CONSIDERATIONS
• See table on testing.	• Eventually, all goals will have to be *decreased* as functional ability declines. • Use short-term goals that can be modified regularly. • Try to avoid excess accumulation of adipose tissue. • Stress that, by doing their own daily living activities, clients are exercising. • Perform all exercise modes as long as possible without causing excessive fatigue. • Frequent rest periods may be necessary throughout the exercise program. • Individuals may be emotionally labile, frustrated, depressed, or discouraged, with little motivation to exercise because of the progressive nature of the disease. • Adapted or support equipment may be needed because of muscle weakness and reduced balance.

CHAPTER 36

Cerebral Palsy

Michael Ferrara, PhD, ATC

Ball State University

James Laskin, PhD, PT

University of Oklahoma Health Science Center

Overview of the Pathophysiology

Cerebral palsy (CP) is defined as a nonprogressive lesion of the brain occurring before, at, or soon after birth that interferes with the normal development of the brain. Cerebral palsy is characterized by limited ability to move and maintain balance and posture because of the damage to areas of the brain that control muscle tone and spinal reflexes. The resulting loss of muscle tone and spinal reflex sequelae depend upon the location and extent of the injury within the brain. The medical classification of CP depends on type of muscle tone and site of injury (see table 36.1).

In the United States, CP is one of the most common physical disabilities, occurring in, depending on the source, 1.5 to 5 of 1000 live births. The brain injury that occurs before, during, or within the first few years after birth has two common etiologies:

- Failure of brain to develop properly:
  - Occurring within the first and/or second trimesters of embryonic development
  - Disruption of normal developmental process, which may be caused by genetic disorder, chromosomal abnormality, or faulty blood supply

- Neurological disorder:
  - Injury to brain before, during, or after birth
  - Lack of oxygen, bleeding in brain, toxic injury or poisoning, head trauma, metabolic disorder, or infection of nervous system

The Cerebral Palsy-International Sport and Recreation Association (CP-ISRA) has developed a classification system based on an individual's "function." This system includes not only those typically medically diagnosed with CP, but also people with other conditions that are characterized by nonprogressive brain lesions (e.g., stroke, traumatic brain injury, and tumor). Many sports (swimming, track and field, and bocci) are moving toward a

Table 36.1 MEDICAL CLASSIFICATION OF CEREBRAL PALSY	
TYPE OF MUSCLE TONE OBSERVED	**SITE OF INJURY**
Spastic paralysis	Cerebrum
Ataxia	Cerebellum
Athetosis	Midbrain
Dyskinesia	Basal ganglia
High spinal spastic	Medulla
Mixed	Diffuse

truly functional classification system that deals with sport-specific abilities and is able to classify athletes across disability groups; however, when discussing CP and exercise the CP-ISRA system allows for the grouping of individuals of similar "abilities":

- CP1: Severe spastic or athetoid quadriplegia—the person is unable to propel a manual wheelchair independently; has nonfunctional lower extremities, very poor to no trunk stability, severely decreased function in upper extremity.

- CP2: Moderate to severe spastic or athetoid quadriplegia—is able to propel a manual wheelchair slowly and inefficiently; has differential function abilities between upper and lower extremities, fair static trunk stability.

- CP3: Moderate spastic quadriplegia or severe spastic hemiplegia—is able to propel a manual wheelchair independently; may be able to ambulate with assistance; has moderate spasticity on the lower extremities, fair dynamic trunk stability, moderate limitations to function in the dominant arm.

- CP4: Moderate to severe spastic diplegia—ambulates with aids over short distances; has moderate to severe involvement of the lower extremities, good dynamic trunk stability, minimal to near-normal function of the upper extremities at rest.

- CP5: Moderate spastic diplegia—ambulates well with assistive devices; has minimal to moderate spasticity in one or both lower extremities; is able to run.

- CP6: Moderate athetosis or ataxia—ambulates without assistive devices; lower-extremity function improves from walking to running or cycling; has poor static and good dynamic trunk stability, good upper-extremity range and strength, poor throwing and grasp and release.

- CP7: True ambulatory hemiplegia—has mild to moderately affected upper extremity, minimal to mildly affected lower extremity.

- CP8: Minimally affected diplegia, hemiplegia, athetosis, or monoplegia.

Effects on the Exercise Response

Specific research examining the exercise responses in the individual with CP is quite limited. Histori-

cally, the person with CP has not participated in any form of structured or unstructured physical fitness program. However, when tested, because of the spasticity/athetosis and the inefficient nature of their mobility, these individuals often present with higher-than-expected exercise response values. In general, the studies that have examined heart rate, blood pressure, expired air, and blood lactate have found that individuals with CP present with higher heart rates, blood pressure, and lactate concentrations for a given submaximal work rate than their able-bodied peers. Individuals with CP are found to have slightly lower peak physiologic responses (10-20%) than able-bodied controls. Reduced mechanical efficiency has also been reported in individuals with CP. This was attributed to the extra amount of energy required to overcome muscle tonus in spastic CP. Physical work capacity has been reported to be as much as 50% lower than that of able-bodied subjects. This appearance of low fitness may be the result of poor exercise habits, difficulty performing skilled movements, contralateral and ipsilateral muscle imbalances, and often poor functional strength. Fatigue and stress are two other factors that have a negative impact on the client's performance. It is not uncommon for a client to report a transient increase in spasticity and discoordination after a strenuous session of exercise.

Effects of Exercise Training

Given the nature of this physical disability, there is no reason to expect that persons with CP cannot benefit from a regular program focusing on muscular strength, flexibility, and/or aerobic endurance. With the understanding that the risk for cardiovascular disease and stroke is greater in the sedentary physically disabled individual than in able-bodied counterparts, it is in fact imperative to counsel this population into some form of regular physical activity.

There is a small but growing body of literature showing that trainability of persons with CP can be achieved. The literature also documents anecdotal evidence of improved "sense of wellness," body image, and capacity to perform activities of daily living, as well as the apparent lessening of severity of symptoms such as spasticity and athetosis. Reports from athletes with CP and their coaches consistently demonstrate improved peak oxygen uptake, lowered ventilatory threshold, increased work rate at given submaximal heart rates, increased range of motion, improved coordination/skill of movements, and increased strength and muscular endurance, including skeletal muscle hypertrophy. These anecdotal reports are supported by the performances of the athletes at national and international competitions.

Management and Medications

As for any client, appropriate physical screening should be performed to rule out any contraindications or precautions with respect to exercise. These factors should be evaluated on typical health screening forms and through a basic physical examination. Before the test battery is selected or the exercise prescription is developed, the client's specific needs, goals, and limitations must be addressed. By using the CP-ISRA classification system, the tester/programmer will gain insight into the type and mode of exercise that should be used as well as any special considerations that will help maximize the individual's performance. It is critical for the tester/programmer to keep under consideration that the symptoms of spasticity and athetosis increase with stress and fatigue.

Medications may be a confounding factor for exercise testing or development of the exercise prescription. The tester or programmer must be aware of the medication the client is currently using. Seizure or seizure tendencies are present in 60% or more of persons with CP. Anti-seizure medications are commonly prescribed for individuals with CP. Three commonly used drugs to control seizures are phenobarbital, phenytoin, and carbamazepine. Some anti-seizure medications have a depressant effect on the central nervous system, thus slowing the physiologic responses to exercise. The use of carbamazepine is recommended, since it has the fewest side effects, which may include mental confusion or irritability, dizziness, nausea, weight loss, and sensitivity to sunburn. It is also important that in some instances the paradoxical effect of hyperactivity may be a result of these medications. Antispasmodic and muscle relaxants are two other classes of medications frequently prescribed to individuals with CP. Often with a decrease in muscle tone, the individual is able to perform physical activities with greater ease. However, a serious side effect of these drugs is drowsiness and lethargy. These medications act systemically; therefore, an already low-tone trunk may be compromised in its ability to act as a base of support, thus further limiting extremity function.

Recommendations for Exercise Testing

There is limited research available to substantiate testing protocols, principles, and techniques for the CP population. The commonly used modalities to test individuals with CP include leg cycle ergometry, Schwinn Air-Dyne ergometry, wheelchair ergometry, and the treadmill. Wheelchair ergometry is the preferred mode of testing the cardiorespiratory fitness of nonambulatory individuals with CP. The treadmill will give the optimal response for ambulatory individuals with adequate balance and coordination.

The selection of testing modalities is dependent on the abilities of the client. The principle of specificity is essential to selection of the test mode that best complements an individual's physical capacities and is easily tolerated. For the wheelchair user, wheelchair ergometry or arm crank ergometry will be the common choice for testing. The use of personal wheelchairs will increase comfort with and tolerance of testing during wheelchair ergometry. Practice time should be allowed with holding gloves and in most cases is necessary to ensure that termination of the exercise test is due to cardiorespiratory and muscular limitations and not the condition itself. Leg cycle ergometry, Air-Dyne ergometry, or treadmill may be the elected testing mode for ambulatory individuals with CP. Balance and coordination are also a concern with ambulatory CP and should be taken into consideration in the choice of the testing mode. Clients may be unable to perform leg cycle ergometry because of inadequate hip flexion due to excessive spasticity, fixed deformities, or both. Practice time should also be allowed when the feet are strapped to the pedals during leg cycle ergometry or Air-Dyne ergometry.

Recommendations for Exercise Programming

The progressive goal of all exercise training programs is to improve health and increase daily functional activities. Traditional contraindications for exercise prescription will also apply to the individual with CP. As with exercise testing, research pertaining to exercise prescription for the individual with CP is limited. Because of the nature and variability in presentation of CP, the practitioner will be required to implement some very creative adaptations. The average individual with CP will benefit most from a balanced program of muscular strength, flexibility, and aerobic endurance. The practitioner must take into consideration the client's abilities, interests, and personal goals. Optimally the specific exercises should be designed such that the client can be independent. As always, progression should be gradual and should increase at the individual's own rate in accordance with the principle of specific adaptations to imposed demands.

Special Considerations

It is imperative for the practitioner to understand that a large proportion of individuals with CP have concomitant cognitive, visual, hearing, speech/ swallowing difficulties, or more than one of these. The practitioner must be very careful not to assume decreased cognitive ability on the basis of the presence of drooling or the quality of the verbal skills of a person with CP. It is important to assess each client as an individual with very specific needs and concerns.

Special considerations for exercise training include strapping the hands or feet to the pedals during arm and leg cycle ergometry, respectively. Also, the use of gloves for wheelchair exercise testing is recommended. Gradual progression is recommended during the initial stages of exercise. Supervising personnel should be present when the treadmill is being used because of the balance problems associated with CP. The importance of spotting on treadmill exercise, because of potential loss of coordination and balance during testing, cannot be overemphasized. Anecdotal experience suggests that when one is collecting expired gases during performance testing utilizing a mouthpiece or mask, it is necessary to be vigilant about checking the quality of the seal. Some individuals with CP present with mouths that have developed in such a way that there is a very acute angle of the mandible, making satisfactory seal difficult.

Suggested Readings

Cerebral Palsy - International Sport and Recreation Association. 1991. *Classification and sports rules manual.* 5th ed. Nottingham, England: CP-ISRA.

Fernandez, J.E., K.H. Pitetti, and M.T. Betzen. 1990. Physiological capacities of individuals with cerebral palsy. *Hum. Factors* 32: 357-466.

Jones, J. 1988. *Training guide to cerebral palsy sports.* Champaign, IL: Human Kinetics.

Lockette, K., and A. Keys. 1995. *Conditioning with physical disabilities*, 65-90. Champaign, IL: Human Kinetics.

Miller, P., ed. 1995. *Fitness programming and physical disability.* Champaign, IL: Human Kinetics.

Paciorek, M., and J. Jones. 1994. *Sports and recreation for the disabled.* Carmel, IN: Cooper Publishing Group.

Pitetti, K.H., J.E. Fernandez, and M.C. Lanciault. 1991. Feasibility of an exercise program for adults with cerebral palsy: A pilot study. *Adapted Phys. Activity Quart.* 8: 333-41.

CEREBRAL PALSY: EXERCISE TESTING

METHODS	MEASURES	ENDPOINTS*	COMMENTS
Aerobic power **If ambulatory: Schwinn Air-Dyne (or any upper/lower limb ergometer)** **If in wheelchair: arm ergometer**	• 12-lead ECG • Blood pressure • Heart rate • RPE • Peak $\dot{V}O_2$, METs	• Serious dysrhythmias • > 2 mm ST-segment depression or elevation • Ischemic threshold • T-wave inversion with significant ST change • SBP > 260 mmHg or DBP > 115 mmHg • Volitional fatigue	• Because of spastic or athetoid complications, straps or wraps may be necessary to keep feet and hands secured. • All the listed measurements are extremely useful in assisting with exercise prescription.
Endurance **If ambulatory: 6-12-minute walk or 1-mile walk** **If in wheelchair: 6-12-minute or 1-mile "push"**	• Distance or time	• Time or distance	• May have to adjust distance trials according to the capacity of the person.
Flexibility **Goniometry** **Sit-and-reach**	• Joint angle • Range of motion		• Range of motion is limited due to spasticity or athetoid complications and contractures.
Neuromuscular **Gait and balance analyses**			• These are useful measurements because CP may affect motor region or pathways in the CNS; also helpful in exercise prescription.

*Measurements of particular significance; do not *always* indicate test termination.

MEDICATIONS

• Anti-seizure medications (including phenobarbital, phenytoin, and carbamazepine) and antispasmodic medications: May decrease aerobic capacity and results from other tests due to a decrease in attention span and/or motivation.

CEREBRAL PALSY: EXERCISE PROGRAMMING

MODES	GOALS	INTENSITY/ FREQUENCY/DURATION	TIME TO GOAL
Aerobic • If ambulatory: Schwinn Air-Dyne (or any upper/lower limb ergometer) • If in wheelchair: Arm ergometer	• Increase aerobic capacity and endurance.	• 40-85% peak $\dot{V}O_2$ or HR reserve. • 3-5 days/week. • 20-40 minutes/session.	
Endurance • If ambulatory: 6-15-minute walks • If in wheelchair: 6-15-minute "pushes"	• Improve distance covered.	• Once or twice weekly.	
Strength • Free weights or weight machines	• Improve muscle strength of involved and uninvolved muscle groups.	• 3 sets of 8-12 repetitions. • 2 sessions/week.	
Flexibility • Stretching (both involved and uninvolved joints)	• Improve range of motion directly related to capacity for daily living activities.	• Before and after aerobic and endurance exercise.	

MEDICATIONS	SPECIAL CONSIDERATIONS
• See table on exercise testing.	• Duration for all of the exercise modes listed is more important than intensity.

CHAPTER 37

Parkinson's Disease

Elizabeth J. Protas, PT, PhD, FACSM
Texas Woman's University

Rhonda K. Stanley, PT, PhD
University of Evansville

Joseph Jankovic, MD
Baylor College of Medicine

Overview of the Pathophysiology

Parkinson's disease is a progressive neurologic disorder involving the extrapyramidal system. The disease is associated with a reduction in the neurotransmitter dopamine primarily in the substantia nigra, a component of the basal ganglia. The dopamine reduction results from the death of dopaminergic cells within the basal ganglia. The loss of dopamine results in the symptoms of resting tremor, bradykinesia (slow movements), rigidity, and gait and postural abnormalities. Symptoms do not occur until there is greater than 80% loss of the dopaminergic cells.

The most common form of Parkinson's disease is an idiopathic neurodegenerative disorder that usually occurs in individuals over the age of 50. It is found slightly more frequently in men than in women and may be less prevalent in African blacks and Asians. There is no known cause of Parkinson's disease; however, both genetics and environment (e.g., exposure to toxins) are thought to be factors in the disease. Other factors that may be contributing mechanisms are aging, autoimmune responses, and mitochondrial dysfunction. Parkinson's disease may be classified in a number of ways:

- Age at onset (< 40 [juvenile]; between 40 and 70; > 70)

- Clinical symptom (tremor predominant, akinetic-rigidity predominant, postural instability-gait difficulty predominant)
- Mental status (dementia present/absent)
- Clinical course (benign, progressive, malignant)
- Disability (Hoehn and Yahr [1967] stage 1.0-5.0)

These classifications are useful for gross categorization of an individual with Parkinson's disease, and some have prognostic implications. For example, a malignant clinical course is the situation in which symptoms have been evident for less than one year but disability has progressed rapidly. The prognosis is poor in this instance.

The motor symptoms that occur with Parkinson's disease affect many aspects of movement. Tremors can be evident both at rest and with action. Rigidity often begins in the neck and shoulders and spreads to the trunk and extremities, making movement difficult. The ability to move fingers, hands, arms, or legs rapidly is drastically reduced (bradykinesia), and motor control to rise from a chair is lessened. Standing posture is characterized by increased kyphosis and flexed knees and elbows, as well as adducted shoulders. Gait is described as slow and shuffling, with shortened, festinating steps (involuntary hurrying), decreased arm swing, and difficulty initiating a step (start hesitation). Postural righting reflexes are compromised and lost (an individual in a Hoehn and Yahr disability level of 3.0 is unable to recover balance on a pull test). Falls can become a recurring problem. Episodes of decreased movement or freezing become more frequent during walking. Passage through doorways or narrowed spaces becomes more difficult. Activities of daily living can be affected by minute, illegible handwriting (micrographia), the inability to cut food or handle utensils, difficulty swallowing food, difficulty turning in and rising from bed, and needing assistance with dressing and bathing. Individuals with Parkinson's disease have problems with both the volume and the understandability of their speech. Communication disorders are exacerbated by a loss of facial expression (hypomimia). The motor symptoms contribute to the impairment displayed by individuals with Parkinson's disease.

Effects on the Exercise Response

The effect of Parkinson's disease on exercise is not well characterized. Considerable intra- and interperson variability exists, increasing the difficulty of generalizing about exercise responses in this population. Symptoms may fluctuate from day to day and week to week regardless of how precise the exercise intervention strategies are.

Autonomic nervous system dysfunction is commonly found in Parkinson's disease. This can cause problems with thermal regulation during exercise, as well as altered heart rate and blood pressure responses with position changes and during exercise. Sweating patterns, heart rates, and blood pressures should be observed during exercise.

Movement disorders and muscular rigidity decrease the exercise efficiency of individuals with Parkinson's disease. Reduced efficiency results in higher heart rates and oxygen consumption responses during submaximal exercise. Walking may be severely impaired, but other exercise responses such as stair climbing are easily accomplished. Freezing and start hesitation may make certain activities more difficult than others. During single sessions of exercise, significant loss of upright posture (increasing kyphosis) can occur.

Effects of Exercise Training

Little is known about aerobic exercise training in individuals with Parkinson's disease. Aerobic training can improve function, can fail to impact function, or can reduce function in individuals with Parkinson's disease. It cannot be assumed that aerobic training will be beneficial in this population because of the complexity of the problem, the progressive nature of the disease, and the impact of medications on the condition.

Management and Medications

Drugs have been the most successful way to treat many of the symptoms of Parkinson's disease. Drug management is aimed at correcting or preventing neurochemical imbalances in relation to the dopamine deficiency, decreased epinephrine and norepinephrine, and a relative increase in the amount of acetylcholine. The most common antiparkinsonian medications are

- dopaminergics (levodopa, levodopa/carbidopa, amantadine, pergolide, bromocriptine),

- anticholinergics (benztropine, trihexyphenidyl), and

- monoamine oxidase type B (MAO-B) inhibitors (deprenyl, selegiline).

Most of the medications have both peripheral and central side effects. The most common side effects are gastrointestinal upsets, confusion, delusional states, hallucinations, insomnia, and changes in mental activity. Long-term use of drug therapies, particularly dopaminergics and MAO-B inhibitors, can result in movement disorders (dyskinesias), dystonias, and clinical fluctuations of motor disability. More than 50% of all persons with Parkinson's disease treated for more than five years with drug therapies have reduced responses to the drugs and display clinical fluctuation of the motor disability.

Most individuals with Parkinson's disease are taking multiple medications to alleviate their symptoms. Sometimes the attending neurologist proceeds by trial and error to determine which combination and dosage of drugs works best for an individual. Levodopa is a key drug for Parkinson's disease. Levodopa is a metabolic precursor to dopamine that can pass through the blood-brain barrier. In the brain, levodopa is metabolized into dopamine and increases the amount of dopamine available in the basal ganglia. Levodopa is also metabolized in peripheral muscle; this can lessen the amount available to cross into the brain's circulation. Carbidopa is added to the levodopa in the drug Sinemet to reduce the peripheral metabolism of levodopa and increase the amount that passes through the blood-brain barrier. The impact of exercise conditioning on the peripheral metabolism of levodopa is not established.

The importance of drug therapy in the medical management of these individuals, the declining effectiveness of the drugs over time, and the variability of individual responses to the drugs make understanding of the influences on drug absorption, metabolism, and effectiveness critical. Most of this has not been carefully studied; however, reduced absorption may be impacted by strenuous exercise, concomitant use of anticholinergic drugs, autonomic dysfunction, recent food intake, amount of protein in the diet, iron supplements, and level of aerobic fitness.

There are a number of implications for graded exercise testing within the context of the antiparkinsonian medications.

- Medication plasma level may influence exercise performance.

- Whenever possible, test at peak dose, usually 45 minutes to one hour after medication has been taken.

- Some individuals who are clinical fluctuators may demonstrate a brief, intense peak-dose tachycardia.

- Some people may have intense and severe dyskinesias at peak dose.

- Some medications are associated with cardiac dysrhythmias.

- Caution should be used in testing an individual who has had a recent change in medications, since the impact may be unpredictable.

- Single sessions of exercise may increase, decrease, or not affect the time to peak dose-response.

- Individuals who are clinical fluctuators should be tested both on and off medications in order to establish performance ranges.

A number of these concerns for exercise testing are equally applicable to exercise training; however, some additional considerations should be noted:

- Some people display a bradycardia in response to an aerobic exercise activity, making it difficult to reach target heart rates.

- Heart rate responses to the same exercise activity may vary greatly from day to day depending upon the medication plasma level.

- Heart rates should be carefully observed during aerobic exercise for evidence of this variability.

- Exercise outcomes may be dependent upon *consistently* exercising at the same time after the last medication dose.

- Observe for changes in Parkinsonian symptoms during exercise training that might be related to changes in drug absorption or metabolism (e.g., increases or decreases in dyskinesias, bradykinesia, dystonias, freezing, tremor).

- Noting the time to peak dose onset may be useful in following an individual's medication response to exercise training.

Recommendations for Exercise Testing

People with Parkinson's disease who have balance deficits or freezing episodes should not be tested on treadmills. An appropriate bicycle ergometer protocol should be selected. Individuals with Parkinson's disease have difficulty maintaining a seal around a mouthpiece during the collection of expired air. A mask is preferable.

There is some evidence that persons in stage 2 on the Hoehn and Yahr disability scale have aerobic capacities comparable to those of healthy individuals. This is probably a reasonable assumption for individuals in stage 1; however, greater variability and lower capacities may be anticipated for stages 3 and 4.

Persons with Parkinson's disease are in an age group that is at high risk for latent cardiovascular disease. This should be considered during testing.

Many of these individuals can ride a leg cycle ergometer or perform an arm-cranking protocol even if they are in an "off" period and unable to walk without assistance. Frequently nonroutine motor behaviors are easily accomplished. Don't make assumptions about what an individual can do. Try the activity.

Recommendations for Exercise Programming

The approaches to exercise for Parkinson's disease fall into five categories: flexibility, aerobic training, functional training, strengthening, and motor control. Any exercise prescription should keep the goals of the exercise clearly in mind. Different interventions will have different outcomes and expectations. Parkinson's disease is a complex problem that is often difficult to evaluate. Schenkman and Butler (1989) have proposed a model that identifies direct, indirect, and composite consequences of Parkinson's disease. This model analyzes the postural, cardiopulmonary, and movement complications leading to associated functional losses in Parkinson's disease. Direct effects are those that occur directly as a result of Parkinson's disease, for example, tremor and rigidity. Indirect effects, such as aerobic deconditioning or loss of range of motion due to inactivity, occur along with the disease. Composite consequences may be a combination of the direct central nervous system changes and compensatory musculoskeletal symptoms such as changes in axial mobility and balance problems. Schenkman (1992) suggests that exercise interventions could have a minimal effect on the symptoms resulting directly from the disease process, but that appropriately designed interventions may alter the indirect and/or mixed effects of the musculoskeletal and cardiopulmonary changes.

Since Parkinson's disease is a chronic progressive condition, exercise interventions should not be short-term, and need to be pursued on a regular basis as part of any individual's lifestyle. Depending upon the focus of the intervention, the frequency of the intervention may vary. For example, general flexibility can probably be maintained with activity that is performed as infrequently as once a week, whereas one should encourage the person to perform postural exercises every day. Individuals with Parkinson's disease can be socially isolated. Group exercise activities may provide social support as well as improve adherence.

Parkinson's disease can interfere with motor planning and motor memory. Repeated demonstrations along with written and visual cues are needed to assure adherence. In some instances, supervision may be necessary for participation in an exercise intervention.

Special Considerations

There is very little objective evidence concerning exercise interventions with Parkinson's disease. Our clinical experience has demonstrated that improvements in function and long-term outcomes occur with exercise. Much more needs to be done to characterize appropriate and worthwhile exercise in this population.

Suggested Readings

Comella, C.L., G.T. Stebbins, N. Brown, and C.G. Goetz. 1994. Physical therapy and Parkinson's disease. *Neurol.* 44: 376-78.

Fahn, S., R.L. Elton, and Members of the UPDRS Development Committee. 1987. Unified Parkinson's disease rating scale. In *Recent develop-*

ments in Parkinson's disease II, ed. S. Fahn, C. D. Marsden, D.B. Caine, and M. Goldstein, 153-63. New York: Macmillan.

Formisano, R., L. Pratesi, F. T. Modarelli, V. Bonifati, and G. Meco. 1992. Rehabilitation and Parkinson's disease. *Scand. J. Rehabil. Med.* 24: 157-60.

Glendinning, D.S., and R.M. Enoka. 1994. Motor unit behavior in Parkinson's disease. *Phys. Ther.* 74: 61-70.

Goetz, C.G., J.A. Thelan, C.M. Macleod, P.M. Carvery, E.A. Bartley, and G.T. Stebbins. 1993. Blood levodopa levels and the unified Parkinson's disease rating scale function: With and without exercise. *Neurology* 43: 1040-42.

Hoehn, M.M., and M.D. Yahr. 1967. Parkinsonism: Onset, progression, mortality. *Neurology* 17: 427-42.

Horak, F.B., J.G. Nutt, and L.M. Nashner. 1992. Postural inflexibility in Parkinson's subjects. *J. Neurological Sci.* 11: 46-58.

Jankovic, J. 1988. Parkinson's disease: Recent advances in therapy. *South. Med. J.* 82: 1021-27.

Koller, W.C., ed. 1992. *Handbook of Parkinson's disease.* New York: Marcel Dekker.

Landin, S., L. Hagenfeldt, B. Saltin, and J. Wahren. 1974. Muscle metabolism during exercise in patients with Parkinson's disease. *Clinical Science and Molecular Medicine* 47: 493-506.

LeWitt, P.A., A. Bharucha, I. Chitrit, C. Takis, S. Patil, A. Schork, and B. Pichurko. 1994. Perceived exertion and muscle efficiency in Parkinson's disease: L-dopa effects. *Clin. Neuropharmacol.* 17: 454-59.

Mouradian, M.M,. J.L. Juncos, C. Serrati, G. Fabbrini, S. Palmeri, and T.N. Chase. 1987. Exercise and the antiparkinsonian response to levodopa. *Clin. Neuropharmacol.* 10: 351-55.

Protas, E.J., R.K. Stanley, J. Jankovic, and B. MacNeill. 1996. Cardiovascular and metabolic responses to upper- and lower-extremity exercise in men with idiopathic Parkinson's disease. *Phys. Ther.* 76: 34-40.

Saltin B., and S. Landin. 1975. Work capacity, muscle strength and SDH activity in both legs of hemiparetic patients and patients with Parkinson's disease. *Scand. J. Clin. Lab. Invest.* 35: 531-38.

Sasco, A.J., R.S. Paffenbarger, I. Gendre, and A.L. Wing. 1992. The role of exercise in the occurrence of Parkinson's disease. *Arch. Neuro.* 49: 360-65.

Schenkman, M. 1992. Physical therapy intervention for the ambulatory patient. In *Clinics in physical therapy: Physical therapy management of Parkinson's disease*, ed. G.I. Turnbull, 137-92. New York: Churchill Livingstone.

Schenkman, M., and R.B. Butler. 1989. A model for multisystem evaluation and treatment of individuals with Parkinson's disease. *Phys. Ther.* 69: 932-43.

PARKINSON'S DISEASE: EXERCISE TESTING

METHODS	MEASURES	ENDPOINTS*	COMMENTS
Aerobic power **Leg or arm ergometry**	• 12-lead ECG • Blood pressure • Heart rate • RPE • Peak $\dot{V}O_2$, METs	• Serious dysrhythmias • > 2 mm ST-segment depression or elevation • Ischemic threshold • T-wave inversion with significant ST change • SBP > 260 mmHg or DBP > 115 mmHg • Hypotensive response • Volitional fatigue	• High prevalence of dysrhythmias. • Autonomic dysfunction is common. • Use HR response to determine impact of medications. • $\dot{V}O_2$ max and METs useful in prescribing exercise.
Submaximal endurance **6-12-minute walk**	• Distance	• Time	• Aerobic training may improve walking velocity.
Strength **Weight machines**	• Maximal voluntary contraction		• Use with electromyography to determine strength deficits.
Flexibility **Goniometry**	• Joint angle		• Especially important to measure neck, trunk, shoulders, hip, and knees.
Neuromuscular **Gait and balance analyses** **Reaction time**	• Balance: pull test, 360° turn, functional turn		• Use gait analysis if functional gait training and/or motor control intervention is necessary. • Classify disability level and define existing balance deficits. • Reaction time is important to determine whether driving competence is questionable.

METHODS	MEASURES	ENDPOINTS*	COMMENTS
Functional performance **Sit-to-stand** **Bed mobility**	• Time		• Multiple attempts in the sit-and-stand may suggest quadriceps weakness and/or poor motor control. Weight training should specifically target quadriceps.

*Measurements of particular significance; do not *always* indicate test termination.

MEDICATIONS	SPECIAL CONSIDERATIONS
• Levodopa/carbidopa: Can produce exercise bradycardia and transient peak-dose tachycardia and dyskinesias. • Pergolide: May exacerbate latent cardiovascular disease. • Selegiline: Associated with dyskinesia; produces mood elevation.	• Orthopedic: Joint dysfunction is common in individuals after age 50 and may interfere with exercise training. Caution against overuse syndromes with exercise training. • Cardiac: High-risk age group; medications can produce dysrhythmia, tachycardia, and bradycardia. • Neurologic: Orthostatic hypotension. • Muscular: Painful dystonia, particularly at night. • Metabolic: Higher resting metabolic rate. • Psychological: Depression is very common. Hallucinations, delusions, and vivid dreaming can occur. Clients report a sense of invincibility when medications are "on" and vulnerability when "off" medications. • Thermoregulatory: Decreased or absent sweating. • Gastrointestinal: GI discomfort is a common side effect of medications. • Environmental: It is critical that testing occur at peak dose of medications, which is usually 45-60 minutes after the first medication dose. • Equipment adaptation: A mask rather than a mouthpiece is recommended for expired air collection.

PARKINSON'S DISEASE: EXERCISE PROGRAMMING

MODES	GOALS	INTENSITY/ FREQUENCY/DURATION	TIME TO GOAL
Aerobic • Leg and arm cycle ergometry • Rowing	• Maintain or improve work capacity.	• 60-85% peak HR. • 3 days/week. • Up to 60 minutes/session.	• As long as 3 months
Endurance • Well-supervised short walking bouts (20-30 meters)	• Increase work capacity.	• Speed dependent on individual. • 4-6 sessions/day.	
Strength • Weight machines	• Maintain strength of arms, shoulders, legs, and hips.	• Use light weights. • 1 set of 8-12 repetitions. • 3 sessions/week.	
Flexibility • Stretching	• Increase or maintain range of motion.	• 1-3 sessions/week.	
Functional performance • Daily living activities • Postural changes	• Maintain capacity to perform as many daily living activities as possible.		

MEDICATIONS	SPECIAL CONSIDERATIONS
• See table on testing.	• Aerobic power: Walking is a problem for individuals with balance deficits; however, some may be able to jog without risk of falling. Heart rate responses to the same power levels may vary from day to day because of autonomic fluctuations. Duration should be increased slowly (every 4-5 weeks). Duration and intensity should receive equal priority. • Orthopedic: Dyskinesia and dystonia can aggravate problems such as degenerative joint disease. There is some evidence that exercise may reduce joint pain. • Cardiac: Use caution with any medication change. • Muscular: Supervised training is recommended to minimize muscular problems. • Metabolic: Observe for changes in medication dosages after 4-5 weeks of aerobic training. • Psychological: Mask-like face makes it difficult to interpret patient's reaction or RPE. • Thermoregulatory: Sweating begins to occur with exercise conditioning. • Environmental: Time of day for exercise and medication should be kept as constant as possible.

SECTION VII

Cognitive, Emotional, and Sensory Disorders

Section Editors:

Kenneth H. Pitetti, PhD, FACSM
Wichita State University

Lorraine E. Bloomquist, EdD, FACSM
University of Rhode Island

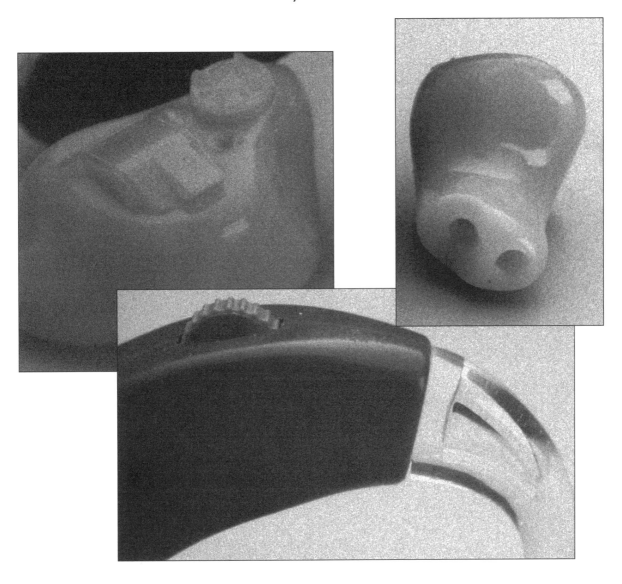

CHAPTER 38

Mental Retardation

Bo Fernhall, PhD, FACSM

George Washington University

Overview of the Pathophysiology

The American Association on Mental Retardation (1992) defines mental retardation as "significantly subaverage general intellectual functioning existing concurrently with related limitations in two or more of the following applicable adaptive skill areas: communications, self-care, home living, social skills, community use, self-direction, health and safety, functional academics, leisure and work" (Sherrill 1993, 518).

There are many potential causes of mental retardation, including genetic and maternal disorders, birth trauma, and infectious diseases. It is also believed that poverty, malnutrition, and severe stimulus deprivation can contribute to mental retardation. With an estimated prevalence of 3%, mental retardation is the most common form of developmental disability in industrialized Western society.

The process of classifying persons with mental retardation by IQ score, used previously, has been replaced by simply determining the presence or absence of mental retardation on the basis of the three criteria of age of onset, significantly subaverage general intellectual function, and limitations in two or more adaptive skill areas. The classification of mild, moderate, severe, and profound is still in wide use but is in the process of being replaced with a classification system based on the determination of level of support needed.

Levels of support are determined across four dimensions: (1) intellectual functioning and adaptive skills, (2) psychological and emotional considerations, (3) physical/health/etiology considerations, and (4) environmental considerations. Levels of support may be needed in any or all of the four divisions at the following levels:

- Intermittent—as needed, short-term support of a high or low intensity
- Limited—a constant need for support of lesser intensity at extensive and pervasive levels
- Extensive—a constant need for support on a daily basis in some environments
- Pervasive—a constant need for high-intensity support across environments

However, all of the reported physical fitness research on persons with mental retardation refers to levels of mental retardation according to the old classifications, as either mild, moderate, or severe and profound. Therefore, the old classification will be used in this discussion of persons with mental retardation.

According to Sherrill, of all individuals classified with mental retardation, approximately 90% fall into the category of *mild mental retardation*. Mild mental retardation can be characterized by

- IQ scores between 52 and 70 on standardized scales (100 points is an average IQ);
- the ability to live independently, work, marry, and rear children; and
- often social isolation and living in or near poverty.

Individuals classified with *moderate mental retardation* comprise approximately 5% of this population and can be characterized by

- IQ scores between 36 and 51 points;
- maladaptive behaviors, including problems with speech, social interaction, and a higher incidence of psychiatric disorders; and
- often the display of physical limitations, including gait problems.

Most individuals with *Down syndrome* fall into this category.

Persons classified with *severe mental retardation* make up approximately 3.5% of this population and those of *profound mental retardation* comprise approximately 1.5%. These persons have the following characteristics:

- IQ scores of 20-35 (severe) or 19 or lower (profound)
- Difficulty with activities of daily living and self-care
- High incidence of physical and motor disabilities
- High incidence of institutionalization

Effects on the Exercise Response

Exercise testing of individuals with mental retardation can be challenging because of difficulties with task understanding, motivation, attention deficits, and motor disabilities. To help control for these factors it is imperative that practice sessions be scheduled before the actual test. The number of practice sessions needed depends on the individuals being tested. The practice session(s) will

- familiarize the person with the test protocol, environment, and staff, and
- allow staff members to adjust the protocol to ensure validity of test results and safety of the person being tested.

For treadmill testing, walking protocols should be selected on the basis of the individual's ability. Selecting a walking speed that is too fast is likely to result in early test termination because of fear rather than fatigue. The practice sessions also help reveal whether or not a given individual is able to perform the intended protocol or exercise mode. Ambulatory limitations or poor coordination, or both, may prevent a person from performing on a treadmill; selecting an alternative exercise mode (e.g., bicycle ergometer) may then become necessary.

People with mental retardation have maximal heart rates that are 8% to 20% lower than expected. Individuals with Down syndrome have 10% lower maximal heart rates than their peers without Down syndrome. It is unknown whether mental retardation per se is the cause of the lower maximal heart rates or whether problems with motivation have produced poor effects, particularly for persons with Down syn-

drome. Furthermore, many individuals with Down syndrome (up to 40%) have congenital heart defects such as aortic arch defects, tetralogy of Fallot, septal defects, and valvular defects. Such defects must be ascertained before testing so that an informed and appropriate decision can be made about testing.

Before exercising, persons with Down syndrome need medical clearance to rule out atlanto-axial instability (lax ligaments/muscles surrounding the joint between vertebrae C1 and C2 that may slip out of alignment and cause spinal cord injury). Approximately 17% of Down syndrome clients have this condition. If atlanto-axial instability exists, or if no x-rays are available, the following activities are contraindicated by the Special Olympics: equestrian sports, gymnastics, diving, pentathlon, butterfly stroke, diving starts in swimming, high jump, alpine skiing, squat lift, and football team competition (soccer). Pretest screening for signs and symptoms of premature coronary heart disease may also be indicated for individuals with mental retardation over the age of 30 years because of a high incidence of sedentary lifestyles, obesity, and very low exercise capacity.

For adult individuals with mental retardation between 20 and 30 years of age without the presence of apparent cardiovascular disease, maximal capacities as low as 4 METs have been reported. Although the mean exercise capacity is usually between 6.5 and 8.5 METs in this population, values as high as 18 METs have been reported. Thus it is not unusual to find very low functional capacity in individuals with mental retardation.

The information on exercise testing, as well as exercise training, applies only to individuals with mild to moderate mental retardation according to the old classification system. People with severe and profound mental retardation have not participated in studies utilizing conventional exercise testing and training. Thus, it is unknown whether or not the protocols discussed in this chapter will apply to that subpopulation.

Effects of Exercise Training

Exercise training has been shown to be beneficial for most people with mental retardation. It is common to observe improvements in functional capacity after cardiorespiratory training and in strength after strength training. However, the increase in functional capacity may not be accompanied by an increase in measured $\dot{V}O_2$max, particularly in persons with Down syndrome. Since motivation and task understanding are common problems, it is important to keep the exercise program simple and to utilize motivational techniques. Token reward systems have been used with some success, and personal supervision is essential. Since obesity is prevalent in this population, weight reduction should be a primary goal in addition to exercise programs. However, exercise alone has not been effective for weight reduction in this population; thus, dietary intervention is necessary. For individuals with Down syndrome, exercise programs have not been as effective as for persons without Down syndrome; however, a physiological reason for this difference has not been identified.

Management and Medications

Because of the very low levels of physical fitness and exercise participation of individuals with mental retardation, the goal is to improve the overall physical fitness profile. Although exercise training cannot impact mental retardation per se, the condition and health profiles of persons with mental retardation can be significantly improved. This is important because individuals with mental retardation have higher rates of cardiovascular mortality at an earlier age than their peers without mental retardation. Furthermore, both cardiovascular fitness and strength are related to job performance in this population, and may be related to the ability to live independently. Considering that the rate of institutionalization is much higher in this population than in groups without mental retardation, improving functional capacity and strength may have important economic and sociologic impact.

Anticonvulsive and antidepressant medications are commonly used in this population. These medications have minimal impact on a single session of exercise or chronic exercise adaptations of the individual, but may impact the level of concentration, motivation, and ability to understand instructions. The use of beta blockers is also not unusual; their effect and the apparent inherently low maximal heart rate responses of persons with mental retardation may produce severely blunted exercise heart rates. Hypnotics are agents used to modify psychotic behavior while neuroleptics induce sleep or dull the senses.

Recommendations for Exercise Testing

Persons with mental retardation, particularly those with Down syndrome, should be evaluated for potential congenital cardiovascular problems prior to exercise testing. To help ensure valid testing, the following recommendations should be followed:

- Provide ample time for laboratory familiarization and practice testing.
- Provide safety features to ensure that participants do not fall or fear falling.
- Tailor the protocol to the individual.
- Provide an environment in which the individual feels like a participating member.

For treadmill testing:

- Walking protocols should be used and the walking speed should be individualized.
- Only grade should be increased, not speed and grade.
- Work stages of one to two minutes should be used.

Since many individuals with mental retardation have ambulatory limitations or poor coordination, treadmill protocols are not always appropriate. However, standard cycle ergometer protocols have not been shown to be valid for this population. Only the Schwinn Air-Dyne has been shown to be both valid and reliable. Exercise testing that uses the Schwinn Air-Dyne should start at 25 watts and increase 25 watts every two minutes.

Strength testing can be performed on most equipment, including isokinetic machines. Standard protocols can be followed, with the low levels of strength of the population kept in mind. Because of safety concerns and problems with motivation, concentration, and task understanding, the use of free weights is not recommended.

Recommendations for Exercise Programming

Exercise programming for individuals with mental retardation can be conducted in a manner similar to that used with other populations, with some important modifications:

- Exercise intensity should be between 60% and 80% of maximal functional capacity.
- Exercise should be supervised, since it is unlikely that most persons with mental retardation will exercise on their own.
- It may take longer than anticipated to produce a training effect (i.e., 16 to 35 weeks may be

needed to improve $\dot{V}O_2$ max), whereas improvements in *functional capacity* have been demonstrated in programs of shorter duration.

- Motivational techniques, such as token rewards, may be necessary to maintain adherence to the program.

- Strength training should be incorporated whenever possible, as this may have important ramifications for vocational productivity and independence.

Special Considerations

The focus of any program for individuals with mental retardation should be on participation and personal enjoyment. It is important to personalize the program as much as possible to keep the individual interested in exercise. Because motivation is a primary obstacle in this population, innovative ideas that increase the enjoyment of the activities for each person become important. Without continuous reinforcement and supervision, it is unlikely that persons with mental retardation will participate in exercise programs. Sport participation in such programs as Special Olympics, while important for other reasons, have not been shown to produce any physiologic training improvements. Large group programs have been equally ineffective. Therefore, the emphasis should be on individualized programs.

Suggested Readings

Fernhall, B. 1993. Physical fitness and exercise training of individuals with mental retardation. *Med. Sci. Sports Exerc.* 25: 442-50.

Fernhall, B., L. Millar, G. Tymeson, and L. Burkett. 1990. Graded exercise testing of mentally retarded adults: Reliability study. *Arch. Phys. Med. Rehabil.* 71: 1065-68.

Fernhall, B., and G. Tymeson. 1987. Graded exercise testing of mentally retarded adults: A study of feasibility. *Arch. Phys. Med. Rehabil.* 68: 363-65.

Fernhall, B., G. Webster, and G. Tymeson. 1988. Cardiovascular fitness of mentally retarded individuals. *Adapted Physical Activity Quarterly* 5: 12-28.

Lavay, B., G. Reid, and M. Cressler-Chavez. 1990. Measuring cardiovascular endurance of persons with mental retardation: A critical review. *Exerc. Sport Sci. Rev.* 18: 263-90.

Pitetti, K.H., and K.D. Campbell. 1991. Mentally retarded individuals: A population at risk? *Med. Sci. Sports Exerc.* 23: 586-93.

Pitetti, K.H., M. Climstein, K.D. Campbell, P.J. Barrett, and J.A. Jackson. 1992. The cardiovascular capacities of adults with Down syndrome: A comparative study. *Med. Sci. Sports Exerc.* 24: 13-19.

Pitetti, K.H., J.H. Rimmer, and B. Fernhall. 1993. Physical fitness and adults with mental retardation: An overview of current research and future directions. *Sports Med.* 16: 23-56.

Pitetti, K.H., and D.M. Tan. 1991. Effects of a minimally supervised exercise program for mentally retarded adults. *Med. Sci. Sports Exerc.* 23: 594-601.

Rimmer, J.H., and L. Kelly. 1991. Effects of resistance training program on adults with mental retardation. *Adapted Physical Activity Quarterly* 8: 146-53.

Sherrill, C. 1993. *Adapted physical activity, recreation, and sport*, 4th ed. 517-518. Madison, WI: Brown & Benchmark.

MENTAL RETARDATION: EXERCISE TESTING

METHODS	MEASURES	ENDPOINTS	COMMENTS
Aerobic power **Treadmill (Naughton-Balke protocol; speed 2-3.5 mph)** **Schwinn Air-Dyne or cycle ergometer (25 watts/2 min stage)**	• Heart rate • Blood pressure • Peak $\dot{V}O_2$, METs	• SBP > 260 mmHg or DBP > 115 mmHg • Volitional fatigue	• Peak HR usually lower than age predicted. • Peak $\dot{V}O_2$ usually lower than age/gender predicted.
Endurance **Rockport mile walk** **1.5-mile run/walk**	• Time	• Distance	• A pacer will be needed along the side of the subject. • Most subjects will walk more than run. • Practice prior to testing is essential.
Strength **Isokinetic** **Free weights or machines**	• Peak torque • 1 maximal repetition		• Speed of 60°/sec should be used with isokinetic testing. • Constant supervision is of utmost importance.

SPECIAL CONSIDERATIONS

• It is essential to familiarize individuals with protocol, staff, and environment.
• Obesity and poor muscle strength and endurance as well as poor cardiovascular capacities are very common for this population.
• Low peak heart rate is common, especially with Down syndrome.
• Congenital heart defects may be found in persons with Down syndrome.
• Motivation can be a problem in attaining maximal effort.
• Seizures are prevalent, and many individuals are on anticonvulsive agents.
• Poor kinesthetic sense could create problems with balance and gait.
• Hyperflexion and hyperextension of the neck are contraindicated for persons with atlanto-axial instability.

MENTAL RETARDATION: EXERCISE PROGRAMMING

MODES	GOALS	INTENSITY/FREQUENCY/DURATION	TIME TO GOAL
Aerobic endurance • Walk, walk/jog • Schwinn Air-Dyne	• Control or lose weight. • Improve cardiovascular fitness.	• 60-80% peak HR. • 3-5 days/week. • 20-60 minutes/session. • Constant supervision is required. Token reward systems should be considered.	• 4-6 months
Strength • Weight machines	• Increase strength of large muscle groups.	• 70-80% of 1 repetition maximum. • 3 sets of 8-12 repetitions. • Monitor closely.	• 10-12 weeks

MEDICATIONS	SPECIAL CONSIDERATIONS
• Clients may be taking antidepressants, anticonvulsants, hypnotics, beta blockers, and neuroleptics. See text for possible side effects.	• Because of motivation problems, constant supervision and encouragement are necessary. • The following activities are contraindicated for persons with atlanto-axial instability: equestrian sports, gymnastics, diving, pentathlon, butterfly stroke, diving starts in swimming, high jump, alpine skiing, squat lift, football team competition (soccer), and any other activity that may cause hyperflexion or hyperextension of the neck.

CHAPTER 39

Alzheimer's Disease

James Rimmer, PhD

Northern Illinois University

Overview of the Pathophysiology

Alzheimer's disease is a chronic degenerative disorder that causes senile dementia. Currently, there is no known etiology or cure. The pathophysiology of Alzheimer's disease includes atrophy of the cerebral cortex, which results in intellectual impairment that progresses from increasing loss of memory to total disability. This deterioration is manifested in the brains of individuals with Alzheimer's disease at autopsy. Coarse and thick neurofibrillary tangles accumulate within the nerve cell. Additionally, *senile plaques,* which contain a core of protein called amyloid-beta protein, are deposited outside the cell. Formation of the senile plaques is the result of neuronal breakdown. In addition to amyloid angiopathy, granulovacuolar degeneration and gliosis (proliferation of neurological tissue in the central nervous system) may also be present.

Alzheimer's disease affects approximately 4 million Americans. It is listed as the primary cause of dementia. The prevalence of Alzheimer's disease rises exponentially with age: it is 0.5% in persons younger than 65 years, 3% in persons aged 75 years, and 10% in persons 85 years of age. Alzheimer's disease is also more common in women than in men.

Despite the great increase in research on Alzheimer's disease over the past decade, the diagnosis of this disease before death remains an enigma. At present, there is no universally accepted set of criteria for a pathologic diagnosis. The disease was first recognized in 1907 by the German psychiatrist, Alois Alzheimer. From 1907 to 1983, the diagnosis of the disease was based solely on exclusion criteria. That is, other conditions such as brain tumors, strokes, infections, head trauma, and so on had to be ruled out before a person was diagnosed as having Alzheimer's disease. In 1980, as stated in the *Diagnostic and Statistical Manual of Mental Disorders (DSM-III),* "the diagnosis (of Alzheimer's disease) required the presence of dementia of insidious onset and a progressive deteriorating course as well as the exclusion of other potential etiologies" (American Psychiatric Association 1980, 124). In 1984, the National Institute for Neurological and Communicative Disorders and Stroke-Alzheimer's Disease and Related Disorders Association (NINCDS-ADRDA) task force formalized and structured the disease into three categories: probable, definite, and possible Alzheimer's disease (McKhann et al. 1984).

In *probable* Alzheimer's disease, dementia is established clinically and confirmed by neuropsychological tests. The subjects show deficits in cognitive functions accommodated by memory loss. In *definite* Alzheimer's disease, the clinical picture of probable Alzheimer's disease is confirmed at autopsy by histopathologic findings of neurofibrillary plaques and tangles. And in *possible* Alzheimer's disease, the major clinical sign is unusual losses of memory.

Gradual progressive memory loss is the hallmark of Alzheimer's disease. Other symptoms include deterioration of language and perception, judgment problems that compromise the person's ability to carry out activities of daily living, and behavioral problems such as agitation and paranoia.

Alzheimer's disease is progressive and degenerative, and it results in a shortened life expectancy. Although the life expectancy among persons with the disease is diverse, early mortality is seen among persons who develop it early in life and in men. At the present time there is no cure for this disease, and treatment, for the most part, has been limited. The course of the illness may extend from 1 to 15 years, with the average duration being 7 to 8 years.

Effects on Exercise Response and Training

The exercise literature is devoid of data on the use of exercise testing and training in persons with Alzheimer's disease. The recommendations on testing and training that follow are based on clinical experiences and practicality.

Management and Medications

A litany of drugs to treat the psychiatric symptoms frequently associated with dementia have been used in the management of Alzheimer's disease. The drugs are used to control depression, psychotic behavior, agitation, aggression, and sleep disturbances. They fall under the headings of antidepressants, hypnotics, and neuroleptics (to modify psychotic behavior). Possible side effects of these drugs include orthostasis, poor balance, and dysrhythmias. As a result of their age, many clients are also on other medications to control hypertension, arthritis, heart disease, Parkinson's, and other conditions often found in elderly populations.

Recommendations for Exercise Testing

Since Alzheimer's disease affects the person's mental capacity, laboratory tests may be difficult or impossible. Many individuals with Alzheimer's disease have a high level of agitation and would probably not tolerate lengthy testing. If a decision is made that testing can be conducted on a client with the disease, it is recommended that several practice sessions be conducted before the actual maximal test. If the client becomes agitated or confused, the test should be stopped and scheduled for another day. Additionally, it is recommended that all testing be conducted in the morning since most persons with Alzheimer's disease usually function better during the early hours of the day.

Guidelines established by ACSM for maximal and submaximal cardiopulmonary testing for the elderly should be followed for this population. Muscle strength and endurance can be assessed with use of standard weight machines or dynamometers, whereas the use of free weights could be dangerous unless the person with Alzheimer's disease is closely supervised. If a sit-and-reach test is used to measure flexibility, it should be modified in the following manner:

- Position client in a straight-backed chair.

- Position the sit-and-reach box in a separate chair of equal height opposite the client.
- Place the client's feet against the box with the knees straight.
- Have the client flex the trunk while arms are extended so that he or she slowly pushes the gauge with the fingertips.

Additionally, since motor coordination is also affected in many persons with Alzheimer's disease, fitness evaluation for this population should include measures of static and dynamic balance to identify those with greater risk of balance problems and falls.

Recommendations for Exercise Programming

During the early stages of Alzheimer's disease, most clients will be able to participate in some form of physical activity. The main problem will involve memory loss. The client may forget to come to the exercise session or may find that he or she has forgotten how to do certain activities. Depression is quite common during the early stage of the disease and may result in the client's withdrawing from the program. The cornerstone of an exercise program for this population is consistency and patience. The exercise leader must constantly provide verbal encouragement and support to maintain the client's interest in the program. During this stage, simple exercises like walking and performing light calisthenics will be easier than more complex routines.

The middle stage of Alzheimer's disease presents a different set of challenges for the exercise leader. The major problem during this stage involves behavior. Since one of the hallmark symptoms of the disease is extreme agitation, it is not unusual for a client to be totally resistant to an exercise program. A client who has been attending exercise classes during the early stage may suddenly drop out. Memory loss during this stage is more pronounced, and the client may need physical assistance in performing the exercise routine. Extreme outbursts of anger and physical aggression are common during this stage. The exercise leader must work through this agitation with the support of the spouse or other family member who is responsible for the client. Often this behavior will last for only a few minutes and the client will immediately forget that the incident occurred. The exercise leader must remember that this is a symptom of the disease and therefore should not take these outbursts personally.

During the advanced and final stage of the disease the client will require constant supervision and physical assistance. Language skills will be greatly diminished and language comprehension extremely limited. The exercise program must be done on an individual basis. Incontinence and limited mobility are common. Range-of-motion and strength exercises will be the major focus at this stage of the disease.

It should be remembered that it is common for persons with Alzheimer's disease to have a higher level of restlessness and agitation at the end of the day, which some investigators have labeled *"sundowning."* Therefore, the exercise program should be conducted during the early hours of the day, preferably in the morning, when the client's agitation level is usually at its lowest.

The cornerstone of the exercise program for this clientele is consistency and patience. Many persons with Alzheimer's disease do not like to participate in new activities, and it is therefore important for the exercise leader to use behavior modification techniques to increase compliance. Often it is necessary to have the spouse/caregiver attend the program to present a familiar face.

The intensity level of the exercise program at all stages of the disease is not as important as the frequency and duration. The key to working with clients with Alzheimer's disease is to keep them active. Fifteen minutes of chair exercises, emphasizing strength and flexibility, may be a good starting point during the early stages of the program. Additionally, because of memory loss, performing the same exercises each day is preferable over changing routines.

If the client is exercising at home with a family member, a daily walk may be the optimal manner of establishing a structured routine. However, if the client refuses to exercise at home, a day care program attended once or twice a week may be a better setting.

Suggested Readings

American Psychiatric Association. 1980. *Diagnostic and statistical manual of mental disorders,* 3rd ed. Washington, D.C.: American Psychiatric Association.

Bowlby, C. 1993. *Therapeutic activities with persons disabled by Alzheimer's disease and related disorders.* Rockville, MD: Aspen.

Breteler, M.M.B, J.J. Claus, C.M. van Duijn, L.J. Launer, and A. Hofman. 1992. Epidemiology of Alzheimer's disease. *Epidemiol. Rev.* 14: 59-82.

Glickstein, J.K. 1988. *Therapeutic interventions in Alzheimer's disease.* Rockville, MD: Aspen.

Groer, M.W., and M.E. Shekleton. 1989. *Basic pathophysiology. A holistic approach.* St. Louis, MO: Mosby.

McKhann, G.D., D. Drachman, M. Folstein, R. Katzman, D. Price, and E.M. Stedlan. 1984. Clinical diagnosis of Alzheimer's Disease: Report of the NINCDS-ADRDA work group under the auspices of the Department of Health and Human Services Task Force on Alzheimer's Disease. *Neurology.* 34:939-43.

Parks, R.W., R.F. Zec, and R.S. Wilson. 1993. *Neuropsychology of Alzheimer's disease and other dementias.* New York: Oxford University Press.

Rimmer, J.H. 1994. *Fitness and rehabilitation programs for special populations.* Dubuque, IA: Brown & Benchmark.

Volicer, L., K.J. Fabiszewski, Y.L. Rheaume, and K.E. Lasch. 1988. *Clinical management of Alzheimer's disease.* Rockville, MD: Aspen.

Wolf-Klein, G.P. 1993. New Alzheimer's drug expands your options in symptom management. *Geriatrics* 48: 26-36.

ALZHEIMER'S DISEASE: EXERCISE TESTING AND PROGRAMMING

See chapter 19 and tables for testing and programming methodologies. If the client has a specific medical problem, see the corresponding chapter in this book (e.g., if the patient has a history of myocardial infarction, see chapter 3 and tables).

MEDICATIONS	SPECIAL CONSIDERATIONS
• Clients may be taking antidepressants, hypnotics, and neuroleptics. See text for possible side effects.	• Emotional instability or outburst may affect exercise test or program. • Constant supervision is of utmost importance. • Range-of-motion and strength exercise should be the main focus with this disease.

CHAPTER 40

Mental Illness

Gary S. Skrinar, PhD, FACSM
Sargent College of Allied Health Professions

Overview of the Pathophysiology

As defined by the American Psychiatric Association (1994, xxi), mental illness is conceptualized as a clinically significant behavioral or psychological syndrome or pattern that occurs in an individual and that is associated with present distress (e.g., a painful symptom) or disability (i.e., impairment in one or more important areas of functioning) or with a significantly increased risk of suffering death, pain, disability, or an important loss of freedom. Whatever its original cause, it must be currently considered a manifestation of a psychological, biological, or behavioral dysfunction in a person.

It is estimated that 5.5 million Americans suffer from severe mental illness, the most common diagnoses being bipolar disorders, personality disorders, and schizophrenia. Of this group, it is estimated that 1.8 million have schizophrenia, a mental illness that has a devastating impact upon people's lives. Historically, schizophrenia has been more resistant to treatment and rehabilitation efforts because of the lack of clear etiological understanding, the residual symptoms, and the debilitating side effects of psychotropic medications. In general, the causal factors responsible for psychiatric disabilities are unclear. Most experts attribute the most common diagnoses of mental illness to a variety of factors—genetic, biological (biochemical, neurophysiological, neuroanatomical), psychosocial, and sociocultural.

Effects on the Exercise Response

Specific diagnosis of mental illness per se (i.e., depression, schizophrenia, personality disorders) does not modulate the exercise response to a single exercise session (i.e., exercise testing) unless concurrent pharmacological therapy has a dual role (e.g., propranolol, which minimizes social phobia but also influences cardiovascular action). In addition, it is not uncommon for persons with psychiatric disabilities to be afflicted with a secondary medical condition. In this case, consideration must be given to the particular secondary problem and its effect on the response to a single session of exercise.

Effects of Exercise Training

Exercise programming has been safely and successfully conducted with diverse populations of persons including individuals with psychiatric disabilities. Changes in *fitness, performance time,* and *body composition* are important and can be expected in this population if standard components of exercise prescription are followed. Programs that include supervision by both exercise and psychiatric rehabilitation personnel are preferred. Possible positive changes in the psychological profile include

- improved mood,
- improved self-concept,
- improved work behavior, and
- decreased depression and anxiety.

The majority of studies reviewed indicate that exercise provides an antidepressive effect and is recommended for inclusion in both inpatient and outpatient treatment programs. A number of studies have substantiated the benefits of exercise in the treatment of depression. From a rehabilitation and health care perspective, it is important to recognize that emotional and physical fitness are central to people's ability to control their lives and create options in living, learning, and working. Exercise is a key component of this process.

Management and Medications

Since people with severe psychiatric disabilities are almost always on some type of pharmacological therapy (e.g., antianxiety, antidepressant, antipsychotic), a review of current medications is of utmost importance, and in situations in which maximal testing is being conducted, physician supervision is advisable. The following is a list of the most common drugs used in pharmacological therapy that usually do not preclude exercise testing:

- *Antipsychotic*—clozapine, fluphenazine, loxapine, trifluoperazine. *Effects*—sedation, nausea, vomiting, weight gain.
- *Antidepressant*—amitriptyline, haloperidol. *Effects*—insomnia, weight gain, dizziness.
- *Antianxiety*—lorazepam, alprazolam. *Effects*—drowsiness, potentiation of alcohol effects, withdrawal.

Some medication used for various diagnoses of mental illness act the same as for other disabilities but are utilized for different purposes. For example, propranolol is a beta blocker employed for individuals with angina and hypertension. For these individuals, propranolol generally reduces the oxygen requirement of the heart at any given exercise intensity, thereby reducing angina. Propranolol is also used to decrease social phobias in individuals with anxiety disorders. In the latter situation the beta blocker reduces the amount of nervous system stimulation and consequently the anxiety associated with social situations. However, propranolol will still have the same cardiovascular effect on the person with social phobias as it does for individuals with angina.

Recommendations for Exercise Testing

When exercise testing is being conducted, both field and laboratory evaluations should be preceded by extensive orientation sessions. The psychological/emotional status of people with psychiatric disabilities varies from day to day and is frequently influenced by the medications being taken. This psychological status may affect the motivation and ability to perform exercise protocols that depend on volitional maximal efforts. People with psychiatric disorders may be either uncomfortable or unaccustomed to treadmill testing, probably as a result of the effects of medication (e.g., fatigue, dehydration, depression), of gait disturbances associated with tardive dyskinesia (side effect of antipsychotic medications), and of anxiety responses associated with certain diagnoses. Because of its stability, the bicycle ergometer offers a less intimidating and more dependable mode of testing for this population. It is recommended that this form of testing be considered whenever possible to reduce the anxiety associated with treadmill testing, which may increase a person's sense of vulnerability and lack of control. It is not necessary, particularly in light of anxiety usually present, to measure oxygen intake via a metabolic cart.

Recommendations for Exercise Programming

Exercise prescription for people with mental illness should follow standard protocol with regard to frequency and duration. Because the achievement of maximal values is infrequent during initial testing, a more conservative approach may be necessary with regard to intensity (i.e., low to moderate) prescription. Since inactivity, high body fat, and low self-esteem are common in this population it is recommended that a structured, supervised program be initially employed to reinforce the elements of exercise programming and exercise education.

Suggested Readings

American Psychiatric Association. 1994. *Diagnostic and statistical manual of mental disorders.* 4th ed. Washington, D.C.: American Psychiatric Association.

Center for Mental Health Services and National Institute for Mental Health. 1992. *Mental health,*

United States, ed. R.W. Manderscheld and M.A. Sonnenschen. DHHS Pub. No. (SMA) 92-1942. Washington, D.C.: Superintendent of Documents.

Greist, J.H., M.H. Klein, R.R. Eschens, J.W. Faris, A.S. Gurman, and W.P. Morgan. 1979. Running as treatment for depression. *Compr. Psychiatry* 20: 41-54.

Martinsen, E.W., A. Medhus, and L. Sandvik. 1985. Effects of aerobic exercise on depression: A controlled study. *British Medical Journal* 291: 109.

Nadel, G., and S. Horvath. 1967. Fitness evaluation of psychiatric patients. *International Neuropsychology* 3: 191.

Plante, T.G., and J. Rodin. 1990. Physical fitness and enhanced psychological health. *Current Psychology: Research and Reviews* 9: 1-22.

Pelham, T.W., and P.D. Campagna. 1991. Benefits of exercise in psychiatric rehabilitation of persons with schizophrenia. *Canadian J. Rehabil.* 5: 159-68.

Skrinar, G.S., K.V. Unger, D.S. Hutchinson, and A.D. Faigenbaum. 1992. Effects of exercise training in young adults with psychiatric disabilities. *Canadian J. Rehabil.* 4: 151-57.

MENTAL ILLNESS: EXERCISE TESTING AND PROGRAMMING

See guidelines for the general population in *ACSM's Guidelines for Exercise Testing and Prescription* for testing and programming methodologies. If the client has a specific medical problem, see the corresponding chapter in this book (e.g., if the patient has a history of myocardial infarction, see chapter 3 and tables).

MEDICATIONS	SPECIAL CONSIDERATIONS
• Beta blockers: Will attenuate heart rate response. • Prolixin: May increase blood pressure. • Haldol: May cause tachycardia and/or hypotension, possible Q-T-interval prolongation on ECG. • Antipsychotic medication: Possible gait disturbances in relation to tardive dyskinesia. Frequently causes dehydration. • Antidepressants: Insomnia, weight gain, dizziness. • Antianxiety: Drowsiness, potentiation of alcohol effects, withdrawal.	• Allow time for the individual to practice mode of test or exercise. Familiarize client with staff and surroundings. Anxiety disorders, social phobia, and lack of motivation are common due to emotional condition and/or medication.

CHAPTER 41

Deaf and Hard of Hearing

Lorraine E. Bloomquist, EdD, FACSM
University of Rhode Island

Overview of the Pathophysiology

Hearing loss is a generic term that applies to people who are hard of hearing or deaf. They can participate in all types of physical activities with some possible minor adaptations.

- **Hard of hearing** is a condition that makes understanding of speech difficult through use of the ears alone, with or without a hearing aid.

- **Deaf** describes a person who is unable to understand speech through use of the ears alone, with or without a hearing aid.

Three major types of hearing loss include *conductive, sensorineural,* and *mixed. Conductive loss* of hearing is a condition in which the sound does not pass through the external and middle ear to reach the inner ear, resulting in the condition of hard of hearing. Conductive loss of hearing is caused

- in the external ear—by build-up of impacted wax, injury, or infection;

- in the middle ear—by otitis media produced by colds, sinus infections, allergies, or small or blocked Eustachian tubes.

Tympanic tubes for ventilation may be surgically inserted to relieve pressure, dry and ventilate the middle ear, and equalize the air pressure on the two sides of the eardrum.

In the more serious *sensorineural loss,* the inner ear hearing apparatus of the cochlea is affected. This is the site at which sensory receptors convert sound waves into neural impulses that are transmitted to the brain for translation. In sensorineural hearing loss, balance is sometimes affected because the vestibular apparatus is also located in the inner ear. Most people who are born deaf have this type of loss. Causes are a result of

- idiopathic (unknown) factors (50% of cases)
- hereditary factors (60 different types have been identified),
- meningitis,
- mumps,
- scarlet fever,
- encephalitis, and
- measles.

Illnesses of the mother during pregnancy, such as herpes viruses, measles, and toxoplasmosis, as well as head trauma and premature birth produce hearing defects. Aging and noise pollution are statistically the most important causes of hearing deterioration. City life, noisy work environments, machinery, rock concerts, and loud personal earphones all cause hearing damage.

Mixed type of hearing loss is a combination of the two conditions already identified and is common in senior citizens.

Effects on the Exercise Response

Hearing loss generally does not change the exercise response to a single session of exercise. However,

233

persons with a hearing loss may exhibit poor balance, have difficulty with spatial orientation and depth perception, have low physical fitness levels, have low self-image, lack self-confidence, and appear restless and hyperactive. As a result of inadequate communication, they may have fewer social skills and grades in school that are lower than normal (if early onset exists).

Effects of Exercise Training

Regular exercise by people with hearing loss produces the same positive physiological and skill benefits as for individuals with no hearing loss. Additional benefits include

- more opportunities to improve socialization skills,
- practice and improvement in balance,
- learning to work with and relate to a new leader in a group
- improving self-image, confidence, and spatial orientation, and
- decreasing nervousness and hyperactivity.

Management and Medications

Depending on the degree of hearing loss, the assistive device used primarily for conductive loss is the hearing aid. Hearing aids have the same component parts as public address systems and amplify in the same way. They do not clarify or make speech sound clearer. A value of the aid is that it helps people to learn to recognize their own names and assist in their speech. Four basic types of hearing aids are available and are named according to the position worn:

- Chest- or body-worn (young children and persons with multiple disabilities)
- Behind the ear (mainly school-aged children)
- In the ear (mainly adults, about 80% of total)
- On the eyeglasses (mainly adults)

There are over 200 other assistive listening devices available to amplify sounds and convert them to light or vibration systems. In large halls or gyms, AM and FM radio frequencies can transmit voice sounds when the speaker wears a special device. Great technological strides are being made in serv-

ing this group of individuals.

In normal healthy adults with deafness or hearing loss, no medications are prescribed. However, if the person has other primary problems (e.g., coronary artery disease), then one should note and consider specific medications when testing and developing the exercise prescription. In some cases, children may have Ritalin prescribed for hyperactivity. Possible side effects of this medication need to be considered:

- Loss of appetite, abdominal pain, weight loss, insomnia, and tachycardia may occur.
- Long-term effects may have implications for the cardiovascular system and normal growth.

Recommendations for Exercise Testing

If the person with a hearing loss does not have any signs or symptoms of other primary conditions, exercise testing can follow standard protocols. When signs or symptoms of other primary disease are present, exercise testing should follow recommended procedures for that particular disorder.

The primary objectives of exercise testing are to

- uncover hidden risk of vascular disease, and
- determine appropriate intensity range for exercise prescription.

Additional considerations for a person with a hearing loss may include

- having all instructions described in writing or on a video,
- allowing the person to describe or demonstrate the test protocol before the test begins,
- giving visual or tactile reinforcement to motivate the participant, and
- taking necessary steps to prevent the individual from tripping or falling.

Recommendations for Exercise Programming

People with hearing loss generally can participate in all types of physical activity. Prescription procedures are the same as for other clients.

Special Considerations

Communication is the major special consideration with prelingually deaf individuals who have never "lost" hearing and have not acquired speech that is understandable to persons with normal hearing. Deaf people may use a variety of manual sign language systems, including American Sign Language (ASL), Conceptually Accurate Signed English (CASE), Signed Essential English (SEE), or gestures only. Use of interpreters may be necessary to facilitate communication and provide access to medical and exercise services and programs. Some interpreters work as oral interpreters; that is, they interpret the speech of the oral deaf person to the hearing person and mouth the words of the hearing person for the benefit of the oral deaf person. Other sign language interpreters specialize in the different sign language systems.

The best speech (lip) readers are able to read only approximately 30% of the words they see. If the deaf individual is having difficulty understanding speech, the speaker should rephrase the wording. If difficulty persists, use paper and pencil to write the message down. The goal is effective communication, no matter how it is achieved.

When communicating with the individual who is deaf, face the person, maintain eye contact, and speak directly to him or her and not the interpreter. Literally, show the person who is deaf what you want from start to finish. Use as many visual cues and concrete examples as possible.

Exercise leaders working with people who have a hearing loss may need to consider the following recommendations and guidelines:

- Show a video demonstrating the routine or activity.

- Remove hearing aids for contact sports, gymnastics, self-defense activities, and aquatics.

- Speak normally if person uses a hearing aid.

- Use visual and tactile cues.

- Keep near the person to maintain eye contact and allow for speech reading.

- Use facial expressions, body language, gestures, and common signs such as thumbs up or down for OK or not OK.

- Orient the client to all aspects of the facility with special attention to exits, use of pool, and fire evacuation procedures.

- If the person's speech is unclear, do not pretend that you understand.

- Strobe visual fire alarms are an important facility addition.

- Swimmers may need to use individualized molded ear plugs if a conductive disorder exits.

- Loud constant background noise or music may cause headaches, reduce hearing aid effectiveness, and prevent hearing aid users from attending to one speaker.

- When tympanic membrane tubes are used, care should be taken to keep water out of the ears, to have swimmers wear individualized ear plugs in water, and to swim under advice from a physician.

Suggested Readings

Butterfield, S. 1988. Deaf children in physical education. *Palaestra* 4 (3): 28-30, 52.

Paciorek, M., and J. Jones. 1994. *Sports and recreation for the disabled.* Indianapolis, IN: Cooper Publishing Group.

Padden, C., and T. Humphries. 1988. *Deaf in America: Voices from a culture.* Cambridge, MA: Harvard University Press.

Sherrill, C. 1993. *Adapted physical activity, recreation, and sport,* 4th ed. 642-60. Madison, WI: Brown & Benchmark.

Sternberg, M. 1987. *American sign language dictionary.* New York: Harper & Row.

Stewart, D. 1991. *Deaf sport: Impact of sports within the deaf community.* Washington, D.C.: Gallaudet University Press.

Stewart, D., J. Robinson, and D. McCarthy. 1991. Participation in deaf sport: Characteristics of elite deaf athletes. *Adapted Physical Activity Quarterly* 8 (2): 136-45.

Tripp, A., and B. Turner. 1986. Hinsdale South High School: A view from the mainstream. *Perspectives for Teachers of the Hearing Impaired* 5: 6-10.

DEAF AND HARD OF HEARING: EXERCISE TESTING AND PROGRAMMING

See guidelines for the general population in *ACSM's Guidelines for Exercise Testing and Prescription* for testing and programming methodologies. If the client has a specific medical problem, see the corresponding chapter in this book (e.g., if the patient has a history of myocardial infarction, see chapter 3 and tables).

MEDICATIONS	SPECIAL CONSIDERATIONS
• Ritalin: Children taking this for hyperactivity may experience tachycardia, appetite loss, abdominal pain, weight loss, and/or insomnia.	• Be aware that clients may have lower-than-average fitness levels. • Show video tape of test before beginning. Show instructions in writing. • Establish signs for "ready," "start," "stop," "faster," or whatever is necessary for the activity. • Speak in a normal voice if the client wears a hearing aid. • Maintain eye contact so that client may speech-read. • Remove hearing aids for contact sports, gymnastics, self-defense, and aquatics. • Review the client's clearance for aquatics. If tympanic tubes are present, require client to wear ear plugs and keep head out of the water. • Keep the same daily routine so the client can adjust quickly.

CHAPTER 42

Visual Impairment

Lorraine E. Bloomquist, EdD, FACSM
University of Rhode Island

Overview of the Pathophysiology

Visual impairment is a generic term that includes a range of visual acuity from legal blindness with partial sight to total blindness. People with a visual impairment can participate in many vigorous physical activities with some adaptations.

- **Legal blindness** is vision of 20/200 or less with the best correction (while wearing glasses). It is the ability to see at 20 feet what the normal eye sees at 200 feet (i.e., 1/10 or less of normal vision)—blind by acuity. Blind by visual field means having a visual field of less than 10° of central vision—having tunnel vision.

- **Total blindness** is lack of visual perception or the inability to recognize a strong light shown directly into the eye and is called *no light perception.*

In approximately 80% of the people who are considered blind, there is some residual vision that needs to be used to allow the person to participate as normally as possible. Uncommon in school-aged children, visual impairment is the second least frequently occurring disability in childhood (next to deaf-blind). It is a major problem of old age, however, with approximately one-half million persons in the United States classified as legally blind.

In younger populations, causes are attributed to birth defects including congenital cataracts and optic nerve disease. Another now uncommon cause is retinopathy of prematurity (excessive oxygen in incubators). Tumors, injuries, and infectious diseases are possible but less common causes. In persons who are elderly, diabetes, macular degeneration, glaucoma, and cataracts are leading causes. Visual impairment may occur concomitantly in people with cerebral palsy and mental retardation.

Effects on the Exercise Response

Visual impairment generally does not alter the exercise response to a single session of exercise. However, some persons may have poor balance, forward head, low cardiovascular fitness, obesity, lack of confidence, timidity, and fewer social skills. Verbal cues are essential during testing. Impairment of loss of field, that is, peripheral vision, may affect mobility.

Effects of Exercise Training

Regular exercise by people with visual impairment produces the same positive physiological and skills benefits as for individuals without a disability. Additional benefits include

- more opportunities to improve socialization skills;

- practice and improvement in balance skills, which may be low;

- improvement in self-image, confidence, and spatial orientation; and

- improvement in cardiovascular fitness and decreasing obesity.

Management and Medications

Depending on the degree of visual impairment, the primary treatment is the use of corrective lenses—wearing eyeglasses, and especially sunglasses for light sensitivity when one is outside.

In normal, healthy adults with visual impairments, no medications are prescribed. People with glaucoma may need to use eye drops. However, if the person has other primary problems (e.g., coronary artery disease or diabetes), then specific medications should be noted and considered in testing and development of the exercise prescription.

Recommendations for Exercise Testing

If the person with a visual impairment does not have any signs or symptoms of other primary conditions, standard exercise testing protocols can be used. When signs or symptoms of other primary diseases are present, exercise testing should follow recommended procedures for that particular disorder.

The exercise professional may need to follow these additional guidelines for a person with a visual impairment:

- Have all instructions described verbally or on audio tape.
- Allow the person to describe or demonstrate the test protocol before the test begins.
- Give tactile and verbal reinforcement to motivate participant.
- Allow the person to lightly touch handrails or tester when necessary.

Recommendations for Exercise Programming

People with visual impairment generally can participate in all types of physical activity. Blind by loss of field leads to greater difficulty in mobility than blind by acuity. The prescription procedure is the same as for any client, but it may be advisable to take one or more of these special steps:

- Manually orient the person to facilities.
- Keep instructions in large print or Braille or use a strong magnifying glass.
- Have an audio tape describing the routine or activity.
- See that eyeglasses are securely held to the face.
- Allow the person to run or exercise with a partner.

- Have the person run with a short tether to partner or holding partner's upper arm.
- Give regular tactile and verbal cues and feedback to prevent boredom.
- Avoid tracking activities such as handball, tennis, and the like.
- Consider offering goal ball, a specialized team sport in which all are blindfolded and a large bell ball is used. Anyone can play.
- Most individual sports, such as swimming, weight training, dance, track and field, golf, and aerobics, are appropriate.

Special Considerations

Exercise leaders working with a person who is visually impaired may need to take these steps:

- See that people with aphakia (absence of natural lens of eye as when a cataract has been surgically removed), detached retina, or high myopia do not engage in high-impact activities such as jumping.
- Orient the person to all aspects of the facility with special attention to exits, use of pool, and fire evacuation procedures.
- Keep areas clear of clutter for safe movement.
- Keep doors either closed or wide open.
- Keep equipment in the same place so the locations can be memorized.
- Using white color, paint or tape floors or walls where changes occur such as stairs, ramps, pool edge, and lockers.
- Keep areas well lighted, especially around stairs, pool, equipment, and so on.
- A handrail or grab bar can be installed for accessing equipment.
- Keep a sound source, radio, or tape recorder at one end of the room or at the shallow end of the pool for direction orientation.

Suggested Readings

Buell, C. 1982. *Physical education and recreation for the visually handicapped*. Rev. ed. Reston, VA: American Alliance for Health, Physical Education, Recreation and Dance.

Buell, C. 1984. *Physical education for blind children.* 2nd ed. Springfield, IL: Charles C Thomas.

Paciorek, M., and J. Jones. 1994. *Sports and recreation for the disabled.* 2nd ed. Carmel, IN: Cooper Publishing Group.

Sherrill, C. 1993. *Adapted physical activity, recreation, and sport,* 4th ed., 661-76. Madison, WI: Brown & Benchmark.

Tapp, K., J.G. Wilhelm, and L.J. Loveless. 1991. *A guide to curriculum planning for visually impaired students,* 197. Bulletin No. 91540. Madison, WI: Wisconsin State Department of Public Instruction.

Winnick, J. 1985. The performance of visually impaired youngsters in physical education activities: Implications for mainstreaming. *Adapted Physical Activity Quarterly* 2 (4): 292-99.

VISUAL IMPAIRMENT: EXERCISE TESTING AND PROGRAMMING

See guidelines for the general population in *ACSM's Guidelines for Exercise Testing and Prescription* for testing and programming methodologies. If the client has a specific medical problem, see the corresponding chapter in this book (e.g., if the patient has a history of myocardial infarction, see chapter 3 and tables).

MEDICATIONS	SPECIAL CONSIDERATIONS
• Moistening eye drops: May be needed by clients with glaucoma.	• Be aware that clients may have lower-than-average fitness levels. • Balance may be poor, so client may need to use handrails for occasional support. • Play audio tape describing the test, activity, or sport. Ask the client to repeat the instructions verbally before beginning. • Manually and verbally orient the client to all testing/training facilities and equipment. • Use verbal cues to reinforce client. • Pair the client with a partner for running, etc. • Avoid jumping or other high-impact activities if the client has had a cataract surgically removed (aphakia), detached retina, or high myopia. • Keep facility clear of clutter.

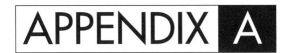
Medications

Table A.1 GENERIC AND BRAND NAMES OF COMMON DRUGS BY CLASS	
GENERIC NAME	**BRAND NAME**
Beta blockers	
Acebutolol	Sectral
Atenolol	Tenormin
Metoprolol	Lopressor, Toprol
Nadolol	Corgard
Pindolol	Visken
Propranolol	Inderal
Timolol	Blocadren
Carteolol	Cartrol
Betaxolol	Kerlone
Bisoprolol	Zebeta
Penbutolol	Levatol
Alpha$_1$ blockers	
Prazosin	Minipress
Terazosin	Hytrin
Doxazosin	Cardura
Alpha and beta blocker	
Lebetalol	Trandate, Normodyne
Antiadrenergic agents without selective receptor blockade	
Clonidine	Catapres
Guanabenz	Wyntensin
Guanethidine	Ismelin
Guanfacine	Tenex
Methyldopa	Aldomet
Reserpine	Serapasil
Guanadrel	Hylorel
Nitrates and nitroglycerin	
Isosorbide dinitrate	Isordil, Diltrate
Nitroglycerin	Nitrostat, Nitrolingual Spray
Nitroglycerin ointment	Nitrol ointment
Nitroglycerin patches	Transderm-Nitro, Nitro-DurII, Nitrodisc
Isosorbide mononitrate	Ismo, Monoket
Pentaerythritol tetranitrate	Cardilate

(continued)

The information for Appendix A was taken from *ACSM's Guidelines for Exercise Testing and Prescription.* (Editors) W. Larry Kenney, R.H. Humphrey, C.X. Bryant. Fifth Edition: Baltimore, Williams & Wilkins, 1995 with permission.

Table A.1   *(continued)*

GENERIC NAME	BRAND NAME
Calcium channel blockers	
Diltiazem	Cardizem
Nifedipine	Procardia, Adalat
Verapamil	Calan, Isoptin
Nicardipine	Cardene
Amlodipine	Norvasc
Felodipine	Plendil
Isradipine	DynaCirc
Nimodipine	Nimotop
Bepridil	Vascor
Digitalis	
Digoxin	Lanoxin
Diuretics	
Thiazides	
Hydrochlorothiazide (HCTZ)	Esidrix
"Loop"	
Furosemide	Lasix
Bumetanide	Bumex
Ethacrynic acid	Edecrin
Potassium-sparing	
Spironolactone	Aldactone
Triamterene	Dyrenium
Amiloride	Midamor
Combinations	
Triamterene and HCTZ	Dyazide, Maxzide
Amiloride and HCTZ	Moduretic
Others	
Metolazone	Zaroxolyn
Peripheral vasodilators (nonadrenergic)	
Hydralazine	Apresoline
Minoxidil	Loniten
Angiotensin-converting enzyme (ACE)	
Captopril	Capoten
Enalapril	Vasotec
Lisinopril	Prinivil, Zestril
Ramipril	Altace
Benazapril	Lotensin
Fosinopril	Monopril
Quinapril	Accupril

GENERIC NAME	BRAND NAME
Antiarrhythmic agents	
Class I	
IA	
Quinidine	Quinidex, Quinaglute
Procainamide	Pronestyl, Procan SR
Disopyramide	Norpace
IB	
Tocainide	Tonocard
Mexiletine	Mexitil
Lidocaine	Xylocaine, Xylocard
IC	
Encainide	Enkaid
Flecainide	Tambocor
Multiclass	
Ethmozine	Moricizine
Class II	
Beta blockers	
Class III	
Amiodarone	Cordarone
Bretylium	Bretylol
Sotalol	Betapace
Class IV	
Calcium channel blockers	
Sympathomimetic agents	
Ephedrine	Adrenalin
Epinephrine	Alupent
Metaproterenol	Proventil, Ventolin
Albuterol	Bronkosol
Isoetharine	Brethine
Cromolyn sodium	Intal
Antihyperlipidemic agents	
Cholestyramine	Questran
Colestipol	Colestid
Gemfibrozil	Lopid
Lovastatin	Mevacor
Nicotinic acid (niacin)	Nicobid, Nicolar, Slo-Niacin
Probucol	Lorelco
Pravastatin	Pravachol
Simvastatin	Zocor
Fluvastatin	Lescol
Others	
Dipyridamole	Persantine
Warfarin	Coumadin
Pentoxifylline	Trental

| Table A.2 | EFFECTS OF MEDICATIONS ON HEART RATE, BLOOD PRESSURE, THE ELECTROCARDIOGRAM (ECG) AND EXERCISE CAPACITY |

MEDICATIONS	HEART RATE		BLOOD PRESSURE	ECG		EXERCISE CAPACITY
	Rest	Exercise	Rest (R) and exercise (E)	Rest	Exercise	
I. Beta blockers (including labetalol)	↓*	↓	↓	↓ HR*	↓ Ischemia#	↑ In patients with agina; ↓ or ↔ in patients without angina
II. Nitrates	↑↑ or ↔		↓ (R) ↓ or ↔ (E)	↑ HR	↑ or ↔ HR ↓ Ischemia#	↑ In patients with angina; ↔ in patients without angina; ↑ or ↔ in patients with congestive heart failure (CHF)
III. Calcium channel blockers Felodopine Isradipine Nicardipine Nifedipine	↑ or ↔	↑ or ↔	↓	↑ or ↔	↑ or ↔ HR ↓ Ischemia#	↑ In patients with angina; ↔ in patients without angina
Bepridil Diltiazem Verapamil	↓	↓	↓	↓ HR	↓ HR ↓ Ischemia#	↑ In patients with angina; ↔ in patients without angina
IV. Digitalis	↓ In patients w/ atrial fibrillation and possibly CHF. Not significantly altered in patients w/ sinus rhythm	↔		May produce nonspecific ST-T-wave changes (rest). May produce ST-segment depression (exercise)		Improved only in patients with atrial fibrillation or in patients with CHF
V. Diuretics	↔	↔	↔ or ↓	May cause premature ventricular contractions (PVCs) and "false positive" test results if hypokalemia occurs. May cause PVCs if hypomagnesemia occurs.		↔, except possibly in patients with CHF (see chapter 8)
VI. Vasodilators Nonadrenergic vasodilators	↑ or ↔	↑ or ↔	↓	↑ or ↔ HR	↑ or ↔ HR	↔, except ↑ or ↔ in patients with CHF
ACE inhibitors	↔	↔	↓	↔	↔	↔, except ↑ or ↔ in patients with CHF
Alpha-adrenergic blockers	↔	↔	↓	↔	↔	↔

MEDICATIONS	HEART RATE		BLOOD PRESSURE	ECG		EXERCISE CAPACITY
	Rest	Exercise	Rest (R) and exercise (E)	Rest	Exercise	
Antiadrenergic agents without selective blockade of peripheral receptors	↓ or ↔	↓ or ↔	↓	↓ or ↔ HR	↓ or ↔ HR	↔
VII. Antiarrhythmic agents				All antiarrhythmic agents may cause new or worsened arrhythmias (proarrhythmic effect)		
Class I Quinidine	↑ or ↔	↑ or ↔	↓ or ↔ (R) ↔ (E)	↑ or ↔ HR May result in "false negative" test May prolong QRS and QT intervals		↔
Disopyramide	↑ or ↔	↑ or ↔	↓ or ↔ (R) ↔ (E)	May prolong QRS and QT intervals; may result in "false positive" test		↔
Procainamide	↔	↔	↔	↔ ↔	↔ ↔	↔
Phenytoin	↔	↔	↔	↔	↔	↔
Tocainide	↔	↔	↔	May prolong QRS and QT intervals		↔
Mexiletine	↔	↔	↔			↔
Flecainide	↔	↔	↔	May prolong QRS and QT intervals		↔
Moricizine	↔	↔	↔	↓ HR	↓ or ↔ HR	↔
Propafenone	↓	↓ or ↔	↔			↔
Class II Beta blockers (see I)				↓ HR	↔	
Class III Amiodarone	↓	↓	↔			↔
Class IV Calcium channel blockers (see III)						
VIII. Bronchodilators						Bronchodilators ↑ exercise capacity in patients limited by bronchospasm
Anticholinergic agents	↔		↔	↔	↔	
Methylxanthines	↑ or ↔	↑ or ↔	↔	↑ or ↔ HR	↑ or ↔ HR	

(continued)

Table A.2   *(continued)*

MEDICATIONS	HEART RATE		BLOOD PRESSURE	ECG		EXERCISE CAPACITY
	Rest	Exercise	Rest (R) and exercise (E)	Rest	Exercise	
Sympathomimetic agents	↑ or ↔	↑ or ↔	↑, ↔, or ↓	May produce PVCs ↑ or ↔ HR	↑ or ↔ HR	
Cromolyn sodium	↔	↔	↔	↔	↔	
Corticosteroids	↔	↔	↔	↔	↔	
IX. Hyperlipidemic agents						
Clofibrate	↔	↔	↔	May provoke arrhythmias, angina in patients with prior myocardial infarction		↔
Dextrothyroxine	↑ or ↔	↑ or ↔	↑ or ↔	May provoke arrhythmias and worsen myocardial ischemia and angina		↔
Nicotinic acid	↔	↔	↓ or ↔	↔	↔	↔
Probucol	↔	↔	↔	May cause QT-interval prolongation		↔
All others	↔	↔	↔	↔		↔
X. Psychotropic medications						
Minor tranquilizers	May ↓ HR by controlling anxiety		May ↓ BP by controlling anxiety	↔	↔	↔
Antidepressants	↑ or ↔	↑ or ↔	↓ or ↔	See text	May result in "false positive" test	↔
Major tranquilizers	↑ or ↔	↑ or ↔	↓ or ↔	See text	May result in "false positive" or "false negative" test	↔
				May result in T wave changes and arrhythmias		
Lithium	↔	↔	↔			↔
XI. Nicotine	↑ or ↔	↑ or ↔		↑ or ↔ HR ↑ or ↔ HR May provoke ischemia, arrhythmias		↔, except ↓ or ↔ in patients with angina
XII. Antihistamines	↔	↔	↔	↔	↔	↔

MEDICATIONS	HEART RATE		BLOOD PRESSURE	ECG		EXERCISE CAPACITY
	Rest	Exercise	Rest (R) and exercise (E)	Rest	Exercise	
XIII. Cold medications with sympathomimetic agents⁺	↑ or ↔	↑ or ↔	↑, ↔, or ↓	↑ or ↔ HR	↑ or ↔ HR	↑ or ↔
XIV. Thyroid medications	↑	↑	↑	↑ HR Levothyroxine may provoke ischemia, arrhythmias	↑ HR	↔, unless angina worsened
XV. Alcohol	↔	↔	Chronic use may ↑ BP	May provoke arrhythmias		↔
XVI. Insulin and oral hypoglycemic agents	↔	↔	↔	↔	↔	↔
XVII. Dipyridamole	↔	↔	↔	↔	↔	↔
XVIII. Anticoagulants	↔	↔	↔	↔	↔	↔
XIX. Antigout medications	↔	↔	↔	↔	↔	↔
XX. Antiplatelet medications	↔	↔	↔	↔	↔	↔
XXI. Pentoxifylline	↔	↔	↔	↔	↔	↑ or ↔ in patients limited by intermittent claudication
XXII. Caffeine	↑, ↔, or ↓, depending on previous usage	↑, ↔, or ↓, depending on previous usage	↑, ↔, or ↓, depending on previous usage	May provoke arrhythmias		↑, ↔, or ↓
XXIII. Diet pills	↑ or ↔	↑ or ↔	↑ or ↔	↑ or ↔ HR	↑ or ↔ HR	

↑ = increase, ↔ = no effect, ↓ = decrease
*Beta blockers with intrinsic sympathomimetric activity (ISA) lower resting HR only slightly
#May prevent or delay myocardial ischemia (see chapter 5)
⁺Effects are similar to those described in sympathomimetic agents (see VIII), although magnitude of effects is usually smaller

APPENDIX B

Case Studies

The examples in this appendix illustrate the use of problem-oriented exercise management in persons with various chronic diseases and disabilities or combinations of chronic disease and disability. The management of each case does not reflect the only approach; alternative solutions may be just as viable. The cases range from simple to complex, and they illustrate how extremely complicated circumstances can be managed by being broken down into multiple problems. Most cases show successful outcomes, though some show that exercise sometimes fails to achieve seemingly reasonable goals. SOAP notes (the organizational technique introduced in chapter 2) accompany each case. Some programs do not reflect recommendations in this text, since the cases predated this manual. These variances from current recommendations are clearly noted. Permission to publish these cases was obtained from the individuals.

Case Study 1 - Low Back Pain

This 41-year-old man had low back pain after slipping while mowing the lawn. The pain radiated down the left lower extremity to the calf and was made worse by activity, and anti-inflammatory medicines did not help. He had no prior back injury. His symptoms had worsened during the previous four months despite conservative care, and his sleep and daily activities were disrupted. He had previously been very active and had participated in competitive and recreational sports. During the last three years, however, he had been less active and had gained 30 pounds.

Height was 6'0" and weight was 190 pounds; the client had no lower-extremity atrophy or fasciculations, but he had a positive straight leg raise (left) at 30°, some (minimal) weakness, and mild sensory losses to touch and pinprick. Magnetic resonance imaging revealed a herniated disk involving the left L-5 nerve root.

The final diagnosis was chronic low back pain radiating to the left lower extremity, secondary to a herniated disk (L 4-5) and nerve root involvement. The man was referred to a conservative care program with the goal of a complete relief of pain and return to his usual lifestyle.

He was given a trial of aggressive nonsurgical therapy, including high-dose anti-inflammatory medications, traction, transcutaneous electrical neural stimulation, ultrasound, and two weeks of rest; he also had diathermy, pelvic exercises, and postural coaching. After this treatment, he was to increase walking and/or stair climbing as tolerated to 30 minutes per day. But after these interventions, he had not improved and was unable to walk. A lumbar diskectomy and hemilaminectomy were performed. Postoperatively, he underwent physical therapy rehabilitation, including no straining or lifting more than 5 pounds for six weeks, trunk musculature strength training, and a gradual reintroduction of aerobic activities/weight training.

Discussion

This person is a professor at a medical center and is very knowledgeable about back injury. The majority of back pain problems get better with conservative care, but some do not, and this is an example. He exhausted all forms of conservative care and physical therapy without relief. A major lesson here is that it is important to recognize when physical activities fail to achieve the desired goal.

S: Back and left leg pain.

O: Weakness, positive straight leg raise on L at 30°.

A: Pain and weakness secondary to herniated disk at L4-5 with L5 nerve root involvement.

P: 1) Conservative care therapy and trunk-strengthening exercises.

2) Surgical evaluation if therapy fails in 4-12 weeks.

3) Pre- and postoperative range of motion/strength training.

Exercise Program

Goal: Pain-free, normal strength, return to previous lifestyle.

Mode: Stretching, spine and abdominal strength exercises.

Intensity: Very low resistance (gravity only).

Frequency: Twice a day, 5-7 days/week.

Duration: 15-20 minutes each set.

Time course: 1-3 months.

Case 2 - Chronic Obstructive Pulmonary Disease

A 74-year-old man with 10-year history of emphysema was having difficulty playing tennis because of shortness of breath. He had smoked for 50 years but had stopped smoking 10 years earlier and had enrolled in a pulmonary rehabilitation program. In recent years he had required oxygen during physical activity (6 $L \cdot min^{-1}$). Medicines included a tapering schedule of oral prednisone and three inhalers: Azmacort, Proventil, and Atrovent. Previous spirometry showed moderately severe obstructive pulmonary disease. His regular activities included a previous pulmonary rehabilitation program, golf, and tennis, but he had been having difficulty with tennis.

Cardiopulmonary exercise testing on a stationary bicycle was performed according to a protocol that continuously ramp-increased by 4 $watts \cdot min^{-1}$. Peak work rate was 56 watts, with a peak heart rate of 103 contractions per minute, peak ventilation of 50 $L \cdot min^{-1}$, and peak $\dot{V}O_2$ of 15 $ml \cdot kg^{-1} \cdot min^{-1}$ (1.21 $L \cdot min^{-1}$). The dead space-to-tidal volume ratio failed to decrease appropriately during exercise, and the alveolar-arterial O_2 gradient widened during exercise (abnormal) as the arterial partial pressure of oxygen (PO_2) fell from 59.4 to 47.8 torr at peak exercise.

A pulmonary rehabilitation program was initiated with a goal of playing tennis again. The program started with 10 minutes each of walking and stationary cycling, with prescribed respiratory rates of 25-35 breaths per minute. The client also did some warmup and cool-down exercises with hand weights. These were well tolerated, and after 12 weeks he was able to do upper- as well as lower-extremity exercise. He continued to improve, and one year after enrollment he had returned to playing tennis.

Discussion

This client had a goal of resuming his tennis play, though his pulmonary disease had seriously limited his exercise tolerance. Since he had a peak work rate of only 56 watts with arterial desaturation, it was not clear that with exercise programming he would ever regain enough functional capacity and return to playing tennis. Nonetheless, he was successful and achieved his goal. A major learning point of this case is that, for most clients, exercise programming is worth a try, because some people can make remarkable advances. Knowing which clients will be successful is not always possible.

S: Shortness of breath on exertion.

O: 1) 15 $ml \cdot kg^{-1} \cdot min^{-1}$ $\dot{V}O_2$max at peak exercise capacity of 56 watts.

A: 2) Arterial desaturation at peak exercise.

P: COPD (emphysema) with severe pulmonary limitation to physical activity.

   1) Lower-extremity aerobic exercise with upper-extremity strength training, and gradual introduction of upper- and lower-extremity exercise.

   2) Supplemental oxygen during activity (initially, monitor with oximeter to keep saturation > 90%).

Exercise Program

Goal: Resume playing tennis.

Mode: Lower-extremity aerobic exercise. Upper-extremity strength exercise.

Intensity: 40% of peak $\dot{V}O_2$max heart rate. 10 repetition maximum.

Frequency: 3 days/week.

Duration: 20 minutes, building to 40 minutes. 2 sets lifting.

Time course: 1-3 months to resume whole-body exercise; 6-12 months for tennis.

Case 3 - Angina, Diabetes, Peripheral Arterial Disease, Arthritis, and Visual Impairment

This 67-year-old man had a long history of diabetes and atherosclerosis involving both coronary and peripheral arteries. He had previously undergone coronary artery angioplasty and femoral-popliteal bypass graft surgery. He had several healed ulcers on the legs and feet from circulatory insufficiency, and claudication pain limited him to walking one block at a time. Walking fast caused him to have "headaches" starting in the back of his head and radiating down to his shoulders and arms and across his chest. Stopping to rest relieved the headaches. These headaches sometimes developed at rest, usually at night. For the nocturnal headaches, sublingual nitroglycerin provided relief but acetaminophen with codeine did not.

He also complained of joint pain, and x-rays showed severe arthritis in the hips and neck. Lastly, he had complete visual disability from retinitis pigmentosa. His major wish was to walk with his guide dog, a Labrador retriever that had been overpowering him since the coronary artery bypass surgery.

Physical examination revealed no heart failure, and near complete sensory loss below the shins. The skin on the legs was intact. Popliteal pulses were strong, but dorsalis pedis and posterior tibialis pulses were absent. Knee jerk and Achilles tendon reflexes were absent on both sides.

A treadmill test was administered that consisted of a modified protocol using 90-second stages, starting at 0.8 mph and 0% grade and increasing the speed to 1.4 mph, which was a comfortable walking speed. The intensity was increased to a maximum of 1.5 mph and 2.5% grade, at which point the client was unable to complete the interval because of severe claudication and a typical "headache." The ECG showed 2 mm lateral ST depression. The chest discomfort was immediately relieved by nitroglycerin; the claudication pain resolved within five minutes. Peak rate-pressure product was 15,600.

A six-minute walk test was performed in a long hallway with a guide. The client walked a total of 686 feet, but had to stop briefly at 462 feet because of claudication pain. He developed no chest pain during this walk. Gait analysis showed remarkably little asymmetry and no evidence of foot drop. Goniometry on forward bend revealed an inability to flex beyond 90° at the hip. Six-minute walk speed was 0.48 m·sec⁻¹.

Clearly, this individual had a multitude of complicating factors, and successful exercise management for him would be quite involved. His problems included

- coronary artery disease with exertional angina and ECG evidence of ischemia,
- severe peripheral arterial disease,
- total loss of vision,
- severe diabetic and ischemic neuropathy below the knees with insensate feet,
- osteoarthritis in the left hip and neck,
- diabetes,
- obesity, and
- limited range of motion (hip flexion).

This man also chose a lofty goal—walking with his guide dog. He was advised that attaining this goal might never be possible, but that he could try. His program included

- supervised treadmill walking three times a week, limited by claudication pain or angina,
- prophylactic and therapeutic sublingual nitroglycerin for angina,
- an interval-oriented exercise program (with claudication and angina as endpoints),
- walking at home on alternate days,
- stretching as a warm-up and cool-down (no specific goal established),
- random blood sugar checks before and after exercise,
- dietary counseling for diabetes (lipid and weight loss given as adjunctive therapy), and
- cholesterol-lowering medications (his primary physician was consulted on this matter).

Several random blood sugars before and after exercise were all normal, so these checks were discontinued. The client progressed to walking for 30 consecutive minutes with no angina or claudication pain. At the beginning of the program, he occasionally required sublingual nitroglycerin for exertional angina, but this need diminished over time and ultimately disappeared. Because of his visual disability, a charitable foundation provided a home treadmill, which he used on days when he did not come to rehabilitation. After six months of exercise training, he had resumed walking with his guide dog. After one year, he suffered a cardiac arrest (unrelated to exercise). He was successfully resuscitated and had a prolonged hospitalization due to vascular complications of a small stroke and leg ischemia.

Discussion

This man presented a complex mixture of multiple chronic diseases (coronary artery disease, peripheral artery disease, diabetes with neuropathy, arthritis) with visual disability. Fortunately, he was highly motivated, accustomed to the discomforts of exercise, and willing to push himself. His ability to overcome a multitude of problems demonstrates his resilience and perseverance, as well as the ability of problem-oriented management to solve highly complex problems.

The exercise was managed primarily with emphasis on the stable angina and claudication. The client initially used prophylactic sublingual nitroglycerin (before exercise), but raised his angina threshold and became able to discontinue this practice. Similarly, he raised his claudication threshold. Fortunately, the severe neuropathy did not cause a profound gait abnormality. Equally fortunately, he was stoic about the arthritic discomfort in his hip. The diabetes was well managed with oral medication and did not require further intervention (other than dietary counseling). The diet was a major problem because this client was a retired chef, and modifying his cooking preferences was difficult. The limited flexibility was treated with stretching, which was familiar to him from his athletic days. The visual disability was largely accommodated by use of a treadmill and the guide dog. His cardiac arrest is very recent and he has not yet returned to rehabilitation.

S: Easy fatigability with cramping calf and headaches.

O: 1) Vital signs normal, body mass index 32, total inability to detect light, no signs of heart failure, markedly decreased sensation and absent pulses below the knees.

2) Medications: lisinopril, glyburide, Mevacor, warfarin.

3) Mild anemia, cholesterol 235 mg·dl⁻¹, triglycerides 220 mg·dl⁻¹.

3) Mild anemia, cholesterol 235 $mg \cdot dl^{-1}$, triglycerides 220 $mg \cdot dl^{-1}$.

4) ECG: left ventricular hypertrophy; chest x-ray: enlarged heart shadow.

5) Aerobic exercise test
  - 4 METs, estimated peak $\dot{V}O_2$ 15 ml·kg⁻¹·min⁻¹, SaO_2 92%.
  - Peak heart rate 118, peak blood pressure 170/105 (rate-pressure product 15,600).

6) Endurance exercise test (6-minute walk)
  - 686 feet, paused for claudication at 462 feet.

7) Gait analysis
  - No foot drop; walking speed 0.48 m/sec; minimal asymmetry.

8) Range of motion
  - Forward bend limited to 90°.

A: 1) Low aerobic power due to multiple contributing factors:
  - Coronary artery disease with ischemia
  - Peripheral arterial disease
  - Diabetic neuropathy
  - Diabetes in fair control
  - Obesity/sedentary lifestyle

2) Low endurance secondary to same.

3) Limited range of motion at hips secondary to sedentariness and arthritis.

4) Complete visual disability.

P: Improve exercise intolerance by several therapies:
  - Increased angina and claudication thresholds with aerobic exercise training.
  - Improved hip flexibility and exercise.
  - Aggressive diabetes and cholesterol management.
  - Weight loss and diabetic diet.

Exercise Program

Goal:	Increase aerobic power and endurance.
Mode:	Walking.
Intensity:	Start at 0.8 mph and 0% grade; increase duration to three 10-minute periods without stopping, then gradually increase speed as tolerated to 1.5-2.0 mph.
Frequency:	3-7 days/week.
Duration:	30 minutes, build to 45 minutes.
Time course:	3-9 months.

Case 4 - Congestive Heart Failure, Coronary Artery Bypass Grafting (CABG), and Chronic Rotator Cuff Tear

A 65-year-old man underwent repeat CABG, had a perioperative heart attack, developed heart failure and ended up spending five weeks in an intensive care unit. He was easily fatigued and had chest pain on exertion. He was unable do his usual activities such as housework, car repair, and playing with his grandchildren, which made him short of breath and easily fatigued upon exertion. He admitted to being sedentary and to 30 pack-years of cigarette smoking, which he had stopped after the most recent hospitalization. He also complained of sharp shoulder pain with an inability to lift his right hand above the shoulder. Medications included an ACE inhibitor, a beta blocker, long-acting nitrates and sublingual nitrates as needed, an anticoagulant, a diuretic, and acetaminophen. He was depressed and felt no one could possibly make him better.

This man's weight was 165 pounds, pulse was 108 contractions per minute, blood pressure was 104/70 mmHg, and there were signs of heart failure (edema and râles). He was unable to abduct his right arm above the shoulder, secondary to pain; internal and external rotation of the shoulder were intact, as were flexion and extension. Laboratory data revealed normal kidney function and total cholesterol of 164 mg·dl⁻¹ (post-infarct); a recent echocardiogram showed a left ventricular ejection fraction of 15% to 20%. No other laboratory data were available.

This client revealed that he took his diuretic only when he thought he needed to, so he was encouraged to take it as directed. Two weeks later, his blood pressure remained stable, his heart failure had improved, and it became appropriate to obtain further objective data. He performed a low-intensity treadmill test, walking for 5 minutes and 55 seconds to a peak of 1.5 mph at 3.5% grade before stopping because of fatigue and chest pain. His peak heart rate was 113, peak blood pressure 100/inaudible; his ECG showed 1 mm of lateral ST depression; oximetry revealed no desaturation. Spirometry tests were normal.

Assessment

1) Congestive heart failure, partially compensated, status post-MI.

2) Aerobic exercise intolerance secondary to heart failure and deconditioning.

3) Rotator cuff tear in right shoulder.

4) Depression.

Plan

The plan was to stabilize the client's loss of function and have him regain fitness (to a sustained aerobic work rate of 3 METs for 30 minutes) and resume previous activities of daily living. He was given a program of walking 5 to 10 minutes at 1 mph at 0% grade, building up to 30 to 45 minutes, a minimum of three times a week; after he achieved 30 minutes three times a week, the intensity was more rigorously controlled to a rate of perceived exertion of 10 to 13. He was encouraged to walk, on his own, at a lower intensity on the other four days of the week.

Passive range of motion, limited by pain, and strengthening exercises using elastic bands were given for the rotator cuff tear. Inoperable coronary artery disease made surgical repair too risky.

Dietary counseling and medication were given to lower cholesterol. The client's primary physician continued medical management of his depression.

Follow-Up

After three months, the client had no change in status and was not sure exercise was helping him.

Discussion

Cases such as this client's are quite common. Several factors contributed to his exercise intolerance: (1) he had congestive heart failure; (2) he had taken a beta blocker after a recent heart attack, which may have worsened his heart failure but helped his angina (although long-term administration of beta blockers sometimes helps heart failure); (3) he was sedentary and deconditioned; (4) he had symptoms of ischemia or worsening heart failure during exertion; (5) possible chronic lung disease from smoking; and (6) he had a rotator cuff tear.

Since this man was not medically stable at the first assessment, exercise testing and programming were deferred until his heart failure was controlled. The beta blocker was prescribed because it improves survival after a heart attack and over the long term may also help heart failure. On the other hand, his heart failure might improve with increased contractility (reducing the beta blocker) and decreased afterload (adding an ACE inhibitor). However, the mainstay of therapy for heart failure is treatment with a diuretic, and he was not taking the diuretic on a regular basis. Resuming the diuretic allowed his heart failure to become compensated; no further medical intervention was necessary, and it became possible to integrate exercise into his medical regimen.

An important lesson from this person is that problems must be solved in steps: (1) evaluation and assessment, (2) an intervention to achieve medical stability, (3) reevaluation and reassessment (to confirm medical stability), (4) an exercise evaluation and assessment—and maybe more reevaluation/intervention/reassessment cycles. In some persons, such cycles may include a therapeutic trial of exercise. Also, note that exercise started with short bouts of low-level exercise and progressed over one to three months to continuous daily exercise at the goal intensity. This was because the dose-response relationship in this patient was limited by early onset of fatigue and a low exhaustion threshold, and he thus required frequent low-dose exercise. In the follow-up, it was unclear whether exercise was truly not helping or whether it was preventing further decline.

S: Chronic fatigue, angina, and shoulder pain.

O: 1) Signs of heart failure (tachycardia, râles, S3 heart sound, edema).

2) Medications: Lasix, metoprolol, Mevacor, aspirin.

3) Echocardiogram: ejection fraction 15-20%.

4) ECG: inferior wall MI.

5) Aerobic exercise test

- 4 METs, estimated peak $\dot{V}O_2$max 15 ml·kg^{-1}·min^{-1}, SaO$_2$ 92%.

- Peak heart rate 113, peak blood pressure 100/- (rate-pressure product 11,300).

- 1 mm ST depression.

- Range of motion: painful elevation of arm beyond 60°, inability to raise hand above shoulder.

A: 1) Low aerobic power due to multiple contributing factors:

- Coronary artery disease with ischemia

- Congestive heart failure

- Sedentary lifestyle

2) Limited range of motion and strength in shoulder secondary to arthritis due to rotator cuff tear.

P: 1) Walking exercise a minimum of 30 minutes three times a week. The client was encouraged to walk, on his own, at a lower intensity on the other four days of the week.

- Increased angina threshold with aerobic exercise training.

- Passive range of motion, limited by pain, and strengthening exercises using elastic bands.

Exercise Program

Goal: Increase aerobic power and endurance.

Mode: Walking.

Shoulder passive resistance/stretching (elastic bands).

Intensity: 5-10 minutes at 1 mph, 0% grade; gradually increase rating of perceived exertion to 10-14.

To limits of range of motion, tolerance of discomfort.

Frequency: 3-7 days/week.

Duration: 30 minutes, build to 45 minutes.

Time course: 2-6 months.

Case 5 - Renal Failure, Diabetes, Congestive Heart Failure, Amputee

A 65-year-old woman knew about the benefits of exercise and wanted to participate in an experimental exercise program offered at her dialysis center. She had long-standing diabetes with multiple complications, including kidney failure. She no longer smoked, but had smoked for over 30 years and had been on dialysis for almost two years. Her blood sugar was controlled on oral medication and diet; her dialysis treatments were administered three times a week and she was sedentary except for travel to the dialysis center.

Examination showed moderate obesity and no signs of heart failure; the client was weak and had a mild sensory loss in the lower extremities. A previous echocardiogram had shown four-chamber enlargement with mitral and tricuspid valve regurgitation. An exercise test was performed with respired gas analysis, cardiac output, and blood gas measurement. The test consisted of unloaded pedaling for two-minute stages of 30, 40, and 50 rpm, after which she stopped because of fatigue. The estimated peak work rate was 10 watts, and the peak $\dot{V}O_2$ was 9 ml·kg^{-1}·min^{-1}. The arterial blood gas at peak exercise showed desaturation.

Assessment

1) Chronic renal failure and bivalvular heart failure, both compensated by hemodialysis.

2) COPD.

3) Aerobic exercise intolerance secondary to #1 and sedentary lifestyle.

4) Diabetes with neuropathy.

Plan

The plan for this client was to facilitate sustained pedaling for 30 to 45 minutes at a 15- to 25-watt work rate by using this program:

- Stationary cycling during dialysis, three times a week.
- Cycling to start at 5 to 10 minutes of unloaded pedaling and increase to 30 minutes as tolerated.
- Adding pedaling resistance after 30 minutes is achieved.

The client did well and progressed rapidly to the target goal. Unfortunately, she had multiple intercurrent medical complications (unrelated to exercise) that caused frequent setbacks. One complication was osteomyelitis, which required a below-the-knee amputation. After her prosthesis was fitted, she wanted to resume cycling.

Reassessment

Below-knee amputation.

Plan

It was decided that the original goal would be modified to accommodate the amputation and that the client would resume the exercise program. The program was modified with the use of a prosthesis mounted onto the pedal by straps during cycling.

The client enjoyed the exercise very much, but she continued to have setbacks that were frustrating and that constantly forced her to have to regain lost ground; she ultimately decided for this reason that the exercise was not worthwhile. She withdrew from the program and died later that year.

Discussion

Exercise management for someone like this client is extraordinarily difficult. She was burdened with severe metabolic disease due to multiple end-stage organ failures, had a leg amputation, and was profoundly deconditioned. There were *disease-dependent* risks and considerations. First, measures were taken to ensure safe blood glucose management during exercise. Second, to avoid arterial desaturation, the exercise sessions were delayed and even deferred when she came to dialysis having gained many pounds of fluid (which worsened her heart failure). Third, the amputation necessitated use of a prosthesis and special straps to hold it onto the pedal.

The interaction of medications with exercise performance must also be considered for such an individual. Erythropoietin is a drug commonly used in persons on dialysis because it improves anemia and exercise capacity. In this case, erythropoietin was not being used because it did not yet have full FDA approval.

The exercise dose-response relationship for such a person is unknown. After years of deconditioning and chronic disease, she was easily exhausted and needed slow, gradual progression of *very* low dose exercise. Her program of stationary cycling was conducted during dialysis; this strategy is safe, effective, and convenient. She started by pedaling against no resistance at a self-chosen rate (30 rpm) and quit from fatigue after about five minutes. Within a few weeks, she was pedaling for 30 minutes and ultimately reached 45 minutes at 50 to 60 rpm against a trace of resistance (about 15 watts). No effect of exercise on blood glucose was observed.

Ultimately, the client abandoned the program in frustration with setbacks from intercurrent illness. This woman thus represents persons for whom exercise training turns out to be more bother than benefit. One must wonder whether her failure to gain any sustained benefit was a marker for her imminent death.

S : No complaint, wants exercise program.

O : 1) Hemodialysis patient, diabetes, valvular heart failure, COPD.

2) Medications: insulin, phosphorus binders.

3) Aerobic exercise test
- 3 METs, peak $\dot{V}O_2$ 9 ml·kg^{-1}·min^{-1}.
- Peak heart rate 144, peak blood pressure 160/100.
- Arterial desaturation at peak exercise.

A : 1) Low aerobic power and endurance due to multiple contributing factors:
- Sedentary lifestyle/deconditioning
- Anemia and low peak heart rate
- "Uremic" myopathy
- Arterial desaturation secondary to COPD

2) Weakness secondary to uremic myopathy/deconditioning.***

P: 1) Aerobic exercise training.

2) (Strength training)***

Exercise Program

Goal:	Increase aerobic power and endurance.***
Mode:	Stationary cycling during dialysis.
Intensity:	30-50 rpm, unloaded (as tolerated); gradual addition of time and resistance.
Frequency:	3 days/week.
Duration:	30 minutes, gradually increasing to 60 minutes.
Time course:	> 3 months.

*** This woman was participating in an aerobic exercise study that did not include strength training. Current recommendations also call for strength training.

Case 6 - Polio

A 28-year-old male athlete was interested in undergoing exercise testing and obtaining guidance on his training program. He had contracted polio as a child and was left with almost complete paraplegia at the T9 level. He competed in wheelchair basketball and athletics (track and field). His best event was the 100 meter, in which he held an American record.

He was given a treadmill wheelchair test with respired gas and blood lactate analysis. The speed of the treadmill was adjusted until wheel pushing was comfortable on a 2% grade; all subsequent work rates were achieved by increasing grade. A safety harness was rigged to prevent the wheelchair from coming off the treadmill. At the end of each work interval, he stopped pushing and rode suspended by the harness while a finger stick was obtained for blood lactate, after which he resumed pushing. Peak $\dot{V}O_2$ was defined as the time when he could no longer keep the wheelchair from being suspended by the harness. An anaerobic capacity test was performed, with use of an investigational format protocol, at a fixed speed of 5 mph and an 8% grade.

The client's peak $\dot{V}O_2$ was 52.9 ml·kg^{-1}·min^{-1}; peak lactate was 8 mmol·dl^{-1}; ventilatory threshold was about 40% of peak $\dot{V}O_2$; anaerobic capacity was estimated at 2.04 L of O_2 debt.

Assessment

1) Complete T9 paraplegia.

2) Excellent aerobic capacity (wheelchair pushing).

3) High anaerobic exercise capacity.

4) Relatively low ventilatory threshold and potential for high performance in middle distance events.

Plan

There was no specific goal. In his program, this client was encouraged to train for and try some longer races, such as the 1500 meter, in order to take advantage of his high $\dot{V}O_2$max.

Discussion

This test shows that with a little ingenuity, anyone can be tested so as to achieve meaningful and useful results. This individual required modification of the treadmill protocol and the testing apparatus, as well as partial interruption at the end of each work period for lactate sampling. The laboratory data were not particularly useful for training purposes, but suggested excellent potential in other events.

S: Wheelchair athlete desires physiologic assessment.

O: 1) Paraplegia at T12 level.

2) Peak $\dot{V}O_2$max 2.64 L·min^{-1} (52.9 ml·kg^{-1}·min^{-1}); peak exercise lactate 8 mM.

3) Anaerobic capacity test: 2.04 L O_2 debt.

4) Strength tests (bench press, handgrip, isokinetic tests of elbow flexor/extensors).***

A: Elite-level aerobic capacity.

P: 1) Endurance and high-intensity interval training to increase $\dot{V}_E$ threshold.

2) Upper-extremity and trunk resistance training.***

Exercise Program***

Goal:	Paralympic Games/Elite Wheelchair competition.
Mode:	Wheelchair cycling.
	Weight lifting.
Intensity:	Complex program in macrocycles

and microcycles through competitive seasons.

40-70% maximum heart rate (submaximal endurance).

90-100% maximum heart rate (intervals).

1-10 repetition maximum resistance training.

Frequency: 7 days/week.

Duration: > 90 minutes/day.

Time course: 6-18 months.

*** This individual was tested in 1987, and no formal exercise program was recommended. These additional studies and program recommendations might reasonably be given in accordance with the current guidelines.

Case 7 - Guillain-Barré Syndrome

A 54-year-old man went to the hospital complaining of weakness, especially in the calves, thighs, and hands. He was found to have the Guillain-Barré syndrome (a demyelinating disorder of the peripheral nervous system that predominantly affects motor nerves and can cause severe paralysis involving the respiratory musculature). His condition worsened and he developed extreme weakness in all extremities, but he escaped respiratory muscle involvement. He was hospitalized for three and one-half months and gradually recovered, but with severe skeletal muscle atrophy. He also had sensory losses in his hands and had bilateral foot drop (inability to raise his toes). He could walk with crutches and ankle braces. Over the next three years, he gradually improved to walking with only one crutch and having minimal weakness in the hands and feet. He presented requesting help with increasing his activities of daily living.

He performed exercise ergometry on an Air-Dyne and underwent isokinetic leg testing. Peak Air-Dyne exercise occurred at 175 watts and a peak $\dot{V}O_2$max of 27.3 ml·kg^{-1}·min^{-1}; right knee extensors developed 56 ft/lb of peak torque and 54 watts average power; left knee extensors developed 65 ft/lb of peak torque and 60 watts average power.

Assessment

1) Guillain-Barré syndrome with residual neuropathy.

2) Aerobic exercise intolerance secondary to deconditioning and #1.

3) Below age-predicted knee flexor/extensor strength secondary to deconditioning and #1.

Plan

The goal was to use a program of Air-Dyne ergometry to increase strength in order to allow independent self-care and capacity to do some yard work. Leg strength training was not specifically prescribed.

Reassessment

Repeat testing after the program revealed 9% and 11% improvements in oxygen uptake and peak work rate. Also, the client had 18% and 24% improvements in right knee peak torque and power, as well as 5% and 13% improvements in left knee peak torque and power, respectively.

Discussion

This individual had exercise intolerance partly due to deconditioning and partly due to permanent neurologic loss. His substantial improvements left him still below normal in aerobic capacity and strength, but did allow him to return to his usual activities of daily living. These improvements reflected not only increased strength, but also equalization of the left-right asymmetry. He became able to climb a flight of stairs without using the banister, felt less fatigued, was able to mow the yard with a push mower, and resumed laborious work such as rototilling and gardening. All goals were successfully achieved, and a home-based maintenance exercise program was started.

S: Weakness and fatigue, prolonged deconditioning.

O: 1) Uses one crutch and ankle brace, residual neurological deficits.

2) Peak $\dot{V}O_2$max 27.3 ml·kg^{-1}·min^{-1}.

3) Right knee extensions: peak torque 56 ft/lb, power 54 watts.

4) Left knee extensions: peak torque 65 ft/lb, mean power 60 watts.

A: 1) Residual motor and sensory deficits from Guillain-Barré.

2) Below-average aerobic capacity.

3) Below-average strength with moderate L-R asymmetry.

P: Submaximal aerobic exercise training on Air-Dyne.

Exercise Program

Goal: Independent self-care activities of daily living, yard work.

Mode: Air-Dyne.

Intensity: 75-80% maximal heart rate.

Frequency: 3 days/week.

Duration: 30 minutes.

Time course: 16 weeks.

INDEX

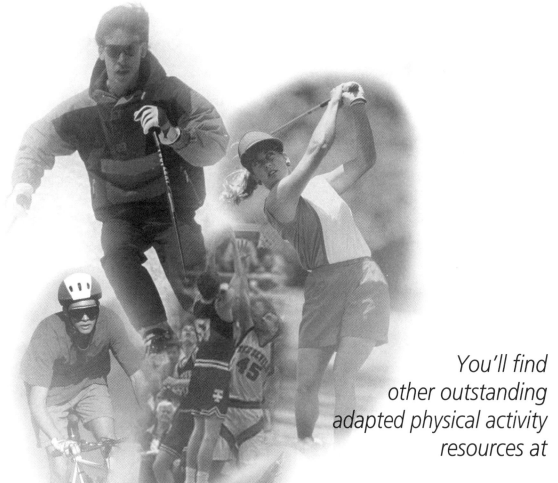